Radioactive Nuclides
in Medicine
and Biology

COMPANION VOLUMES

RADIOACTIVE NUCLIDES

★ ★ **Medicine**—by SOLOMON SILVER

★ ★ ★ **Chemistry and Biology**—by JOHN C. BUGHER

3rd Edition

Radioactive Nuclides
in Medicine
and Biology

BASIC PHYSICS AND INSTRUMENTATION

EDITH H. QUIMBY, Sc.D.
Professor Emeritus of Radiology, College of Physicians and Surgeons, Columbia University

SERGEI FEITELBERG, M.D.
Late Director, Andre Meyer Department of Physics, The Mount Sinai Hospital

and

WILLIAM GROSS, Ph.D.
Associate Professor of Radiology (Physics), College of Physicians and Surgeons, Columbia University, New York

THIRD EDITION · *94 Illustrations*

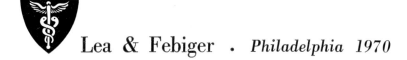 Lea & Febiger · *Philadelphia 1970*

First Edition, 1958
Second Edition, 1963
Third Edition, 1970

Published in Great Britain
by Henry Kimpton, London

Library of Congress Catalog Card Number: 68–18868

Printed in the United States of America

ISBN 0–8121–0197–9

Preface to Volume I of Third Edition

CHANGES in the medical radionuclide field were rapid in the years immediately following the publication of the second edition of this book. Within five years it was apparent that the medical volume needed complete revision, and that new techniques and instrumentation ought to be treated in the physical volume. Dr. Silver, stimulated by the fact that his volume was about to go out of print, met the hoped-for publication date of 1968. The sudden and untimely death of Dr. Feitelberg in September 1967 upset any time table for the present volume, especially since he had not actually started on his revision. We regret the inevitable delay.

In preparing the new volume we have endeavored to adhere to the objectives of the earlier editions. We hope that the book will continue to serve as a basis for study, both for classes and individuals, but we realize that it is no longer possible to cover the field, even at the elementary level. Nor is it possible to furnish complete bibliographies, but it is hoped that the listed references will point the way to further library work when it is necessary.

In Part I, on basic physics, and in the appendix tables, every effort has been made to provide the most recent numerical data. Brief sections have been inserted on certain types of calculations, and some chapters have been somewhat amplified, but no appreciable increase in the size of the volume has been necessary.

For Part II, on instrumentation, it has been possible to retain a good deal of Dr. Feitelberg's basic material, but in many chapters considerable rewriting has been necessary. A chapter on scanning equipment has been added and new sections on the more sophisticated electronic instrumentation now in common usage have had to be prepared.

We wish to express our appreciation to the many colleagues who have made helpful suggestions. Miss Ellen Ewald has prepared the new illustrations, and our secretary, Mrs. Gerda Osborn, has given invaluable aid with the manuscript. The encouragement of the publishers, and their patience with unavoidable delays, have contributed greatly to the completion of the book.

EDITH H. QUIMBY

WILLIAM GROSS

New York, New York

Preface to the First Edition

THE artificial production of radioactive isotopes was announced twenty-five years ago, and caused a tremendous sensation among physicists and chemists, but aroused little attention among physicians. However, within a short time physiologists found that the new substances provided powerful tools for metabolic studies, and then some more truly clinical applications became apparent. In 1939 radioactive phosphorus was used as a substitute for whole-body x-irradiation in the treatment of certain blood dyscrasias. About the same time the value of radioactive iodine in the study of thyroid function was demonstrated, and within another three years this material was used in the treatment of toxic goiter. Radioactive iron was simultaneously employed by other groups in various studies relating to red blood cells and iron reserves. By 1940 there was a considerable literature dealing with medical uses of artificially radioactive isotopes, but there was no suggestion that they would eventually provide standard diagnostic and therapeutic procedures. They were obtainable only from cyclotrons, usually at great cost, and frequently in such form as to require considerable chemical manipulation before they could be used.

The discovery of the chain-reacting pile or nuclear reactor changed this picture, but it was not until 1946, after the end of World War II, that even one reactor could be used to provide isotopes for non-military purposes. In July of 1946, the Atomic Energy Commission announced a limited availability of certain isotopes for medical use, at much lower costs than cyclotron products, and in the next six months about 100 shipments were made for medical research in 38 institutions. Ten years later a thousand medical institutions were authorized to obtain the materials, and doctors in some of them were using very large quantities of radioactive isotopes.

At the beginning of this period, each individual or group had to enter an almost uncharted field. Some information was available in the literature, but in general, procedures were developed independently; all studies were essentially on a research basis. However, as their value became known many physicians wanted to avail themselves of the new tools. There were demands for instruction courses and for textbooks; these were intensified by the fact that the Atomic Energy Commission required the physician to have a certain amount of training before issuing him an authorization to obtain radioactive isotopes from their reactor. Few people or groups felt that they had the time or the qualifications to give a comprehensive course, and the books that appeared dealt mainly with limited parts of the field. In any case, progress was being made so rapidly that a book was out of date almost by the time it was published.

In June of 1954, the present authors, with the generous cooperation of physicians and physicists throughout New York City, undertook to offer a four-week full-time comprehensive course in clinical uses of radioactive isotopes. The response was so enthusiastic that they were forced to present the course twice a year, once as originally planned, for non-residents of the city, and once on a basis of one afternoon a week for eight months, for those living within commuting distance. It has now been given eight times, naturally with modifications from year to year. This book is the outgrowth of our experience in lectures, laboratory exercises, and conferences with the approximately 225 students who have completed the course.

It has been written as three quite separate parts, each by the author who has the most to do with that field in teaching the course. But each author owes much to the collaborators who have given so freely of their time and interest. It is hoped that the book will serve as a basis for study both by classes and by individuals, but no claim is made to completeness. In fact, it is certain that considerable supplementary reading will be necessary for every one who wants a really comprehensive survey of even the generally used procedures. References have been supplied for this purpose, but no effort has been made to assemble a complete bibliography. For any particular type of study, recent papers of the survey type, which are listed, will provide complete sets of references.

We wish to express our grateful appreciation to our colleagues in the presentation of the course, for their generous sharing of their information, and to those other friends who have freely permitted us to use their published material. A special acknowledgment is due to Miss Ellen Ewald, who prepared all the illustrations from sketches supplied by the authors. To our secretaries, Miss Judith M. Weinberg, Mrs. Katherine Johanny, and Miss Blanche Lipkowitz, who have typed and re-typed the manuscript, looked up references, and generally been indispensable, we give our thanks. The publishers' enthusiasm in getting the book under way, and their patient but persistent attention to its progress should receive a large share of the credit in bringing it to completion.

EDITH H. QUIMBY

NEW YORK, NEW YORK   SERGEI FEITELBERG

SEPTEMBER, 1958   SOLOMON SILVER

Contents

PART I.—BASIC PHYSICS

By EDITH H. QUIMBY

Introduction 3

A time-table of significant events leading up to the present radionuclide picture.

Chapter 1.—Atoms. 7

History of atomic concept. Atomic building-blocks. Present picture of atomic structure. Periodic table. Isotopes. Nuclear nomenclature. Classification of stable nuclei. Dimensions of atoms and nuclei. Nuclear forces.

Chapter 2.—Radioactivity 17

Historical introduction. Nature of the radiations. Atomic disintegration. Artificial or induced radioactivity. Characteristics of radioactive disintegration. Mathematical expression of disintegration law. Half life and average life. Determination of decay constants. Units of activity of radioactive nuclides. Carrier, specific activity.

Chapter 3.—Disruption of Stable Nuclei—Induced Radioactivity . 33

First artificial transmutation. Discovery of the neutron. Discovery of the positron. Artificially produced radionuclides. The cyclotron.

Chapter 4.—Nuclear Reactions 39

Energy of a reaction. Equivalence of mass and energy. Notation for nuclear reactions. Mechanisms of nuclear reaction. Yield of nuclear reaction. Reactions in neutron, proton, deuteron and alpha particle bombardment. Nuclear reactions produced by photons. Energy considerations.

Chapter 5.—Nuclear Fission and Fusion 52

Discovery. Fission products. Nuclear chain reaction. Atomic pile or nuclear reactor. Transuranic elements. Radionuclide production in the pile. Nuclear weapons. Nuclear fusion.

Chapter 6.—Sources of the Radiations; Modes of Radioactive Decay   60

> Structure of the nucleus. Alpha decay. Beta decay. The neutrino. Average and maximum beta energy. K-electron capture. Gamma decay. Internal conversion. Nuclear isomers. Other modes of decay. Radioactive series. Radioactive equilibrium. Growth of radionuclide in neutron flux.

Chapter 7.—Interaction of Radiation and Matter 78

> Characteristics of the radiations. Energies of the radiations. Possible types of interactions of radiation and matter. Interactions of alpha particles with matter. Interactions of beta particles with matter. Interaction of neutrons with matter. Interactions of photons with matter. Ionization, recombination and production of characteristic radiation. Wilson cloud chamber. Absorption of beta radiation. Range of beta rays. Scattering of beta particles. Self-scattering and self-absorption of beta particles. Absorption and scattering of photon beams.

Chapter 8.—Basic Considerations Regarding Medical Uses of Radioactive Nuclides 98

> Tracer and therapeutic uses. Limitations for tracers—type of radiation, half life, chemical effects. Types of tracer studies. Therapy with nuclides encapsulated and under control; with nuclides administered internally and out of control. Need for knowledge of radiation dose.

Chapter 9.—Dosage Calculations for Radioactive Nuclides . . . 102

> Units of radiation dose. External (controlled) alpha, beta and gamma ray sources. Nuclides administered internally (out of control). Alpha and beta-emitting nuclides in the body. Dose in objects floating in radioactive solution. Gamma ray emitting nuclides in the body. Effective and biological half life. Addition of beta and gamma ray doses. Examples of dosage problems. Approximate formula for thyroid dose with [131]I. Calculation of quantity of nuclide to administer for delivery of a specified dose. Non-uniformity of irradiation. Special dosage problems.

Chapter 10.—Biological Effects of Ionizing Radiations 141

> I. Grossly observable effects. General phenomena. Units of radiation dose. Factors influencing radiation effects. Sources of information regarding radiation effects. Radiation doses to produce particular effects. Effects on skin. Effects on blood. Induction of cancer. Induction of cataract. Effects of exposure during pregnancy. Sterility. Shortening of life span. Genetic effects of radiation. The doubling dose.
> II. Effects at molecular level. Direct and indirect effects. Activated water. Mean lethal dose.

Chapter 11.—Radiation Hazards and Their Avoidance 155

Historical introduction. Present point of view. Maximum
permissible dose recommendations for occupational conditions
(MPD'S in controlled areas). Maximum permissible dose
recommendations for the whole population. (MPD'S for the
general public.) Dosage due to internal emitters. Safety procedures with external beta-particle emitters. Safety procedures
with external gamma ray emitters. Handling of bodies containing radioactive material. Safety considerations for radionuclides
administered internally. General safety routines.

Chapter 12.—Disposal of Radioactive Waste and Removal of Contamination 178

General considerations. Atomic Energy Commission Rules.
Disposal in sewage. Stable isotope dilution. Disposal in
garbage. Disposal by incineration. Soil burial and sea disposal.
Return to Atomic Energy Commission. Bodies containing
appreciable quantities of radioactive material. Radioactive
contamination and decontamination. Special case of internal
personnel contamination.

PART II—INSTRUMENTATION AND LABORATORY METHODS

By Sergei Feitelberg and William Gross

Chapter 13.—Radiation Detectors: Principles of Operation . . . 185

Ionization chambers. Proportional counters. Geiger-Mueller
counters. Scintillation counters. Solid state detectors. Photographic emulsions.

Chapter 14.—Auxiliary Instruments 201

Ionization chambers: dose rate meters, total dose meters.
Counting circuits: high voltage supply, amplifiers, preamplifiers,
discriminators; counting mechanisms, timing mechanisms,
preset time and preset count features; time and count printers.
Rate meters and recorders. Coincidence and anti-coincidence
circuits. Pulse height analyzers.

Chapter 15.—Statistical Considerations of Radiation Counting . . 221

Basic principles. Statistics of nuclear counting: principles;
sample and background counting. Preset time and preset count
methods of counting. Resolving time. Counting statistics in
rate meters and recorders. Efficiency and sensitivity of radiation
detectors.

Chapter 16.—Quantitative Measurements *in Vitro*   257

   Standardization of radionuclides: handling of radioactive
   samples. Selection of electronic circuits and control settings
   with Geiger-Mueller, proportional, and scintillation counters.
   Sample measurements *in vitro:* gamma ray counting, beta ray
   counting, self-absorption. Shielding of counting set-ups. Use of
   pulse height discrimination for background reduction. Identification of nuclides. Specialized methods: chemical purification,
   gas counting, radiochromatography; double nuclide techniques.

Chapter 17.—Quantitative Measurements *in Vivo*   299

   Basic principles. Measurement of thyroidal uptake; influence
   of gland size and location, role of backscatter, counter sensitivity.
   Body background. Other *in vivo* measurements.

Chapter 18.—Observation by Radioactive Tracers of the Time
   Factor in Physiological Processes   307

   Slow changes. Intermediate speeds. Rapid changes. Printing
   counters and rate recorders. Shielding problems.

Chapter 19.—Determination of Distribution of Radioactive Material
   within the Body   314

   Collimation. Scanning. Instrumentation; fixed and moving
   detector systems. Nuclides for scanning.

Chapter 20.—Autoradiography   338

   Contact autoradiography. Emulsion painting. Section flotation. Emulsion flotation.

Chapter 21.—Use of Radiation Detectors for Health Protection   .   346

   Total dose meters. Dose rate meters. Portable Geiger-Mueller
   counters. Application of instruments to monitoring problems:
   personnel monitoring, area monitoring, process monitoring.

Chapter 22.—Laboratory Design   352

   Space requirements. Location. Equipment. Personnel.

Appendices.—Useful Physical Constants.   359

   Convenient conversion tables. Physical data for a number of
   radionuclides. Characteristics of standard man. Radiation
   dose in critical organs. Fluorescent yields; critical absorption
   edges. Four-place logarithms. Exponentials. Table for
   decay calculations.

Author Index   397

Subject Index   381

Radioactive Nuclides in Medicine

Part I

BASIC PHYSICS

Edith H. Quimby

Introduction

A TIME-TABLE OF SIGNIFICANT EVENTS LEADING UP TO THE PRESENT RADIONUCLIDE PICTURE

1808. John Dalton (England) presented the first experimental basis for an atomic hypothesis.

1811. Amadeo Avogadro (Italy) distinguished between atoms and molecules.

1815. Wm. Prout (England) suggested hydrogen (protyle) as a basic component of all matter.

1869. D. I. Mendeleev (Russia) set up a periodic table of chemical classification of elements.

1895. Wilhelm Conrad Roentgen (Germany) discovered x rays.

1896. Henri Becquerel (France) discovered radioactivity of uranium.

1897. J. J. Thompson (England) discovered that the electron is a constituent of all atoms.

1898. Marie and Pierre Curie (France) discovered polonium and radium.

1900. P. Curie (France) found that the rays from radium consisted of two kinds, of very different penetrating power and deviated in different directions in a magnetic field. These later became known as alpha (α) and beta (β) rays.

1900. P. Villard (France) discovered a third type of radiation from radioactive substances, called it gamma rays (γ), and stated it to be identical with x rays.

1905. Albert Einstein (Switzerland) proposed the theory of equivalence of mass and energy.

1910. F. Soddy (England) identified isotopes and isobars in naturally radioactive substances.

1911. Ernest Rutherford (England) discovered the atomic nucleus.

1911. C. G. Barkla (England) demonstrated the existence of extranuclear electrons.

1911. Victor Hess (Austria) discovered cosmic rays.

1912. J. J. Thompson (England) demonstrated the existence of isotopes in stable elements.

1912. C. T. R. Wilson (England) invented the cloud chamber for studying ionization tracks.

1913. Niels Bohr (Denmark) proposed an atom model with a central positively charged nucleus and a system of negative orbital electrons.

1913. H. G. J. Moseley (England), from a study of x-ray spectra, developed the system of atomic numbers.

1919. E. Rutherford (England) produced nuclear transmutation by bombarding nitrogen with α particles. He identified one product of the transmutation as a proton.

1932. Harold Urey (USA) discovered heavy hydrogen or deuterium.

1932. James Chadwick (England) discovered the neutron (whose existence Rutherford had suggested in 1919).

1932. J. D. Cockroft and E. T. S. Walton (England) produced nuclear transmutation by artificially accelerated protons.

1932. C. D. Anderson (USA) discovered the positron.

1932. E. O. Lawrence (USA) invented the cyclotron.

1934. F. Joliot and I. Curie-Joliot (France) discovered induced radioactivity in light elements by bombardment with natural α particles.

1934. E. O. Lawrence (USA) produced artificially radioactive nuclides by bombardment with artificially accelerated particles.

1934. Enrico Fermi (Italy) produced transformation of nuclei by neutron capture.

1939. O. Hahn and F. Strassman (Germany) discovered nuclear fission.

1939. Lise Meitner and O. Frisch (Sweden) calculated the huge energy release to be expected in nuclear fission.

1939. Enrico Fermi (USA) suggested the possibility of a chain reaction in nuclear fission. This was experimentally verified in several laboratories in USA and France.

1939. "Manhattan Project" (USA) was organized for military development of atomic energy.

1940. E. M. MacMillan and P. Abelson (USA) discovered two "transuranic" elements, neptunium and plutonium, following the bombardment of uranium by slow neutrons.

1942. (USA) First self-maintaining nuclear chain reaction in a uranium graphite "pile" or reactor, was initiated in Chicago.

1945. Atomic bombs were exploded July 16th in New Mexico, August 6th and 11th over Hiroshima and Nagasaki, Japan.

1946. (USA) "Manhattan Project," becoming Atomic Energy Commission, announced availability of pile-produced radioactive nuclides for medical, industrial and scientific research. Three hundred shipments made during first year.

1956. Atomic Energy Commission (USA) made over 15,000 shipments of radioactive nuclides to more than 5000 institutions in the United States and 32 other countries during this 10th year of distribution.

1968. In addition to the Atomic Energy Commission's direct shipments, a considerable number of firms are dispensing purified and calibrated radionuclides and labeled compounds. It is almost impossible to estimate the total amount being distributed.

A LIST OF USEFUL REFERENCE BOOKS

ATTIX, FRANK H. and ROESCH, WILLIAM C.: *Radiation Dosimetry*, 2nd Ed., Vol. II, New York, Academic Press, Inc., 1966.

BRUCER, MARSHALL: *Trilinear Chart of the Nuclides*. St. Louis, Mallinckrodt Nuclear, 1968.

CHASE, GRAFTON D. and RABINOWITZ, JOSEPH L.: *Principles of Radioisotope Methodology*, 3rd Ed. Minneapolis, Burgess Publishing Company, 1967.

COMAR, C. L.: *Radioisotopes in Biology and Agriculture*, New York, McGraw-Hill Book Co., Inc., 1955.

EISENBUD, MERRILL: *Environmental Radioactivity*, New York, McGraw-Hill Book Co., Inc., 1963.

ELMORE, WILLIAM C. and SANDS, MATTHEW: *Electronics, Experimental Techniques*, New York, McGraw-Hill Book Co., Inc., 1949.

EVANS, ROBLEY D.: *The Atomic Nucleus*, New York, McGraw-Hill Book Co., Inc., 1955.

FERMI, LAURA: *Atoms in the Family*, Chicago, Chicago University Press, 1954.

FRIEDLANDER, GERHART, KENNEDY, JOSEPH W. and MILLER, JULIAN M.: *Nuclear and Radiochemistry*, 2nd Ed., New York, John Wiley & Sons, Inc., 1964.

General Electric Chart of the Nuclides, Latest Revised Edition, Knolls Atomic Power Laboratory, Knolls, New York.

GLASSER, OTTO, QUIMBY, EDITH H., TAYLOR, LAURISTON S., WEATHERWAX, JAMES and MORGAN, RUSSELL H.: *Physical Foundations of Radiology*, 3rd Ed., New York, Paul B. Hoeber, 1961.

HALLIDAY, D.: *Introductory Nuclear Physics*, New York, John Wiley & Sons, Inc., 1950.

HINE, G. J. and BROWNELL, G. L.: *Radiation Dosimetry*, New York, Academic Press, Inc., 1956.

HULL, GORDON F.: *Elementary Nuclear Physics*, Revised Ed., New York, The Macmillan Co., 1949.

International Commission on Radiological Protection: *Report of Committee II on Permissible Dose for Internal Radiation* (contains also *Permissible Dose for External Irradiation*). New York, The Pergamon Press, 1959.

International Commission on Radiological Units and Measurements, *Complete Report, 1961.* National Bureau of Standards Handbook 78, Washington, U. S. Government Printing Office, 1962.

Introduction

JOHNS, H.: *The Physics of Radiology*, 2nd Edition. Springfield, Charles C Thomas, 1964.

KAMEN, M.: *Radioactive Tracers in Biology*, 3rd Ed., New York, Academic Press, Inc., 1957.

LAPP, R. E. and ANDREWS, H. L.: *Nuclear Radiation Physics*, 3rd Ed., New York, Prentice-Hall, Inc., 1963.

LEDERER, C. M., HOLLANDER, J. M. and PERLMAN, I.: *Table of Isotopes*, 6th Ed., New York, John Wiley & Sons, Inc., 1967.

MORGAN, R. H. and CORRIGAN, K. E.: *Handbook of Radiology*, Chicago, Year Book Publishers, Inc., 1955.

POLLARD, E. C. and DAVIDSON, W. L.: *Applied Nuclear Physics*, 2nd Ed., New York, John Wiley & Sons, Inc., 1951.

QUIMBY, EDITH H.: *Safe Handling of Radioisotopes in Medical Practice*, New York, The Macmillan Co., 1960.

Radiochemical Manual, Part One, Physical Data. The Radiochemical Centre, Amersham, England, 1962.

Radiological Health Handbook. U. S. Department of Health, Education, and Welfare, Washington, D.C., 1960.

RUTHERFORD, E., CHADWICK, J. and ELLIS, C. D.: *Radiations from Radioactive Substances,,* Cambridge, England University Press, 1930; reissued 1951.

SEMAT, H.: *Introduction to Atomic and Nuclear Physics*, 4th Ed., New York, Holt, Rinehart, & Winston, 1962.

SLACK, L. and WAY, K.: *Radiations from Radioactive Atoms in Frequent Use*, Washington, U.S. Atomic Energy Commission, 1959.

WAGNER, H. N., Editor: *Principles of Nuclear Medicine.* Philadelphia, W. B. Saunders Co., 1968.

WHITE, H. E.: *Introduction to Atomic and Nuclear Physics*, New York, D. Van Nostrand Co., Inc., 1963.

Useful Handbooks of the National Bureau of Standards, available from the Superintendent of Documents, Government Printing Office, Washington, D.C. 20402.

59. Permissible Dose from External Sources of Ionizing Radiation.
69. Maximum Permissible Body Burdens and Maximum Permissible Concentrations of Radionuclides in Air and Water for Occupational Exposure.
80. A Manual of Radioactivity Procedures.
84. Radiation Quantities and Units. (ICRU Report 10a)
85. Physical Aspects of Radiation. (ICRU Report 10b)
86. Radioactivity. (ICRU Report 10c)
87. Clinical Dosimetry. (ICRU Report 10d)
88. Radiobiological Dosimetry. (ICRU Report 10e)
92. Safe Handling of Radioactive Materials.

Useful Reports of the National Council on Radiation Protection and Measurements. NCRP Publications, P.O. Box 4867, Washington, D. C. 20008.

8. Control and Removal of Radioactive Contamination in Laboratories.
28. A Manual of Radioactivity Procedures.
36. Precautions in the Management of Patients Who Have Received Therapeutic Amounts of Radionuclides.

1

Atoms

RADIOACTIVITY is a characteristic of certain atoms, hence the approach to the study of radioactive substances should begin at the atomic level.

History of Atomic Concept. The idea of atoms as basic particles of matter is very old, but through the ages the concept of their nature has undergone many modifications. At the beginning of the last century Dalton organized ideas then current in this field. It was accepted that all matter was built up of components called *elements,* of which there were a large but limited number. The smallest fundamental particles of each element were its *atoms;* atoms of a particular element were all exactly alike, and different from atoms of all other elements; they were indivisible and unalterable.

With the discovery of radioactivity by Becquerel in 1896 and of the electron as a constituent of matter by J. J. Thompson in 1897, it became evident that the atom must have structure and even be capable of undergoing some sort of breakdown. During the next 15 years various atomic models were suggested, to be crystallized in the Rutherford-Bohr picture about 1913. According to this, the atom is described as basically like a miniature solar system; there is a central *nucleus* containing most of the atomic mass and carrying a positive electric charge; this is surrounded by a system of orbital negative *electrons.*

Atomic Building-Blocks. At first the nucleus was believed to be a mixture of basic positively charged particles and electrons, since the net number of units of positive charge on the nucleus was less than the number of units of atomic mass. The number of orbital electrons was accepted as being the same as the excess of positive charges in the nucleus, after the nuclear electrons had balanced out a certain number of them. This model was theoretically difficult to justify, and a new particle was postulated which should be of essentially the same mass as the unit positively charged particle, but have no electric charge. The positive particle was called the *proton;* the uncharged one was the *neutron.* Later, as will be seen, both particles were experimentally identified.

In the currently accepted model, neutrons replace nuclear electron-proton combinations and the number of orbital electrons is the same as that of the nuclear protons, so that the complete atom is electrically neutral. Protons and neutrons are called *nucleons.*

7

Masses of nuclei, or of atomic components, are specified in terms of mass units, whose derivation will be discussed later (page 13). One mass unit is 1.66044×10^{-24} grams.*

$$1 \text{ proton weighs } 1.007825 \text{ mass units} = 1.67252 \times 10^{-24} \text{ gm.}$$
$$1 \text{ neutron } \qquad 1.008665 \qquad\qquad 1.67482 \times 10^{-24}$$
$$1 \text{ electron } \qquad 0.0005486 \qquad\qquad 9.1091 \ \times 10^{-28}$$

Present Picture of Atomic Structure. The simplest atom is that of ordinary hydrogen, with one proton for its nucleus and a single orbital electron. Next comes helium, with two protons and two neutrons in the nucleus and two orbital electrons, and then lithium with three protons, four neutrons and three electrons, as indicated in Figure 1–1. The electrons of

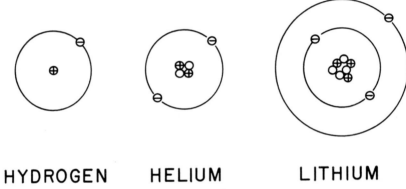

HYDROGEN   HELIUM   LITHIUM

FIG. 1–1.   Structure of simple atoms.

hydrogen and helium travel in a single orbital region, but with lithium, the third electron starts a new orbit. Through the next seven elements (beryllium, boron, carbon, nitrogen, oxygen, fluorine, neon) the nucleus successively adds one proton and one or two neutrons, and an additional electron appears in the second orbit. Sodium, the eleventh element, starts a third orbit, which in turn fills up for succeeding elements; further orbits are added as the number of nuclear protons increases. All known elements fall into this type of build-up pattern.

Periodic Table. This periodicity offers an explanation for the classification by Mendeleev, who found in 1869 that when the known elements were listed according to their ascending atomic weights, certain properties recurred in regular cycles. Thus members of related chemical families appeared in the same column, when the elements were arranged in eight

* The use of positive and negative powers of 10, as abbreviations for very large and very small numbers is standard procedure and will be employed throughout this book.

For example, $3 \times 10^6 = 3{,}000{,}000$. $3 \times 10^{-6} = \dfrac{3}{10^6} = \dfrac{3}{1{,}000{,}000} = 0.000003$.

groups, if hydrogen and helium were omitted and some places left vacant. This listing of the elements is known as the Periodic Table, and in its present form it is shown in Figure 1-2. Vacant spots in the earlier tables were assumed to correspond to undiscovered elements, and, in fact, by permitting deductions as to atomic weight and chemical properties of missing elements, led to their discovery.

If now the elements are arranged according to content of electron orbits, the same periodicity appears (Fig. 1-3). Thus the chemical behavior of an element seems related to the number of electrons in its outermost electron orbit. If that orbit is completely filled, the element is an inert gas, entering into no chemical combinations. If it has only one electron, the element is chemically active (hydrogen, lithium, sodium). Mendeleev's periodic table contained some uncertainties, but the orbital periodic table is complete and accurate up to the heaviest known elements.

Isotopes. A question which troubled early students of the atom was why atomic weights were not whole numbers. An early (1815) suggestion by Prout that all atoms were built up out of hydrogen had to be discarded for this reason, although, as will be seen, he was not far wrong. Later (1886) Crookes suggested that possibly atoms of a single element need not be identical, and that the atomic weight was that of a mixture of somewhat different atoms. This was heresy and little attention was paid to it. In 1910 J. J. Thompson developed an apparatus using electric and magnetic fields for accurate determination of relative nuclear charges and masses, and a year later Soddy showed experimentally that certain elements were in fact composed of atoms chemically identical but physically differing slightly in weight. He proposed the term *isotopes* for such atoms. Isotopes, then, are atoms of the same chemical element, but having atomic weights differing from each other by small whole numbers.* If the chemical properties depend on the number of orbital electrons, this must remain the same for isotopes of a particular element, and mass differences must be due to different numbers of nuclear neutrons. Diagrams of some isotopes are shown in Figure 1-4.

It now becomes evident that atoms of an element are not completely identified by the chemical symbol, but that the number and type of the nuclear components should also be indicated. Therefore the notation has been adopted which is used in Figure 1-4. The chemical symbol carries a left-hand subscript denoting the number of nuclear protons (or of orbital electrons). This is the *atomic number* and chemically characterizes the element. There is one element and only one for every number from 1 to 104† The symbol also carries a left-hand superscript denoting the total number of nuclear mass particles, protons plus neutrons. This is the *mass number* and physically characterizes the particular isotope. Some

---

* Actually it is the *mass numbers* which differ by small whole numbers.
† For elements found naturally, atomic numbers go from 1 to 92: the others are man-made and will be discussed later.

Period	Group I	Group II	Group III	Group IV	Group V	Group VI	Group VII
1	1 1.008 **H** 2 1						
2	3 6.940 **Li** 2 2	4 9.012 **Be** 1 5	5 10.82 **B** 2 3	6 12.011 **C** 2 6	7 14.007 **N** 2 5	8 16.000 **O** 3 5	9 19.00 **F** 1 4
3	11 22.990 **Na** 1 7	12 24.31 **Mg** 3 7	13 26.98 **Al** 1 7	14 28.09 **Si** 3 5	15 30.974 **P** 1 6	16 32.08 **S** 4 6	17 35.453 **Cl** 2 9
4	19 39.102 **K** 3 8	20 40.08 **Ca** 6 8	21 44.96 **Sc** 1 12	22 47.90 **Ti** 5 5	23 50.94 **V** 2 7	24 52.00 **Cr** 4 6	25 54.94 **Mn** 1 12
	29 63.54 **Cu** 2 11	30 65.38 **Zn** 5 10	31 69.72 **Ga** 2 13	32 72.59 **Ge** 5 13	33 74.92 **As** 1 17	34 78.95 **Se** 6 16	35 79.91 **Br** 2 22
5	37 85.48 **Rb** 2 20	38 87.62 **Sr** 4 15	39 88.91 **Y** 1 24	40 91.22 **Zr** 5 17	41 92.91 **Nb** 1 25	42 95.94 **Mo** 7 13	43 (99) **Tc** 0 23
	47 107.87 **Ag** 2 25	48 112.40 **Cd** 8 16	49 114.82 **In** 2 35	50 118.7 **Sn** 10 24	51 121.8 **Sb** 2 36	52 127.6 **Te** 8 28	53 126.9 **I** 1 25
6	55 132.9 **Cs** 1 22	56 137.3 **Ba** 7 20	57-71 **Rare Earths**	72 178.5 **Hf** 6 16	73 180.95 **Ta** 2 17	74 183.9 **W** 5 16	75 186.2 **Re** 2 24
	79 197.0 **Au** 1 29	80 200.59 **Hg** 7 23	81 204.4 **Tl** 2 25	82 207.2 **Pb** 4 24	83 209.0 **Bi** 1 20	84 (210) **Po** 0 33	85 (211) **At** 0 24
7	87 (223) **Fr** 0 18	88 226.05 **Ra** 0 13	89 (227) **Ac** 0 11	90-102 **Actinides**			
Rare Earths (Lanthanides)	57 138.9 **La** 2 18	58 140.1 **Ce** 4 17	59 140.9 **Pr** 1 17	60 144.2 **Nd** 7 11	61 (145) **Pm** 0 18	62 150.4 **Sm** 7 10	63 152.0 **Eu** 2 21
Actinides	90 232.0 **Th** 0 13	91 (231) **Pa** 0 15	92 238.0 **U** 0 15	93 (237) **Np** 0 14	94 (242) **Pu** 0 16	95 (243) **Am** 0 12	96 (247) **Cm** 0 13

Fig. 1–2. Periodic Table of the Elements (after Mendeleev).

Group VIII

2 4.003 — **He** — 2 | 2		
10 20.183 — **Ne** — 3 | 6		
18 39.948 — **Ar** — 3 | 6		
26 55.85 — **Fe** — 4 | 6	**27** 58.93 — **Co** — 1 | 17	**28** 58.71 — **Ni** — 5 | 7
36 83.80 — **Kr** — 6 | 22		
44 101.1 — **Ru** — 7 | 9	**45** 102.91 — **Rh** — 1 | 21	**46** 106.4 — **Pd** — 6 | 15
54 131.3 — **Xe** — 9 | 24		
76 190.2 — **Os** — 7 | 15	**77** 192.2 — **Ir** — 2 | 24	**78** 195.09 — **Pt** — 6 | 27
86 (222) — **Rn** — 0 | 26		

64 157.25 **Gd** 7 | 12	**65** 158.9 **Tb** 1 | 27	**66** 162.5 **Dy** 7 | 15	**67** 164.9 **Ho** 1 | 31	**68** 167.3 **Er** 6 | 14	**69** 168.9 **Tm** 1 | 20	**70** 173.0 **Yb** 7 | 17	**71** 175.0 **Lu** 2 | 25
97 (247) **Bk** 0 | 9	**98** (249) **Cf** 0 | 11	**99** (254) **Es** 0 | 13	**100** (253) **Fm** 0 | 16	**101** (256) **Md** 0 | 3	**102** (254) **No** 0 | 7	**103** (257) 0 |	**104** 2 | 2

Upper Left—Atomic Number
Lower Left—Number of Stable Isotopes
Upper Right—Atomic Weight of Normal Isotopic Mixture
Lower Right—Number of Radioactive Isotopes (as of 1967, according to Lederer, Hollander, and Perlman, Table of Isotopes).

Atomic Element	Element	Electrons in Orbits						
		K	L	M	N	O	P	Q
1	H	1						
2	He	2						
3	Li	2	1					
4	Be	2	2					
5	B	2	3					
6	C	2	4					
7	N	2	5					
8	O	2	6					
9	F	2	7					
10	Ne	2	8					
11	Na	2	8	1				
12	Mg	2	8	2				
13	Al	2	8	3				
14	Si	2	8	4				
15	P	2	8	5				
16	S	2	8	6				
17	Cl	2	8	7				
18	A	2	8	8				
19	K	2	8	8	1			
20	Ca	2	8	8	2			
21	Sc	2	8	9	2			
22	Ti	2	8	10	2			
23	V	2	8	11	2			
24	Cr	2	8	13	1	(Note Irregularity)		
25	Mn	2	8	13	2			
26	Fe	2	8	14	2			
27	Co	2	8	15	2			
28	Ni	2	8	16	2			
29	Cu	2	8	18	1	(Note Irregularity)		
30	Zn	2	8	18	2			
31	Ga	2	8	18	3			
32	Ge	2	8	18	4			
33	As	2	8	18	5			
34	Se	2	8	18	6			
35	Br	2	8	18	7			
36	Kr	2	8	18	8			
37	Rb	2	8	18	8	1		
38	Sr	2	8	18	8	2		
39	Y	2	8	18	9	2		
40	Zr	2	8	18	10	2		
41	Cb	2	8	18	12	1	(Note Irregularity)	
42	Mo	2	8	18	13	1		
43	Tc	2	8	18	14	1		
44	Ru	2	8	18	15	1		
45	Rh	2	8	18	16	1		
46	Pd	2	8	18	18	—	(Note Irregularity)	
47	Ag	2	8	18	18	1		
48	Cd	2	8	18	18	2		
49	In	2	8	18	18	3		
50	Sn	2	8	18	18	4		
51	Sb	2	8	18	18	5		
52	Te	2	8	18	18	6		
53	I	2	8	18	18	7		
54	Xe	2	8	18	18	8		

Fig. 1–3.   Partial table of electron configuration of the elements.

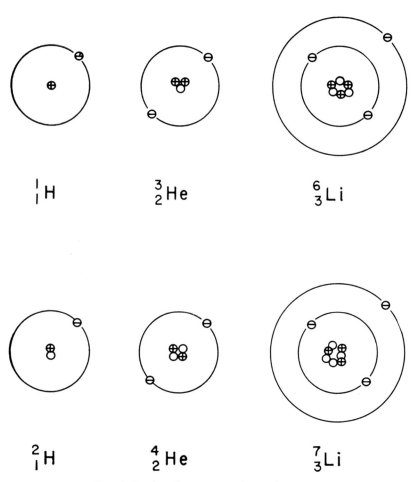

FIG. 1-4.   Atomic structure of some isotopes.
(Nucleus of $^1_1$H is the *proton*, of $^2_1$H the *deuteron*.)

elements, such as phosphorus and iodine, have only one stable isotope. Many have two or three and some have several; tin has 10.

Atomic masses are specified in terms of the *atomic mass unit*, which is $\frac{1}{12}$ of the mass of an atom of $^{12}_{6}$C.   According to Avogadro's hypothesis, one gram-atomic weight of any element contains 6.02252×10^{23} atoms. This, then, is the number of atoms in 12 grams of ^{12}C.   One twelfth of one atom would weigh

$$\tfrac{1}{12} \times \frac{12 \text{ gm}}{6.02252 \times 10^{23}} = 1.66044 \times 10^{-24} \text{ gm},$$

which is the value of one atomic mass unit.   (It should be noted that until recently the mass of $\frac{1}{16}$ of an atom of $^{16}_{8}$O was taken as the standard.

Atomic masses based on this are found in older publications; they differ very slightly from those given in the present volume. The differences are not large enough to be of concern in medical radionuclide problems.) An extensive table of atomic masses may be found in Nuclear and Radiochemistry, by Friedlander, Kennedy, and Miller.

Nuclear Nomenclature.   In addition to isotopes, there are also *isobars*, atoms having the same number of mass particles, but different numbers of protons and neutrons, and hence different atomic numbers. Another group is that of *isotones*, atoms having the same number of nuclear neutrons; they have both different mass numbers and different atomic numbers.

The definitions and classifications just discussed may be summarized as follows:

Atomic Number—number of protons in nucleus—symbol Z;
Neutron Number—number of neutrons in nucleus—symbol N;
Mass Number—number of mass particles in nucleus—symbol A.

$$A = Z + N.$$

Neutron Excess—Excess of neutron number over proton number—$(N-Z)$
For ^2_1H and ^3_2He there is no neutron excess, but a deficit; in each case $N - Z = -1$. For elements of atomic number 1 to 20, one isotope has $N - Z = 0$, or $N = Z$. After helium all elements have at least one isotope for which $N - Z$ is greater than 0.

The symbol used for a particular nuclear species, or *nuclide* is
^A_ZChemical Symbol, *e.g.* $^{23}_{11}$Na.

Isotopes—atoms have same Z's, different A's, and hence different N's:
$^{35}_{17}$Cl, $^{37}_{17}$Cl.

Isobars—atoms having same A's, different Z's and hence different N's:
$^{64}_{28}$Ni, $^{64}_{30}$Zn.

Isotones—atoms having same N's, different Z's and different A's:
$^{40}_{18}$A, $^{41}_{19}$K, $^{42}_{20}$Ca.

Isomers—Atoms having same Z's and same A's, but different energy states in the nucleus. (These will be discussed later, page 66.)

Classification of Stable Nuclei.   There are known to be 274 stable nuclides of 81 elements; they are classified as follows:

Z even, N even—162
Z even, N odd — 56
Z odd, N even — 52
Z odd, N odd — 4 ($^2_1$H, $^6_3$Li, $^{10}_5$B, $^{14}_7$N.)

As Z increases, N increases a little faster, so that above $Z = 20$, there are always more neutrons than protons. A chart of all known stable nuclides, according to neutron and proton content, is shown in Figure 1–5. It is seen that they are grouped along a smooth curve, with neutron content increasing steadily with regard to proton content.

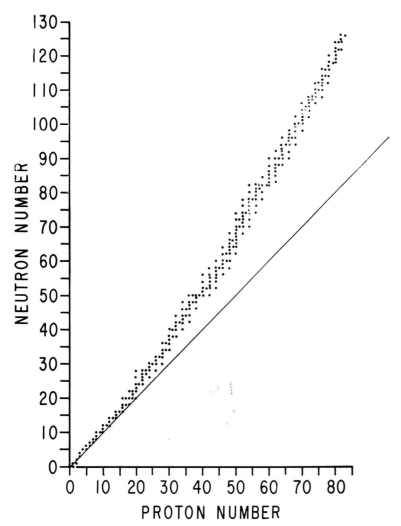

FIG. 1-5.   Proton-neutron plot of known stable nuclei.
Note the gradual increase in ratio of neutron numbers to proton numbers.   The 45°
line indicates a neutron-proton ratio of 1.

Dimensions of Atoms and Nuclei.   The dimensions of atoms and nuclei
are very small.   Diameters of outer electron orbits are of the order of
10^{-8} cm.   Diameters of nuclei themselves are of the order of 10^{-12} to
10^{-13} cm.   Thus the atom is almost all empty space; the actual part of its
volume occupied by the nucleus and the electrons is extremely small.   The
simile of a fly and a few gnats in a large cathedral is suggestive.   The very
small nucleus must have an extremely high density; in fact, it is of the order
of a hundred million tons per cubic centimeter!

Nuclear Forces.   The nature of forces holding the nuclear components
together has been the subject of much speculation.   Protons would be

expected to repel each other according to classical electrostatic behavior of charged particles. Evidently the nuclear forces contain an additional factor besides electrical and gravitational components. The presently accepted idea is of so-called *exchange forces* based upon the existence within the nucleus of small sub-atomic particles called *mesons*. Such particles are known to exist. The pi mesons, or *pions* have a mass about 276 times that of the electron; some have positive charges, some negative, and some are uncharged. It is suggested that two nuclear particles share such a pion so that it is sometimes part of one and sometimes of the other; that is, they *exchange* it back and forth. Symbolically the force between a proton and a neutron could then be described as

$$p_1 + n_1 \rightarrow n_2 + \pi^+ + n_1 \rightarrow n_2 + p_2,$$

where the p's denote protons, the n's neutrons, and the π^+ the shared pion. The original proton emits a positive pion and becomes a neutron. The pion is quickly absorbed by another neutron, which thereby becomes a proton. Thus the proton and the neutron have *exchanged* the pion. Similarly a neutron turns into a proton by emitting a negative pion, whereas two protons or two neutrons may share a neutral pion. These exchanges must take place at excessively high frequencies, so that the pion never really escapes from either particle; they are "bound together." It is not within the scope of this book to elaborate further on this topic. The nature of the nucleus will be further discussed in Chapters 4 and 6.

REFERENCES

GLASSER, O., QUIMBY, E. H., TAYLOR, L. S., WEATHERWAX, J. and MORGAN, R. H.: *Physical Foundations of Radiology*, 3rd Ed., Chap. 2. New York, Paul B. Hoeber, Inc., 1961.

NEEDHAM, J. and PAGEL, W.: *Background to Modern Science*, Chaps. 1, 2, 3, 4, and 7. New York, The Macmillan Co., 1938.

SEMAT, H.: *Introduction to Atomic and Nuclear Physics*, 4th Ed., New York, Holt, Rinehart & Winston, 1962.

2

Radioactivity

Historical. The discovery of x rays by Wilhelm Conrad Roentgen in 1895 stimulated the imagination of physicists in many countries. Henri Becquerel, in France, observed that x-ray tubes fluoresced brilliantly when emitting x rays, and wondered whether substances which fluoresced under sunlight might also emit invisible radiations. Fortunately among the first materials he tested were some uranium compounds, and in 1896 he announced that these did in fact give off radiations, and furthermore that fluorescence had nothing to do with the phenomenon. Mme. Marie Curie took up the study of these substances, coining the words "radioactive" and "radioactivity" to describe the process. She investigated systematically the known elements and compounds, and found that all compounds of uranium and thorium possessed this property, and no other substances. She found also that some of the natural ores of uranium were much more active than the element itself, and so concluded that they must contain a hitherto unknown and very radioactive element.

At this point her husband, Pierre Curie, became so interested in her work that he gave up his own researches to join her, and they worked together until his untimely death in 1906. In 1898 they announced the discovery of not one, but two new radioactive elements, which they named *polonium* and *radium*.

The radiations emitted by these radioactive substances possessed the same properties as x rays, of darkening photographic plates and of discharging electrically charged bodies. It was early observed that most of the rays were very unpenetrating, and could be stopped by a sheet of paper. A large part of those passing through the paper could traverse a few millimeters of wood or paper, but no more. A very small part of the original beam was very penetrating, traversing considerable thicknesses of metal.

Nature of the Radiations. At first the rays were thought to be all alike, differing only in penetrating power, and little was known of their nature. However, extensive series of researches by Becquerel, Pierre Curie, and Villard showed that there were three quite distinct types of ray. This may be demonstrated by a simple experiment, as in Figure 2–1. When a beam of moving, electrically charged particles is passed between the poles of a magnet, their paths are bent into circles whose radii depend on the strength of the field, the magnitude of the charge, and the kinetic energy of the particles. The direction of the deflection depends on the sign of the charge. In the figure, the magnetic field is perpendicular to the page, with the south pole above and the north pole below. The very unpenetrating radiation is deflected clockwise, and the paths are circles of rather large radius, indicating that these are positively charged particles, and rather heavy. The moderately penetrating radiation is deflected in the opposite direction and the paths are much more strongly bent. These are therefore lighter, negatively charged particles. The heavier component was called the alpha (α) radiation, or more properly, α particles; the lighter, beta (β)

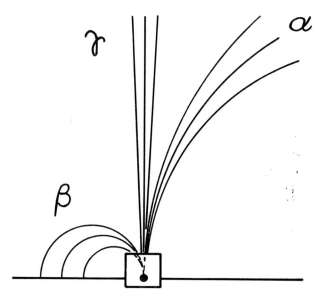

Fig. 2–1. Diagrammatic representation of deviation of alpha and beta rays in a magnetic field, while gamma rays are not affected. The field is perpendicular to the plane of the paper, the south pole being above and the north pole below.

radiation, or β particles. The undeflected component obviously does not consist of charged particles; its real nature was demonstrated by Villard, who showed that these rays were identical with those emitted by an x-ray tube. They were called gamma (γ) rays. Both x and γ rays are called *photons.*

Further study showed that the alpha particles have a mass about four times that of the hydrogen atom, and two unit positive charges. They are really nuclei of helium atoms, stripped of their orbital electrons and traveling with speeds of 8 to 15,000 miles per second. The beta particles have a mass about $\frac{1}{1800}$ that of the hydrogen atom, a single negative charge, and travel with speeds up to almost that of light. They are actually electrons. The gamma rays are electromagnetic radiations of the same sort as x rays. These radiations will be considered further in Chapter 6.

Atomic Disintegration. It had been found that radioactivity was a property of the *atoms* of the radioactive elements. For a given quantity of such an element, the radiation was always the same, regardless of the chemical composition of the compound under study. Therefore it appeared that the actual atoms must be breaking down in some manner, to eject material particles. It has been mentioned in the previous chapter that this was the starting point for the development of the ideas of atomic structure.

The radioactive elements which were first discovered were all high up in the atomic table, $^{238}_{92}$U, $^{232}_{90}$Th, $^{226}_{88}$Ra, $^{210}_{84}$Po. Their nuclei obviously contain large numbers of particles and are apparently too complicated to be completely stable. It is now known that every element with atomic number greater than 83, or mass number greater than 209, possesses the property of spontaneous emission of radiation, or is radioactive. These nuclei contain in a very tiny volume large numbers of charged and uncharged particles, all in motion and hence exerting electric, magnetic, gravitational, and intranuclear forces upon one another. It is not surprising that at some time a configuration is produced which is unstable, so that the nucleus breaks down.

This breakdown, or *disintegration* is not, however, complete destruction. It consists always of the expulsion of a relatively small charged particle (α or β, never both simultaneously) accompanied by energy. The remaining nuclear components then rearrange themselves and settle down (temporarily or permanently) as the nucleus of an atom of a different element. The removal of an alpha particle decreases the nuclear charge by two units and its mass by four. The removal of a (negative) beta particle increases the positive nuclear charge by one unit; the mass is essentially unchanged:

$$^{A}_{Z}X - ^{4}_{2}\alpha = ^{A-4}_{Z-2}X.$$

$$^{A}_{Z}X - _{-1}\beta = ^{A}_{Z+1}X.$$

If the product element has Z greater than 83, or A greater than 209, it will in turn be radioactive. Thus the disintegration of radium is followed by a series of further disintegrations:

$$^{226}_{88}Ra - \alpha = ^{222}_{86}Rn,$$

$$^{222}_{86}Rn - \alpha = ^{218}_{84}Ra\ A,$$

$$^{218}_{84}Ra\ A - \alpha = ^{214}_{82}Ra\ B,$$

$$^{214}_{82}Ra\ B - \beta = ^{214}_{83}Ra\ C,$$

and so on through four further transformations until the final stable product is reached, $^{206}_{82}$Pb. Radioactive series will be considered in more detail in Chapter 6.

Artificial or Induced Radioactivity. Before considering the behavior of naturally radioactive substances, the field should be expanded to those elements in which radioactivity is induced artificially.

In 1919 Rutherford demonstrated the disruption of stable nitrogen nuclei by bombarding them with natural alpha particles, with the production of hydrogen and a heavy isotope of oxygen (see page 33 for details). This was not an induced radioactivity; the instant the bombardment stopped the production of new particles also stopped. However, in 1934 the Curie-Joliots discovered that when they bombarded aluminum with alpha particles a radiation appeared which continued after the removal of the source, and which died away in the same manner as radiation from known radioactive substances. They had actually produced a radioactive isotope of phosphorus by introducing extra mass and charge into the aluminum nucleus.

Since that time artificially produced radioactive isotopes of every stable element have been prepared. The subject of induced radioactivity will be considered in detail in subsequent chapters. At present it is sufficient to know that such substances do exist, and that their disintegration follows the same rules as those applying to the natural radioelements.

Characteristics of Radioactive Disintegration. Nuclei of any particular radioelement always disintegrate in the same way. It is apparently not possible, for instance, for radium sometimes to emit an alpha particle and sometimes a beta. There are a few instances in which a nuclide appears to have more than one mode of disintegration, such as, for instance, emission of both positive and negative beta particles; in these cases a fixed percentage of the material disintegrating always goes by each path. Furthermore, the energy accompanying the disintegration of atoms of a particular nuclide is always the same. It will be seen later that alpha particles from a specific nuclide either all have the same energy, or fall into a very few monoenergetic groups. The beta particles present a continuous range of energies up to a definite maximum, but this *spectrum* is constant for any one nuclide. The gamma rays, if there are any, are also emitted in one or a few monoenergetic groups. (This whole topic is treated in more detail in Chapter 6.) This *constancy of type and energy of radiation emitted* is one specific characteristic of radioactivity.

The other specific characteristic is *constancy of rate of disintegration*. The amount of any radioactive element is always gradually decreasing; this gradual decrease is the result of many sudden disintegrations of individual nuclei. In any measurable quantity of an element there is always an enormous number of atoms (6×10^{23} per gram-atomic weight). During any instant, a relatively small fraction of these achieve instability and disintegrate. For every radioactive nuclide *a fixed percentage of all the atoms present disintegrate per unit of time*. There is no way of knowing *which* atoms will disintegrate in a given interval, but statistically it is possible to know *how many* will change. Actual rates vary enormously among various radioactive nuclides, in some cases only a small fraction of 1 per cent of all the atoms decays or disintegrates in a century, in others a high percentage is transmuted per second. Most of those of interest in medicine fall far within these two extremes.

Mathematical Expression of Disintegration Law. This type of activity can be described mathematically. If N represents the number of radio-active atoms present at any instant, $-\dfrac{dN}{dt}$ represents the decrease in this number during a very short interval of time. This decrease is a fixed percentage of all the atoms present. Hence

$$\frac{dN}{dt} = \lambda N, \qquad\qquad 2-(1)$$

where λ is the decay constant, or the fraction transformed per unit time, when the time unit is chosen short enough so that only a small fraction of the total number of nuclei disintegrate in that interval. λ is then the fraction *per second, per day*, etc., it expresses a *rate* of disintegration. This differential equation can be integrated,

$$N_t = N_o\, e^{-\lambda t}. \qquad\qquad 2-(2)$$

N_t is the number of atoms remaining from an initial number N_o after a period t; λ is the decay constant for the unit of time in terms of which the interval t is expressed; e is the base of natural logarithms, 2.71828. This is the expression of an "exponential decay law." The decay constant is characteristic of the nuclear species and cannot be changed by any means known at present. Great variations in temperature, pressure, chemical state, magnetic, electric, and gravitational fields, have been without effect.

Half Life and Average Life. Instead of using the decay constant it is possible to express the rate of radioactive transformation by specifying the period during which half of all the atoms initially present will disintegrate. This *half period* or *half life* can be obtained from a knowledge of the decay constant. In equation (2), N_t at the end of a half period is $\frac{1}{2}$ N_o. The half period is indicated by T. The equation then becomes

$$\tfrac{1}{2} N_o = N_o\, e^{-\lambda T}. \qquad\qquad 2-(3)$$

Solving this equation by natural logarithms,

$$\ln \tfrac{1}{2} = -\lambda T,$$

$$\text{or } \lambda T = \ln 2,$$

$$\text{whence } T = \frac{0.693}{\lambda}, \text{ or } \lambda = \frac{0.693}{T} \qquad\qquad 2-(4)$$

Thus the decay constant and the half period bear a fixed relation to each other; if one is found by any means, the other can be calculated.

Then equation 2—(2) can be written

$$N_t = N_o\, e^{-0.693t/T}. \qquad\qquad 2-(5)$$

3

During the first half period, half of all the atoms initially present will decay, in the second half period, half of those remaining at the end of the first, or one-fourth of the original amount, and so on. Thus at the end of two half periods, three-fourths of the original will be gone; after seven half periods less than 1 per cent will remain.

In general, if N_t represents the number of atoms remaining after time t, $N_o - N_t$ represents the number which have decayed, or

$$\text{Number of atoms decayed, } N_o - N_t = N_o (1 - e^{-\lambda t}). \qquad 2-(6)$$

Another useful concept is that of the *average life* of all the atoms of a particular radionuclide. Just as insurance statistics can specify the average life expectancy of all members of a particular group of individuals, so radioactivity statistics can specify the average life expectancy of all atoms of a certain element.

Let N_o represent the original number of atoms, and N_{t_1} the number at any time t_1, where $N_{t_1} = N_o e^{-\lambda t_1}$. During a very short interval after t_1 the number disintegrating is $\dfrac{dN_{t_1}}{dt}$. This is the number of atoms of lifetimes between t_1 and $t_1 + dt$, or, if dt is vanishingly small, the number of lifetime t_1.

$$\frac{dN_{t_1}}{dt} = \lambda N_{t_1} = \lambda N_o e^{-\lambda t_1}$$

or

$$dN_{t_1} = \lambda N_o e^{-\lambda t_1} dt. \qquad 2-(7)$$

The *total* lives of the atoms in any group are the number in the group multiplied by the age of each, or, for the group of age t_1, $dN_{t_1} \times t_1$. The summation of groups for all values of t_1 from zero to infinity gives the total lives of all the atoms in the system. This sum, divided by the total number of atoms, give the *average life of any atom*.

$$\int_o^\infty t \, dN_t = N_o \lambda \int_o^\infty t \, e^{-\lambda t} \, dt = \frac{N_o}{\lambda}. \qquad 2-(8)$$

$$\frac{N_o}{\lambda} \div N_o = \frac{1}{\lambda}. \qquad 2-(9)$$

Thus *the average life is the reciprocal of the decay constant.* Since the decay constant has been shown to be $\dfrac{0.693}{\text{half life}}$, the average life is $\dfrac{T}{0.693}$ or 1.443 T.

It is usually denoted by the Greek letter τ.

The average life is a quantity based on statistical analysis. It does not represent the lifetime of most of the atoms, as is sometimes erroneously supposed. Actually during this period, which is 1.443 T, the number of atoms initially present, N_o, will be reduced to $1/e \times N_o = 0.37 N_o$, as will be seen by introducing 1.443 T for t in equation 2—(2).

Half periods or decay constants of radioactive nuclei are listed in many places. Data concerning some of the more useful ones will be found in the appendix. By use of the decay constant and equation 2—(2) the amount of any radioactive material remaining at any time can be calculated. It is often convenient to plot "decay curves" for individual nuclides as shown in Figure 2-2. The curves of Figure 2-2A, plotted on linear graph paper, require the determination of a considerable number of points, and the drawing of a smooth curve through them. The use of semi-logarithmic paper, as in Figure 2-2B, simplifies the procedure. It is a property of exponential expressions of the type $N_t = N_o e^{-\lambda t}$ that their graphs on semi-logarithmic paper are straight lines. For this reason it is only necessary to establish two points on the curve and draw a straight line through them.

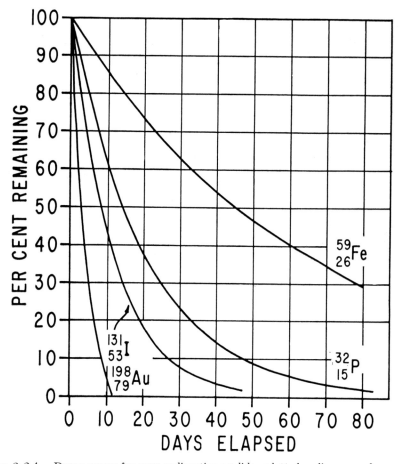

FIG. 2–2A.   Decay curves for some radioactive nuclides, plotted on linear graph paper.

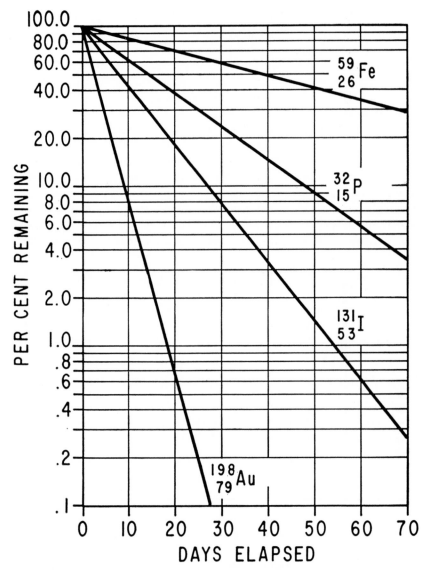

Fig. 2–2B.   Decay curves for the same radioactive nuclides plotted on semi-logarithmic graph paper.

Activity.   In practical work with radioactive nuclides the number of atoms N is not directly measured, nor usually is the rate of change $\dfrac{dN}{dt}$. What is actually measured is something proportional to the number of disintegrations per unit time, that is, something proportional to λN. This is usually termed the *activity*, and denoted by A when A = cλN, c being a constant of proportionality. The value of this constant will depend on the nature and efficiency of the measuring and recording instruments, and on the geometrical arrangement of sample and detector. Great care must be exercised to keep these constant during any series of measurements. A is directly proportional to N, and the decay law may be written

$$A = A_o \, e^{-0.693t/T}. \hspace{3cm} 2\text{—}(10)$$

Hence a plot of experimentally determined values of A will give values for T and τ for the nuclide in question, from which such curves as those of those of Figure 2–2 may be prepared.

Units of Activity of Radioactive Nuclides. The amount of a radioactive nuclide is specified in terms of its disintegration rate, or its *activity*. The unit of activity is the *curie* (Ci), which is 3.7×10^{10} disintegrations per second (d/s). The millicurie (mCi) and the microcurie (μCi) are disintegration rates one-thousandth and one-millionth respectively of the curie. Larger and smaller units are also used:—

1 kilocurie	. . .	3.7×10^{13} d/s
1 curie	. . . .	3.7×10^{10}
1 millicurie	. . .	3.7×10^{7}
1 microcurie	. .	3.7×10^{4}
1 nanocurie	. . .	3.7×10
1 picocurie	. . .	3.7×10^{-2}

It has been customary to use the curie and its fractions as units of quantity of radioactive material rather than of activity. To be strictly correct, instead of saying "so many curies" of a specified nuclide, the form should be "a quantity of the specified nuclide having an activity of so many curies." This is awkward and really unnecessary; for convenience the old form will be used in this book.

Obviously there is no simple relationship between curies and total number of atoms or weight of material. A nuclide with a short half period will not require such a large reservoir of its atoms to supply them at the needed disintegration rate as will one with a long half period. However, it will be shown below that either the number of atoms or the weight per curie can be calculated when the half period and the atomic weight are known.

Total Number of Radioactive Atoms. The actual *number* of atoms of a nuclide is seldom specified; it is rather the *quantity* or the *activity* in terms of the units just specified. Actual calibration or measurement of such activities will be discussed in Chapter 16. If Q_o and Q_t represent the quantities of a nuclide with decay constant λ, initially and after a period of time t, then from equation 2—(2)

$$Q_t = Q_o \, e^{-\lambda t}.$$

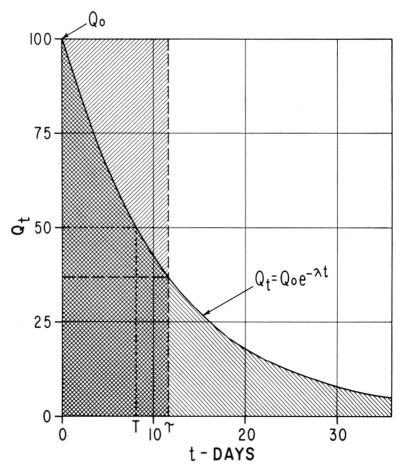

FIG. 2–3.   Curve showing relationships among various constants involved in disintegration expressions.

The relationship among the various constants Q_o, Q_t, λ, T, and τ are shown in Figure 2–3.   Any point on the curve represents the quantity Q_t of radioactive nuclide at time t.   The amount by which this will be diminished in the next instant is given by $\lambda Q_t = \lambda Q_o\, e^{-\lambda t}$.   The sum of all these small decrements from t = 0 to t = ∞ is, of course, equal to Q_o, and is represented by the area under the curve.

Now if instead of the exponential type of decay, it be imagined that in each unit of time the initial quantity is diminished by the same *amount* as the first day's decay (not the same per cent as the first day's decay), up to the period of the average life, it will be totally destroyed.   An example may make this clear.   Assume a nuclide with a half life of 8 days, then λ/day is 0.693/8 = 0.086, or 8.6 per cent of whatever is present decays in the next day, until all is gone.   But if instead 8.6 per cent *of the original amount* decayed each day, for the time of the average life, namely $1/\lambda$, or 11.6 days, again all would have gone. $0.086 \times 11.6 = 1$.

The actual number of atoms, N_o, in a quantity Q_o mCi, can readily be calculated. For 1 mCi, in the first second 3.7×10^7 nuclei disintegrate. That is, in the expression $\dfrac{dN_o}{dt} = \lambda N_o$, when λ is the decay constant per second,

$$\frac{dN_o}{dt} = 3.7 \times 10^7, \qquad \text{or,} \quad \lambda N_o = 3.7 \times 10^7 \text{ per mCi} \qquad 2\text{---}(11)$$

$$\text{and} \qquad N_o \text{ per mCi} = \frac{3.7 \times 10^7}{\lambda} = 3.7 \times 10^7 \times 1.443 \text{ T} \qquad 2\text{---}(12)$$

where T is the half period in seconds. In other words, the total number of atoms in a curie is the number disintegrating per second times the average life in seconds. The constant which is usually known is the half life T in days. The average life, τ, in seconds $= 1.443\text{T} \times 86,400$. Whence the number of atoms per curie is

$$3.7 \times 10^{10} \times 86,400 \times 1.443 \text{ T} = 4.6 \times 10^{15} \text{ T (days)}. \qquad 2\text{---}(13)$$

The weight of one curie depends on the number of atoms per curie and the weight of each one. Since one gram atomic weight of the element contains 6×10^{23} atoms (Avogadro's hypothesis), the weight of one atom of atomic

$$\text{weight G} = \frac{G}{6 \times 10^{23}} \text{ gm} = \frac{G \times 10^3}{6 \times 10^{23}} \text{ mg.}$$

Whence the weight of one curie of the element is

$$\frac{4.6 \times 10^{15} \times T \times G \times 10^3}{6 \times 10^{23}} \text{ mg} = 7.65 \text{ T G} \times 10^{-6} \text{ mg.} \qquad 2\text{---}(14)$$

For example, for ^{131}I, T $= 8.04$ days, G $= 131^*$, weight of 1 curie $= 7.65 \times 8.04 \times 131 \times 10^{-6} = 8 \times 10^{-3}$ mg.

Weights of some common radionuclides, in milligrams per curie, are given in Table 2–1.

Determination of Half Periods and Decay Constants. The method of determining the decay constant for a radioactive nuclide, whose rate is neither very long nor very short, is to prepare a sample which can be maintained in a fixed form for the necessary period, and make measurements at successive intervals. It is not necessary to determine the abso-

---

* G and A are not strictly identical. A is always a whole number, the total number of mass particles in the nucleus; while G is the actual atomic weight of the particular nuclide. In practice they are not very different, and the use of A in the formula is justified.

Table 2–1. Weights of One Curie of Some Radionuclides

Nuclide	Half Period	Weight—Mg per Ci
^{24}Na	15.0 hours	0.000114
^{131}I	8.1 days	0.0081
^{32}P	14.2 days	0.0035
^{89}Sr	54 days	0.0368
^{45}Ca	164 days	0.0566
^{60}Co	5.26 years	0.88
^{14}C	5530 years	216

lute activity at any time, relative values are sufficient. These relative values are plotted, the half period determined, and the decay constant calculated. For example, a series of daily measurements on a sample of radioactive gold were as follows:

Hour	Counts per Minute
0	5600
24	4330
48	3340
72	2680
96	2000
120	1540
144	1190
192	710

These values, plotted in Figure 2–4, indicate a half period of 64 hours, or 2.7 days. The decay constant then is $\dfrac{0.693}{64} = 0.0108$, or 1.08 per cent per hour. Thus each day there will be about 25 per cent less than on the preceding day.

For nuclides of very short or very long half period, successive measurements within a reasonable time are not practicable, and other methods have been devised. These will be found described in the literature.

A mixture of two or more nuclides with different decay rates will give decay data which will not fall on a straight line. However, by plotting and analyzing the complex decay curve, decay constants for the components can often be determined. For example, a sample supposed to be ^{133}I with a half period of 20.8 hours gave the following readings:

Day	Counts per Minute	Day	Counts per Minute
0	800	6	66
1	414	8	52
2	235	10	42
3	144	12	36
4	101	14	30

These values, plotted in Figure 2–5, give the solid curve. The last part of this is a straight line, which can be extrapolated backward as shown by the dotted line, and indicates an exponential decay with a half period of just

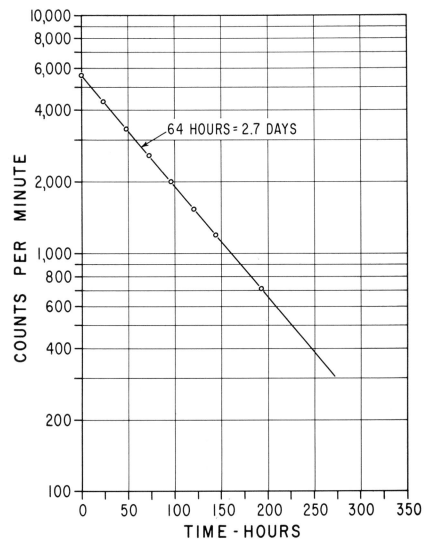

FIG. 2-4. Experimental determination of decay constant for radioactive gold, $^{198}_{79}$Au.

over 8 days, corresponding to ^{131}I. For each day, the ^{131}I contribution indicated by this dotted line should be subtracted from the measured value. The results are the crosses shown in the figure; a straight line drawn through these indicates exponential decay with a half period of about 0.9 day, corresponding to ^{133}I. Apparently the material was a mixture of these two isotopes of iodine; at the initial reading one-eighth of the total counts were due to the longer-lived component.

It must be remembered that in a mixture of two isotopes of an element, with different half lives, as time goes by the percentage of the longer-lived

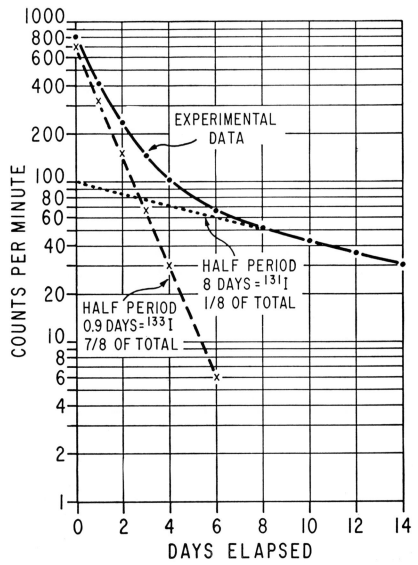

FIG. 2–5. Analysis of complex decay curve obtained from mixture
of two radioactive isotopes of iodine.

one will increase relative to the shorter. A practical example arises in the
case of ^{203}Hg and ^{197}Hg. The ^{197}Hg as supplied normally has some contamination with ^{203}Hg. Suppose that at the time of receipt of a supposedly
100 mCi sample, the contamination was 2 per cent (relatively low). That
is the batch contains 98 mCi ^{197}Hg (T = 65 hours), and 2 mCi ^{203}Hg
(T = 47 days). Two days later there are 57 mCi of ^{197}Hg and 1.94 mCi
of ^{203}Hg; the percentage of the latter in the total has risen to 3.4. At 5 days

there are only 25 mCi of ^{197}Hg, but 1.8 mCi of ^{203}Hg; the percentage is now 7. By 10 days it has risen to 20. Obviously, from the point of view of radiation to the patient, use of the old sample may present problems.

In addition to curves prepared by the individual worker, usually by calculation from published data rather than from individual measurements, large-scale curves for the most common radioelements are commercially available, and some new slide rules with special scales for radionuclide decay are now on the market.

A convenient table for finding values of the decay factor $f = e^{-0.693\ t/T}$ is given in Appendix, where, as usual, t is the decay time in question and T the half life. Values for T for a large number of nuclides are listed in Appendix C. Values of t/T must be calculated by the user; three significant figures will usually be satisfactory, although more can be used if interpolation is employed. The steps between the tabulated values of f have a constant fractional increment of 0.7 per cent. When fractional half life is calculated "exactly," the largest error in f when using the table will be about 0.5 per cent, which is sufficient for all practical purposes.

Carrier, Specific Activity. A particular radioactive sample may consist entirely of the radioactive nuclide in question, or it may contain stable isotopes of the same element. In the first case, the radioactive material is said to be *carrier-free*. In the second, if the stable and radioactive isotopes are in the same chemical form, it is said to be *with carrier*.

The term "carrier" arose from radiochemistry. Where chemical precipitations are carried out involving very small quantities of material, as is the case with a few microcuries of a short-lived nuclide, it is sometimes impossible to carry the reaction to completion. Almost all compounds are soluble to some extent, and minute quantities of radioactive material may remain in the solution. By adding a relatively large amount of the stable isotope in the same chemical form, essentially all of the mixture can be "carried" down.

In some biological work, the total quantity of the element involved must be kept small, if normal physiological conditions are to be maintained. In this case, carrier-free radioactive material is highly desirable. An example of this is in the study of thyroid function with radioactive iodine. The body's normal daily intake of iodide is of the order of 100 to 200 micrograms, and administration of more than a few additional micrograms might alter the delicate physiological balance in the function of the thyroid gland. Accordingly radioactive iodine, carrier-free or at least containing very little carrier, is essential. On the other hand, in such studies as determination of fluid volume by isotope dilution the existence of carrier is seldom important unless it is chemically toxic.

The *specific activity* of an isotope preparation is usually stated as the number of millicuries of radioactive isotope per gram of the total mixture of radioactive and stable isotopes of the element in question. In carrier-free material the specific activity is, of course, the highest possible; in radionuclide catalogs such material is simply denoted by CF.   When stable isotopes are also present, specific activity may vary from thousands of millicuries per gram to any small fraction of this proportion.

REFERENCES

CURIE, EVE.:   *Madam Curie*, New York, Doubleday Doran & Company, 1938.

CURIE, MARIE: *Pierre Curie*, New York, The Macmillan Co., 1923.

FRIEDLANDER, G., KENNEDY, J. W. and MILLER, J. M.:   *Nuclear and Radiochemistry*, 2nd Ed., New York, John Wiley & Sons, Inc., 1964.

GLASSER, O., QUIMBY, E. H., TAYLOR, L. S., WEATHERWAX, J. and MORGAN, R. H.: *Physical Foundations of Radiology*, 3rd Ed., Chapter 14.   New York, Paul B. Hoeber, Inc., 1961.

LAPP, R. E. and Andrews, H. L.:   *Nuclear Radiation Physics*, 3rd Ed., New York, Prentice-Hall, Inc., 1963.

3

Disruption of Stable Nuclei—Induced Radioactivity

First Artificial Transmutation. As mentioned in the preceding chapter in 1919 Rutherford demonstrated the disruption of ordinary nitrogen nucle as a result of their bombardment by alpha particles from naturally radio-active material. A diagram of his simple apparatus is shown in Figure 3–1. Particles coming from the alpha particle source at S traversed the gas in the tube, and on striking the fluorescent screen F, gave rise to scintillations which could be observed as individual points of light, by means of the telescope. The source was mounted on a movable support with a scale. When the gas in the tube was oxygen, no scintillations were observed at a

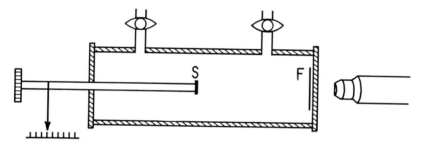

Fig. 3–1. Diagram of apparatus used by Rutherford to demonstrate disintegration of nitrogen nuclei by alpha particle bombardment.

source-screen distance greater than a few centimeters. When hydrogen was used, the distance was about four times as great, but again there was a definite limit. However, when pure nitrogen was introduced into the tube, some scintillations were observed at distances up to 40 centimeters. Study of the deflections of the paths of these long-range particles in electric and magnetic fields demonstrated that each had a single positive charge and unit mass; they were *protons.*

The nature of the complete transformation was not obvious. It might be a shattering of the nitrogen nucleus, although only one type of fragment was observed. It might just be a breaking off of part of the nucleus, or it might be a new kind of "nuclear chemical reaction." The matter was

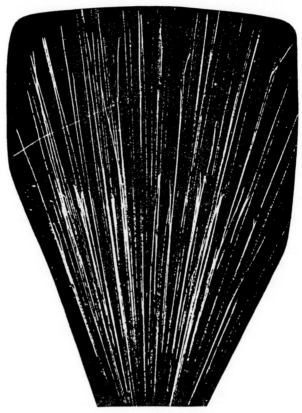

Fig. 3–2. Cloud track photograph of alpha particles traversing air. The heavy white lines are tracks of two sets of alpha particles from the Thorium (C + C′) source. In the center of the picture an alpha particle has hit a nitrogen nucleus. The long thin track extending to the left is made by the released proton, the short stub by the new heavy oxygen nucleus. (Courtesy of P. M. S. Blackett and D. S. Lees, and of the Royal Society of London.)

finally settled by actual photographs of the reaction taken by means of the Wilson cloud chamber (see Chapter 7, p. 87). Figure 3–2 is a reproduction of such a photograph taken by Blackett. The heavy white lines are tracks of two sets of alpha particles from the Thorium (C + C′) source. In the center of the picture an alpha particle has hit a nitrogen nucleus. The long thin track extending to the left is made by the proton; the short stub is made by the remaining nuclear fragment. Evidently there are only two fragments. Since there must be conservation of total charge and mass, it is apparent that the heavier particle must have atomic number 8 and mass number 17. It is therefore a heavy isotope of oxygen, and the nuclear reaction can be written

$$^{14}_{7}\text{N} + ^{4}_{2}\text{He} = ^{17}_{8}\text{O} + ^{1}_{1}\text{H}.$$

As soon as Rutherford announced this discovery, the procedure was repeated in other laboratories and alpha particles were used to bombard many elements. It was found that atoms of all elements with atomic numbers from 4 to 19 (beryllium to potassium) with the exception of oxygen, could be made to disintegrate; in all cases one product was a proton. The natural alpha particles did not have sufficient energy to get inside heavier nuclei than these.

A further disadvantage in these experiments was the relatively small number of alpha particles available for bombardments. Rutherford had estimated that only one alpha particle in a million of those passing through nitrogen gas resulted in a disintegration. The desire for sources emitting larger numbers of particles more energetic than natural alphas led to the development of powerful electrical instruments for accelerating charged particles. The *cyclotron*, the most useful of these in production of radioactive nuclides, will be described later in this chapter.

Discovery of the Neutron. In the course of alpha particle bombardment of various substances, the neutron, whose existence was postulated by Rutherford as described in Chapter 1, was discovered. Three groups of physicists in three countries contributed to this. In 1932, Bothe and Becker in Germany, shot alpha particles into beryllium, $^9_4$Be, and found a very penetrating radiation given off. They supposed that the alpha particle had entered the beryllium to make $^{13}_6$C and that the extra energy had been given off as penetrating gamma rays. The Curie-Joliots in Paris studied this radiation, and found that after it was passed through paraffin there was *more* activity instead of *less* as there should have been. They identified protons in the radiation coming from the paraffin, but could not account for them. Then Chadwick, at Cambridge University in England, put forth the assumption that what came from the beryllium was a particle, with mass about the same as the proton, but no charge. Such an electrically neutral particle could go a long way through matter; it would not be affected by nuclei unless it really collided with them. In paraffin, which is very rich in hydrogen, the neutral particle, making head-on collisions with the hydrogen nuclei, would knock them out as protons. Many experiments since that time have verified the existence of the *neutron*. The correct equation for Bothe and Becker's reaction (excluding energy transfer) is

$$^9_4\text{Be} + ^4_2\alpha = ^{12}_6\text{C} + ^1_0\text{n}.$$

Discovery of the Positron. About this time another particle was discovered in cosmic ray research, that was destined soon to play a part in nuclear physics; this was the *positron*. It has been seen (p. 18) that when charged particles traverse a magnetic field their paths are bent into circles. Many cloud chamber photographs had been made of tracks of electrons following such curved paths. In 1932, Anderson, in southern California, in a cloud chamber record of cosmic rays, found a track curved in the "wrong" direction. The particle making it had apparently the same mass as the electron, but a positive instead of negative charge. Since then, positrons have been frequently photographed, and have been found to be emitted in some radioactive disintegrations.

Artificially Produced Radionuclides. In fact, the first artificially produced radioactive nuclide was a positron emitter. By 1934 many elements had been disintegrated under alpha particle bombardment, but in all cases the products were stable, as were the hydrogen and oxygen of Rutherford's first experiment. Once the alpha particle source was removed, no further particles or radiations were observed. In that year the Curie-Joliots, bombarding aluminum with alpha particles, discovered something new. They observed neutrons emitted during the bombardment. But after the alpha source was removed, the irradiated aluminum foil continued to emit some kind of radiation, which decreased exponentially with time! Apparently they had created a radioactive substance, with a half period of three and a quarter minutes:

$$^{27}_{13}Al + ^{4}_{2}\alpha = ^{30}_{15}P + ^{1}_{0}n,$$

and

$$^{30}_{15}P \rightarrow ^{30}_{14}Si + ^{0}_{+1}\beta.$$

Immediately after the announcement of this discovery the hunt was on for new radioactive nuclides, or possibly for other new nuclear phenomena. By this time several types of accelerators for charged particles had been developed but the cyclotron was, and still is, the most useful in this field. It can supply bombarding particles in tremendously greater numbers than any source of naturally radioactive material and with greater energies than the natural alpha particles.

The Cyclotron. The first cyclotron was built by E. O. Lawrence in 1932. The essential parts of the instrument are shown in Figure 3–3. The acceleration chamber consists of two hollow, semi-circular parts called Dees, because of their shape. Top, bottom, and outer circumference are closed, but the inner straight faces are open. These straight faces are parallel and slightly separated. The Dees are coupled into a very high frequency electrical system so that they are oppositely charged and the charge on each is alternately positive and negative, changing sign about 10^7 times per second. The whole chamber, in a shield that can be evacuated to a very low pressure, is placed between the pole pieces of a large electromagnet. At the center of the space between the Dees some arrangement is made for releasing protons or deuterons (Point S). Consider a proton released at S just at the instant that Dee A is at its peak negative charge, and B at its peak positive. The proton, being positively charged, will be repelled by B and attracted by A, and will enter the interior of A, with a

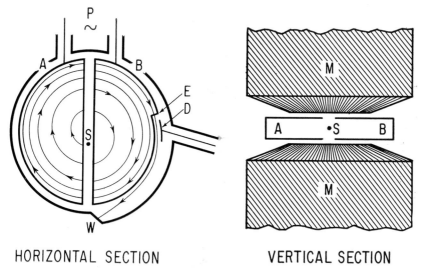

P
~
A
B
E
D
S
W

HORIZONTAL SECTION

M
A •S B
M

VERTICAL SECTION

Fig. 3–3. Diagram of central part of cyclotron.
A and B, Dees; S, ion source; P, alternating potential; D, deflecting plate; E, exit slit; W, window; MM, magnet poles.

definite velocity due to the potential difference between A and B. The electric charge on the Dee remains on the outside; the interior is field-free, so that once the particle is inside the charge ceases to act. However, the magnetic field does act on the moving, charged particle, bending its path into a circle. If the particle travelling in this circular path arrives back at the space between the Dees just at the instant that their charges have been reversed, it will again be accelerated across the gap, and will enter B with a higher velocity than it had while in A. Therefore, the radius of its new circular path will be larger. However, since it is moving faster, it will again arrive at the gap at the instant of charge reversal, receive an additional impulse, and re-enter Dee A at still higher velocity. If each individual impulse is 200 keV, by the time the particle has made 50 revolutions, with two accelerations in each, it will have reached a total energy of 20 MeV.* By this time it will be far out toward the periphery of the Dee. An exit slit is provided at E, with a charged deflector plate D to pull the particle out of the circular path; it can then escape through the window W.

The stream of high energy protons or deuterons emerging through the window can be used as nuclear bombarders for any target introduced into its path. If neutrons are desired as bombarders, they can be produced by deuteron bombardment of beryllium:

$$\mathrm{^{9}_{4}Be + {}^{2}_{1}d = {}^{10}_{5}B + {}^{1}_{0}n.}$$

* One electron volt (eV) is the energy acquired by an electron in falling through a potential difference of one volt. Here the individual potential differences are each 200 kilovolts, and the final energy is twenty million electron volts. See Chapter 4, p. 40 for further discussion of energy units.

4

The beryllium target is placed in the deuteron beam, and a neutron beam emerges on the far side of the beryllium.

Thus the cyclotron provides positive or neutral particles, at any desired energy (within limits) and in relatively large quantities, for use in nuclear bombardment, disruption, and production of radioactive nuclides.

Machines to accelerate electrons to high energies have also been developed. Except in very special circumstances the electrons themselves, even at the highest available energies, are not able to produce nuclear transmutation. However, the x rays produced by these energetic electrons in the betatron or synchrotron can sometimes bring about nuclear reactions. The phenomenon is not of practical importance in the production of radioactive nuclides, but has been valuable in studying energy relations.

REFERENCES

FRIEDLANDER, G., KENNEDY, J. W. and MILLER, J. M.: *Nuclear and Radiochemistry*, 2nd Ed., Chapters 1–3. New York, John Wiley & Sons, Inc., 1964.

GLASSER, O., QUIMBY, E. H., TAYLOR, L. S., WEATHERWAX, J. L. and MORGAN, R. H.: *Physical Foundations of Radiology*, 3rd Ed., Chapters 9 and 14, New York, Paul B. Hoeber, Inc., 1961.

LAPP, R. E. and ANDREWS, H. L.: *Nuclear Radiation Physics*, 3rd Ed., Chapters 12 and 13, New York, Prentice-Hall, Inc., 1963.

MORGAN, R. H. and CORRIGAN, K. E.: *Handbook of Radiology*, Section 4, Chicago, Yearbook Publishers, Inc., 1955.

POLLARD, E. C. and DAVIDSON, W. L.: *Applied Nuclear Physics*, 2nd Ed., Chapters 4, 5, and 7, New York, John Wiley & Sons, Inc., 1951.

4

Nuclear Reactions

AT the present time over a thousand nuclear reactions are known; hundreds of radioactive nuclides have been prepared artificially. Transmutation is brought about by bombardment of nuclei with positively charged alpha particles, deuterons, or protons, with uncharged neutrons, and with photons (x rays) of pure energy. These phenomena will be discussed in detail, but first certain general considerations should be developed.

The Energy of a Reaction. In a chemical reaction, heat is either used up or given off; the reaction is called endothermic or exothermic. The complete reaction equation contains an expression for the heat of the reaction. For instance, instead of writing simply

$$C + O_2 = CO_2,$$

the complete form is

$$C + O_2 = CO_2 + 94,000 \text{ calories.}$$

That is, when one gram mol of carbon and two of oxygen combine to form carbon dioxide, 94,000 calories of heat are evolved. Similarly, in a nuclear reaction, energy is either used up or given off; the term analogous to "heat of reaction" is "nuclear energy change." The complete equation for Rutherford's first nuclear reaction should be

$$^{14}_{7}N + ^{4}_{2}He = ^{17}_{8}O + ^{1}_{1}H + Q,$$

where Q represents the energy change. In a particular reaction, Q may be positive or negative. Positive Q means energy release; the reaction is *exoergic*. Negative Q, energy absorption, denotes *endoergic* reaction.

Exoergic reactions, those releasing energy, have attracted great attention. The energy liberated in a reaction with a large positive Q value is the "atomic energy" so widely discussed in recent years.

Equivalence of Mass and Energy. To understand the source of this energy it is necessary to accept a new idea, the equivalence of mass and energy. In 1905, as part of his special relativity theory, Einstein advanced this hypothesis and supplied the transformation equation

$$E = Mc^2, \qquad\qquad 4\text{—}(1)$$

where E is the energy in ergs equivalent to a mass of M grams, c being the velocity of light (2.997925×10^{10} cm per sec). Therefore the mass of a nucleus is a direct measure of its *total* energy content, the energy which would be released if the mass were totally destroyed. Such total destruction is seldom found, but partial mass disappearance can readily be detected.

It is found that the measured mass of a nucleus is always less than the sum of the masses of its constituent nucleons. The difference between the two represents loss of mass in consolidating the nucleons into the nucleus; its energy equivalent is called the *binding energy* of the nucleus.

The energy equivalent of one mass unit (1.66044×10^{-24} gm) is

$$E = 1.66044 \times 10^{-24} \times (2.997925 \times 10^{10})^2$$
$$= 1.492 \times 10^{-3} \text{ erg.}$$

An energy unit more useful in nuclear study is the *electron volt*, the energy acquired by an electron in falling though a potential difference of one volt.

$$1 \text{ ev} = 1.602 \times 10^{-12} \text{ erg}$$
$$\text{or } 1 \text{ erg} = 0.624 \times 10^{12} \text{ ev.}$$

Correspondingly

$$1 \text{ keV (kiloelectron volt)} = 1.602 \times 10^{-9} \text{ erg,}$$
and $\quad 1 \text{ MeV (million electron volts)} = 1.602 \times 10^{-6} \text{ erg.}$

In these terms,

$$1 \text{ mass unit} = 931.48 \text{ MeV}$$
and $\quad 1 \text{ electron mass } (0.0005486 \text{ mu}) = 0.511006 \text{ MeV.}$

The binding energy of the ^{4}He nucleus may be calculated from the known values of the mass of the helium atom and of its components. The mass of the ^{4}He atom is 4.002604 mu. The two orbital electrons account for 0.001097 mu, leaving 4.001507 as the nuclear mass. The masses of a proton and a neutron are 1.007277 and 1.0086654 mu respectively. Then

$$\text{Nucleus } ^4\text{He} = 2 \text{ p} + 2 \text{ n}$$
$$4.001507 = 2 \times 1.007277 + 2 \times 1.0086654 + Q$$
$$Q = 0.030377 \text{ mu.}$$

Therefore 0.030377 mass units, or 28.3 MeV of energy is used up in binding together the components of the helium nucleus. This is 7.1 MeV per nucleon. The average binding energy per nucleon in general is from 6 to 9 MeV throughout the periodic table. The maximum occurs for elements in the region A = 55.

In making calculations for nuclear reactions in which beta particles are emitted, there is sometimes confusion as to what nuclear masses to use. In general masses of complete neutral *atoms* are tabulated, for convenience of workers with mass spectrographs. In this case the total mass of all the orbital electrons must be subtracted from the atomic mass to obtain the nuclear mass. In dealing with a radioactive disintegration it must be remembered that the number of orbital electrons for parent and daughter is not the same. An exhaustive table of nuclidic, or atomic, masses is given in Friendlander, Kennedy, and Miller, *Nuclear and Radiochemistry*, page 535 ff.

When Einstein proposed his hypothesis, no experimental evidence of the equivalence of mass and energy was available. However, by careful measurement of masses and energies in nuclear reactions, abundant evidence has now been accumulated. For instance, radioactive sodium disintegrates according to the equation

$$_{11}^{24}\text{Na} = {}_{12}^{24}\text{Mg} + e^- + 2\gamma \ (1.368 \text{ and } 2.754 \text{ MeV}).$$

$$23.990967 = 23.985045 + Q.$$

$$Q = 0.0059 \text{ mu} = 5.5 \text{ MeV}.$$

The two gamma rays account for 4.1 MeV, and the maximum energy of the beta particles is 1.4 MeV, bringing the sum to the calculated value of Q, 5.5 MeV.

Notation for Nuclear Reaction. A nuclear reaction evidently proceeds in two stages. The first is the formation of a very unstable compound nucleus containing all the material of both target and bombarder nuclei; this is followed very promptly by a rearrangement to a more stable state, with the emission of energy, and frequently of particles. To aid in visualizing the two-stage nature of a nuclear reaction, a compact notation has been devised, which can be illustrated by Rutherford's original transmutation. Thus, instead of writing

$$_{7}^{14}\text{N} + {}_{2}^{4}\text{He} = {}_{8}^{17}\text{O} + {}_{1}^{1}\text{H},$$

the shorter form would be

$$^{14}\text{N} \ (\alpha,\text{p}) \ ^{17}\text{O}.$$

The target nucleus is placed before the parentheses, the bombarder just inside, the expelled particle next, and finally, outside the parentheses, the product nucleus. Here the α stands for the alpha particle, p for the ejected proton. The process is referred to as an α-p reaction, indicating that an α particle goes in and a proton comes out.

Corresponding symbols for neutron, deuteron, and photon are n, d, γ. The common forms of reaction are (n,p), (n,α), (p,n), (p,α), (d,p), (d,n),

(d,α), (α,p), and (α,n). Simple "capture" of neutrons or protons also occurs; in this case energy is emitted and the reaction is written (n,γ) or (p,γ).

Mechanisms of Nuclear Reaction. The actual mechanisms by which nuclear processes take place are not firmly established, but Bohr, in 1936, developed a concept of nuclear reactions which explains many of these phenomena. He pictures the nucleus as a densely packed but systematic arrangement of protons and neutrons, with distances between the nucleons of the same order of magnitude as the range of the nuclear forces, and inter-action energies between nucleons of the same orders of magnitude as the kinetic energies needed by bombarders in order to penetrate the nucleus, namely a few MeV. A particle comparable in size to the nucleons, coming into the aggregate with a definite kinetic energy, would lose most of this energy in the first few collisions with nucleons, would then become indistinguishable from them, and would thus be amalgamated into the nucleus, forming a new nucleus whose atomic and mass numbers would depend on the nature of the bombarding particle. This new nucleus contains an extra allotment of energy, the kinetic energy which was brought in by the bombarding particle, plus its binding energy. Thus a 5 MeV proton, bringing in a new binding energy of about 7 MeV, gives rise to a new nucleus with atomic and mass numbers each greater by one than the original, and containing about 12 MeV more energy. This happens in a period of the order of 10^{-20} seconds. Now in haphazard motions energy is transferred among nucleons until one by chance finds itself with enough extra energy to escape from the nuclear binding forces. It is not necessary for the escaping nucleon to accumulate *all* the extra energy, but only enough to get away. This takes place in perhaps 10^{-12} seconds, a much longer period than the first step, but still extremely short. Thus there are two distinct steps in the nuclear reaction. The formation and the breaking up of the compound nucleus are independent of each other and may take place in various ways. If the escaping nucleon does not carry all of the extra energy from the nucleus, this is said to be left in an excited condition, and will return to normal with the emission of energy in the form of a gamma ray. (See Chapter 6, p. 63.) This is not radioactivity; the escaping nucleon is simply the second stage in the development of the new nucleus. The ejected unit may be a proton or a neutron, or occasionally a deuteron or an alpha particle. The new nucleus may be stable or radioactive.

In order to initiate the reaction, it is necessary for the bombarder to get into the nucleus. The neutron, having no charge, can enter readily; it is only necessary for it to encounter the nucleus, which occupies a small space. However, the positively charged protons, deuterons, and alpha particles must overcome the electrical repulsion of the positively charged nucleus. This nuclear potential barrier is usually depicted in the form of a potential "well" as in Figure 4–1. The nucleus is imagined as having its center at point O, and a radius equal to R. The internal potential energy

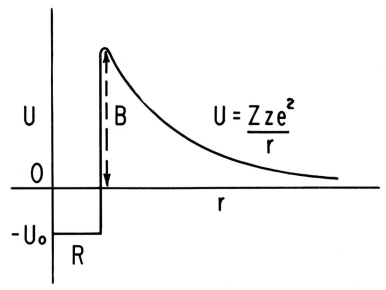

Fig. 4–1. Assumed form of potential energy curve in neighborhood of nucleus. R, nuclear radius; r, distance between center of nucleus and center of bombarding particle; $-U_0$, internal potential energy of nucleus; U, total potential energy; B, height of potential barrier, $= \dfrac{Z z e^2}{R}$.

of the nucleus is constant, and equal to $-U_0$ over the distance from $r = 0$ to $r = R$. At this point the potential energy increases suddenly to the value B, here the maximum repulsion will be exerted on an external charged particle. If the nucleus and the bombarder have atomic numbers Z and z respectively, the electrostatic potential energy between the charges at any distance r is $\dfrac{(Ze)\,(ze)}{r}$, e being the magnitude of a unit charge. The nucleus and the particle are considered as spheres, r being the distance between their centers. As r decreases, the potential energy increases, as indicated by the rising curve, to the maximum value at B. If the kinetic energy of the particle is great enough to overcome this potential energy repulsion, it can "get over the barrier" and enter the nucleus. In general, with smaller energy it cannot, although in special cases it may "leak through." (Discussion of this phenomenon is outside the scope of this book.)

The entire region from $r = R$ to $r = \infty$ is called the *coulomb region*, since here only coulomb or electrostatic forces operate between Z and z. The rising curve of U against r is called the *nuclear potential barrier*. The peak of this curve, at the nuclear radius, is the value $B = \dfrac{(Ze)\,(ze)}{R}$. Thus the height of the barrier depends on the charge on the bombarding particle.

It can be shown that the height of any nuclear coulomb barrier is approximately B $= 0.762$ z $Z^{2/3}$MeV. Thus for an alpha particle to penetrate a sodium nucleus (Z $= 11$), its energy would have to exceed $0.76 \times 2 \times 11^{2/3} = 7.5$ MeV.

Production of Radioactive Nuclides by Nuclear Bombardment. As described above, the entrance of any bombarding particle into a nucleus results in the rearrangement of nuclear material to form a new substance. The particle may simply be absorbed into the nucleus, and the superfluous energy emitted as a gamma ray, or a particle may be ejected. Bombardment by a sufficient number of projectiles will result in the accumulation of a quantity of the product nuclide. The various interactions are described in the following sections.

Alpha Particle Bombardment. Although alpha particles were the first bombarders, they are not used at present to as great extent as other particles. Complete alpha capture apparently does not exist. The (α,n) reaction gives rise to positron emitters:

$$^A_Z X \ (\alpha,n) \ ^{A+3}_{Z+2} X.$$

The first artificially radioactive reactions observed by the Curie-Joliots were of this type:

$$^{10}_5 B \ (\alpha,n) \ ^{13}_7 N.$$
$$^{27}_{13} Al \ (\alpha,n) \ ^{30}_{15} P.$$

Not all products of this reaction are radioactive, some are stable nuclides as in

$$^9_4 Be \ (\alpha,n) \ ^{12}_6 C.$$

This is the first reaction by which neutrons were produced in usable quantity, and is still often employed for small sources. A mixture of powdered beryllium and radium or radon produces about 25,000 neutrons per second per millicurie of radium or radon. This is very small compared to the output that can be achieved in a cyclotron, but much valuable research has been done with such sources.

Proton Bombardment. The proton was the first bombarder used in experiments with artificially accelerated particles. Simple capture of the proton (p, γ), is a common reaction:

$$^A_Z X \ (p,\gamma) \ ^{A+1}_{Z+1} X.$$

An atom of mass A has captured a proton to form an isotope of the element with the next higher atomic number. This reaction has a good yield and many of the products are positron-emitting radioactive nuclides. Examples are

$$^{12}_6 C \ (p,\gamma) \ ^{13}_7 N \text{ and } ^{46}_{20} Ca \ (p,\gamma) \ ^{47}_{21} Sc.$$

The (p,n) reaction is important:

$$^A_Z X \ (p,n) \ ^{A}_{Z+1} X.$$

It will proceed only if the proton has relatively high energy. The product, an isobar of the target and an isotope of the element of the next higher atomic number, is always radioactive and a positron emitter. This reaction can be used to yield neutrons as secondary bombarders: $^9_4$Be (p,n) $^9_5$B. It is frequently used in cyclotrons when an intense neutron beam is desired.

The (p,d) reaction

$$^A_Z X \ (p,d) \ ^{A-1}_{Z} X$$

might be expected, but is known in only one instance, $^9_4$Be (p,d) $^8_4$Be, and the product disintegrates in a fraction of a second into two alpha particles.

The (p,α) reaction

$$^A_Z X \ (p,\alpha) \ ^{A-3}_{Z-1} X$$

occurs rather readily, but the products are almost always stable isotopes of the element of the next lower atomic number.

Deuteron Bombardment. Since deuterons, being twice as heavy as protons, have twice the kinetic energy for the same velocity, they are now much more generally used for bombarders. Simple deuteron capture does not occur. The deuteron consists of a proton and a neutron not too tightly bound together, and in most deuteron bombardments one or the other component is rejected. The (d,n) reaction

$$^A_X X \ (d,n) \ ^{A+1}_{Z+1} X$$

gives the same type of products as the (p,γ) reaction. Yields are good if the deuterons are sufficiently energetic. Products are frequently positron-emitting isotopes of the next higher element: $^{12}_6$C (d,n) $^{13}_7$N. A very useful reaction of this type is the bombardment of deuterons by deuterons: $^2_1$H (d,n) $^3_2$He. This proceeds readily at relatively low bombarding energies, and supplies a good yield of neutrons; the end product, helium, is not radioactive.

In the (d,p) reaction

$$^A_Z X \ (d,p) \ ^{A+1}_{Z} X$$

a heavier isotope of the target element is formed. This is a beta-emitter. $^{23}_{11}$Na (d,p) $^{24}_{11}$Na is a good example.

Neutron Reactions. Only one nuclide is known that will not react with neutrons of moderate energy; this is $^4_2$He. The most usual process is simple neutron capture, (n,γ):

$$^A_Z X \ (n,\gamma) \ ^{A+1}_{Z} X.$$

This reaction always has a very good yield. Products are frequently radioactive, emitting beta particles. Examples are $^{107}_{47}Ag$ (n,γ) $^{108}_{48}Ag$, and $^{127}_{53}I$ (n,γ) $^{128}_{53}I$.

Other reactions which may occur are (n,p) and (n,α); there is also a less common (n, 2n).

$$^A_Z X \text{ (n,p) } ^{\ \ A}_{Z-1}X.$$

$$^A_Z X \text{ (n,}\alpha\text{) } ^{A-3}_{Z-2}X.$$

$$^A_Z X \text{ (n,2n) } ^{A-1}_{\ \ Z}X.$$

The first two usually yield beta emitters, the third positron emitters. Examples are:—

$$^{32}_{16}S \text{ (n,p) } ^{32}_{15}P \qquad\qquad ^{27}_{13}Al \text{ (n,}\alpha\text{) } ^{24}_{11}Na \qquad\qquad ^{14}_{7}N \text{ (n,2n) } ^{13}_{7}N.$$

By comparing the above sections it will be seen that the products of the (n,γ) and (d,p) reactions are the same; likewise those of the (d,n) and (p,γ).

Nuclear Reactions Produced by Photons. Photon-induced reactions (γ,n) and (γ,p) can be produced by photons of sufficient energy to overcome the nuclear binding energy of the neutron or proton, that is, about 9 MeV. The first produces positron emitters, the second electron emitters. Yields are always low, and the process is not important from the point of view of radionuclide production.

Energy Considerations. For any of the reactions described above, certain conditions must exist. The mass of the two reacting particles plus the mass equivalent of the kinetic energy of the bombarding particle must exceed the mass of the resulting products. All bombarders must have sufficient energy to surmount or penetrate the potential barrier, which becomes greater the higher the atomic number of the target. There will always be competition among possible reactions, depending on energy conditions. For instance, the bombardment of $^{27}_{13}Al$ by energetic neutrons may result in any of the following:

$$^{27}_{13}Al \text{ (n,}\gamma\text{) } ^{28}_{13}Al$$

$$^{27}_{13}Al \text{ (n,p) } ^{27}_{12}Mg$$

$$^{27}_{13}Al \text{ (n,}\alpha\text{) } ^{24}_{11}Na$$

$$^{27}_{13}Al \text{ (n,2n) } ^{26}_{13}Al$$

In general, the simpler reactions start at lower bombarding energies and produce better yields.

With higher energies even more complicated reactions may occur, such as (p,2n) or (p,p2n), and at energies of 100 or 200 MeV or more complete break-up of the target nucleus (spallation) may occur. However, it is not likely that these processes will be of importance in radionuclide production.

Yield of a Nuclear Reaction. The individual nuclear reaction can always be written as described in the preceding sections. However the *yield* in a particular bombardment cannot be predicted without more information. It obviously depends on the number of bombarding particles and the number of target nuclei, and further on some factor having to do with the probability of a collision. In considering the bombardment of relatively large objects such as tennis racquets by smaller objects such as balls, the actual cross-section areas of the target and the bombarder are factors. A similar concept is useful in describing nuclear reactions. A target area, or "cross-section" is assigned to each nucleus for each type of reaction. This may be close to the physical area of the nucleus, but this is not necessarily so. Nuclear cross-sections are established by experiments outside the scope of this book, and tabulated in various places.* The unit of cross-section, the *barn*, is 10^{-24} sq cm.

The chance of encounters in a bombardment can then be described as follows: The target has an area A sq cm, and thickness X cm. It contains n nuclei per sq cm of surface. The cross-section for the reaction in question is σ barns per nucleus, hence the area which may be struck, per sq cm of actual surface, is n σ. If the flux of bombarding particles is I per sq cm per second, the number of reactions occurring per sq cm of surface is given by

$$N = I \, n \, \sigma \text{ per second.} \qquad\qquad 4\text{---}(2)$$

From this, the total number of product nuclei in a given bombardment can be calculated.

As an example, consider the bombardment of stable gold, ^{197}Au, by slow neutrons in the nuclear reactor, to produce radioactive gold, ^{198}Au. As a target, a gold foil will be used, 5 sq cm in area, and 0.3 mm thick, a volume of 0.15 cu cm. This foil will be folded or crumpled to slide into an irradiation tube of 1 sq cm cross-section, whence the *average* thickness of gold in the tube will be 0.15 cm. The density of gold is 19.3 gm per cu cm, and its atomic weight is 197.2. From these values and Avogadro's hypothesis, the number of atoms in the gold foil is n $= \dfrac{6.02 \times 10^{23}}{197.2} \times 19.3 \times 0.15 = 88$ $\times 10^{20}$, in a mass of 2.9 gm, with an area of 1 sq cm exposed to the neutron beam.

The foil is to be exposed to a flux of 10^{12} neutrons per sq cm per sec. For ^{197}Au, σ is tabulated as 98 barns. Then the number of radioactive nuclei produced per second should be given by

$$N = 88 \times 10^{20} \text{ target atoms/sq cm} \times 10^{12} \text{ neutrons/sq cm/sec} \times$$
$$98 \times 10^{-24} \text{ sq cm/atom} = 86 \times 10^{10}/\text{sq cm/sec.}$$

* See Friedlander, Kennedy, and Miller: *Nuclear and Radiochemistry*, Appendix C.

The above calculation is based on the assumption that every gold atom has an equal chance of receiving a neutron; this is true only for *very thin* targets. Otherwise the effective neutron flux will decrease as the deeper layers of the target are reached, and a different approach is necessary. The attenuation $-dI$ of the neutron flux is an infinitesimal thickness of the target, containing dn nuclei is given by the equation

$$-dI = I\,\sigma\,dn. \qquad\qquad 4\text{—}(3)$$

This expression can be integrated in the same manner as that for radioactive decay (see page 21), giving

$$I = I_o\,e^{-n\sigma} \qquad\qquad 4\text{—}(4)$$

where I is the neutron flux after it has traversed a target containing n nuclei per sq cm, and I_o is the incident flux. Then the number of neutrons lost, that is used up in producing ^{198}Au, is $I_o - I$, or

$$I_o - I = I_o\,(1 - e^{-n\sigma})\ \text{per second.} \qquad\qquad 4\text{—}(5)$$

The number obtained from this relation is the number of radioactive nuclei actually produced in a second, rather than that obtained by N in formula 4—(2), and hence should be used to find the actual production. For the problem under consideration

$$I_o - I = 10^{12}\,(1 - e^{-88\,\times\,10^{20}\,\times\,98\,\times\,10^{-24}}) = 10^{12}\,(1 - e^{-0.862})$$
$$= 0.58 \times 10^{12} = 58 \times 10^{10}\ \text{per second.}$$

Accordingly the number of radioactive atoms actually produced in the foil in 58×10^{10} per second, instead of 86×10^{10}, a reduction to 2/3 of the original estimate.*

In an hour, then, there would be $58 \times 10^{10} \times 3600 = 2.1 \times 10^{15}$ radioactive atoms, if there were no decay. However decay sets in as soon as any of the nuclide is formed, and if the irradiation time is appreciable, an allowance must be made for this. The appropriate formula will be developed in Chapter 6; at present it will be accepted.

$$N_t = \frac{R}{\lambda}\,(1 - e^{-\lambda t}) \qquad\qquad 4\text{—}(6)$$

where N_t is the net number of atoms produced after time t, R is the rate of production per unit time (in same units as t), and λ the decay constant.

---

* In practice, when a sample is introduced into a reactor, it is assumed that the the neutron flux comes from all directions and the absorption correction is made on this basis.

For ^{198}Au the half period is 64.5 hours, so $\lambda = \dfrac{0.693}{64.5} = 0.0107$ per hour

(see page 22).

R (above) $= 2.1 \times 10^{15}$ per hour; then the amount in 24 hours is

$$N_{24} = \frac{2.1 \times 10^{15}}{0.0107} (1 - e^{-24 \times 0.0107}) = 45 \times 10^{15} \text{ atoms,}$$

instead of 50.5×10^{15} which would be obtained by multiplying the rate per hour by the number of hours. This is a decay correction of about 12 per cent.

The fact must not be over looked that the radioactive product is also subject to the neutron bombardment, and may give rise to a secondary interaction. In practice this sometimes has to be taken into account. Calculations are complicated and beyond the scope of this book.

It is usual to think of radionuclide production in terms of millicuries rather than in terms of numbers of atoms. It has been shown (page 26) that 1 mCi of any radioactive nuclide contains 4.6×10^{12} T atoms, where T is the half life in days. Therefore 1 mCi of ^{198}Au contains $4.6 \times 10^{12} \times \dfrac{64.5}{24} = 12.4 \times 10^{12}$ atoms. The above hourly and daily production rates then become 169 and 3600 mCi respectively.

In one half period, $N_{64.5} = 7500$ mCi, and for an infinite period, $N_\infty = 15{,}000$ mCi. Thus one-half of the maximum is produced in an irradiation of one half period, three-fourths in two half periods, and so on.

The specific activity of the ^{198}Au in the sample after irradiation of two half periods is $\dfrac{11{,}250 \text{ mCi}}{2.9 \text{ gm}} = 3880$ mCi per gm.

The actual number of atoms which have been activated during this period (including those which have already decayed) is
58×10^{10} (atoms per second) $\times (2 \times 64.5 \times 3600)$ seconds in two half lives $= 27 \times 10^{16}$. The percentage of the initial number in the foil is $\dfrac{27 \times 10^{16}}{88 \times 10^{10}} \times 100 = 0.0031$. In other words, one atom in 32,000 has been transformed.

Neutron Activation Analysis. In most elements introduced into a neutron reactor, radioactive isotopes will be produced. The technique known as neutron activation analysis has been developed for the detection of very small amounts of stable elements in fairly large quantities of extraneous matter. This is applicable to the measurement of so-called "trace" elements* in human tissues. Such elements as zinc, copper, molybdenum and

---

* Not to be confused with "tracer" elements which are usually radioactive.

arsenic may exist in extremely minute amounts in certain organs or tissues. They seem to take no part in normal metabolism, but may exert some sort of catalytic action.   Changes in these very small amounts may be related to some diseases.

A sample of tissue, thought to contain the trace element, is put in a known neutron flux for a known period, and the resulting radioactivity measured. Of course there may be a number of activities induced in various tissue components, but a chemical separation can be used to isolate the one of interest, or it can be identified by spectrometer analysis.   (Stable carrier can be added to prevent the loss of the minute quantity of the element in the sample.)   Simultaneously with the unknown, a small sample of the stable element, of known weight, is irradiated.   In this, the expected number of radioactive atoms can be calculated by the method outlined above, and the radioactivity per unit weight of stable element determined. The same degree of activity will be expected in the unknown, hence the initial weight of the stable element in this unknown can be calculated.

For example, to detect the amount of copper present in one gram of tissue, using 1 mg of thin copper foil as control.   (Technical details of preparation of samples are omitted.)   Normal copper contains 69 per cent ^{63}Cu and 31 per cent ^{65}Cu. The (n,γ) reactions on these two stable isotopes produce ^{64}Cu and ^{66}Cu respectively.   The half life of ^{64}Cu is 12.8 hours; that of ^{66}Cu is 5 minutes.   Therefore the latter can be ignored, if more than an hour elapses between the end of the irradiation and the measurement.   The cross section for ^{63}Cu for slow neutrons is 4.3 barns.   The foil is to be exposed to a flux of 10^{12} neutrons per second, for several days (until a convenient time for opening the reactor).   After 3 days, or 6 half lives, essentially the maximum possible amount of ^{64}Cu will be present.

The decay constant is $\dfrac{0.693}{12.8} = 0.054$ per hour.

The rate of production per hour is

$$0.69 \times \frac{6.02 \times 10^{23} \times 0.001}{63.54} \times 10^{12} \times 4.3 \times 10^{-24} \times 3600 = 10^{11} \text{ atoms}$$

of ^{64}Cu. [formula 4—(2)]

From 4—(6) the maximum production is $\dfrac{10^{11}}{0.054} = 18.5 \times 10^{11}$ atoms.

One millicurie of ^{64}Cu contains [formula 2—(10)] 2.5×10^{12} atoms.   Therefore the sample at the end of the irradiation contains 0.74 mCi ^{64}Cu in 1 mg copper.   The unknown, measured against the standard, shows a content of

10^{-4} μCi of ^{64}Cu $(= 10^{-7}$ mCi$)$. Then $\dfrac{\text{mg Cu in unknown}}{1 \text{ mg Cu in standard}} = \dfrac{10^{-7} \text{ mCi}}{0.74 \text{ mCi}}$

and the copper in the tissue sample is 1.35×10^{-7} mg per gram of tissue.

REFERENCES

FRIEDLANDER, G., KENNEDY, J. W. and MILLER, J. M.: *Nuclear and Radiochemis ry*, 2nd Ed., New York, John Wiley & Sons, Inc., 1964.

LAPP, R. E. and ANDREWS, H. L.: *Nuclear Radiation Physics*, 3rd Ed., New York, Prentice-Hall, Inc., 1963.

SAYRE, E.: *Methods and Applications of Activation Analysis*, Ann. Rev. Nuclear Science, *13*, 145–162, 1963.

SEMAT, H.: *Introduction to Atomic and Nuclear Physics*, 4th Ed., New York, Holt, Rinehart & Winston, 1962.

WHITE, H. E.: *Introduction to Atomic and Nuclear Physics*, New York, D. Van Nostrand Co., Inc., 1963.

5

Nuclear Fission

In the last chapter the neutron as a bombarder in nuclear reactions was discussed. When sources of neutrons became available by the

$$^{9}_{4}\text{Be} \ (\alpha,\text{n}) \ ^{12}_{6}\text{C}$$

reaction there described, several physicists systematically studied the results of bombarding many elements with these particles. One of these experiments was destined to have extremely far-reaching consequences since it led to the discovery of nuclear fission.

Discovery of Nuclear Fission. Like the discovery of the neutron, this is a complicated story. Fermi, in Italy in 1934 and 1935, exposed practically all the known elements to neutron bombardment and discovered a large number of new radioactive substances. The usual reaction was simple neutron capture, (n,γ) with the production of a heavier isotope of the target element, which is frequently a beta-emitting radioactive nuclide. The emission of a beta particle has been shown (p. 19) to result in formation of a new nucleus with atomic number greater by unity than the parent atom. Fermi wondered whether by such bombardment of uranium, with atomic number 92, the highest known in nature, he could produce a new element with atomic number 93. If such an element fell into its proper place in the periodic table, it should be chemically like manganese. Accordingly, a manganese salt was added to a solution of a uranium salt which had been irradiated with neutrons, and then the manganese precipitated as the oxide. A considerable amount of the newly formed radioactive material came down with the manganese. It was demonstrated that neither uranium nor any element between $Z = 86$ and $Z = 92$ could be precipitated in this manner. Other experimenters found radioactivity associated with elements of other chemical families, and assumed that they were producing nuclides of several atomic numbers greater than 93. These were called "transuranic elements"; they were named and their half periods determined. Yet there were many irregularities in the experimental findings, and some of the energy relations were difficult to explain. Three German scientists, Hahn, Meitner, and Strassman, initiated a systematic study to identify these elements and organize the knowledge concerning them.

One method of study which was used was co-precipitation of an unknown with various known substances, to find the chemical family, as in the manganese precipitation just mentioned. In one such precipitation the Curie-Joliots had brought down a radioactive substance with lanthanum (Z = 57). This might have been actinum (Z = 89), since this is in the same chemical family; it could not well be fitted into the transuranic group, and in fact its discoverers presently abandoned it.

Hahn and Strassmann repeated this work. (By this time Lise Meitner had been obliged to leave Germany and had not yet started more experimental work in Sweden.) They found not only the lanthanum-like precipitate, but one like barium. This, they thought, was radium, since these two elements are chemically much alike. But by differential tests they found that it was not radium but was truly barium. This news reached Meitner in Sweden, and she and Frisch developed the hypothesis that the neutron entering the uranium atom had produced a new kind of instability. Instead of forming a radioactive nucleus which would eventually expel an alpha or a beta particle, it had formed a nucleus so unstable that it instantly split into two nearly equal fragments, or underwent *fission* (adopting a term from biology for the dividing nucleus). This hypothesis was quickly proved experimentally by groups in several countries, including the United States. It was also demonstrated that every fission was accompanied by the release of about 200 MeV of energy—much more than in any previously known nuclear reaction.

Fission Products. There are three isotopes of natural uranium (Z = 92), with mass numbers 234, 235, and 238. It was found that ^{235}U was the nucleus involved in the fission phenomenon. If an isotope of barium (Z = 56) is one of the products, then the other must be an isotope of krypton (Z = 36). However, it was soon demonstrated that many different elements were to be found in the fission products. In fact, practically every element from selenium (Z = 34) to lanthanum (Z = 57) was identified. Each individual fission results in two nuclei, one usually definitely heavier than half the uranium atom and one definitely lighter. The two new atomic numbers must add up to 92; the new masses, however, do not quite add up to 235, because two or three neutrons are "spilled out" at each fission. It will be recalled that the neutron-proton ratio constantly increases as higher atomic numbers are reached (Fig. 1–5), so that in one atom of uranium there would be too many neutrons for two atoms of about half its atomic number. Even with the "spilling out" of some of the extra neutrons, the fragments still have too many, and have to return to stability by one or more, probably several, radioactive disintegrations. For instance, one product might be $^{139}_{53}$I and the other $^{94}_{39}$Y, two extra neutrons having been lost. The iodine disintegration series would be $^{139}_{53}$I $\rightarrow$ $^{139}_{54}$Xe $\rightarrow$ $^{139}_{55}$Cs $\rightarrow$ $^{139}_{56}$Ba $\rightarrow$ $^{139}_{57}$La, a beta particle being emitted at each step. The lanthanum is stable. At least 75 such series are known.

The Nuclear Chain Reaction. If the fission process is initiated by the entrance of a neutron into a uranium atom, and if in undergoing fission

5

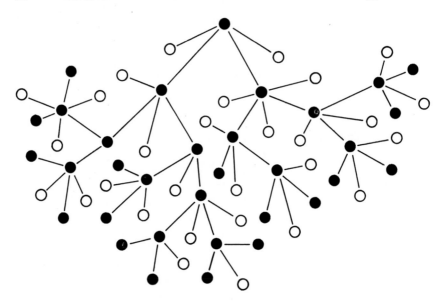

●- Fission fragments

○- Extra neutrons

FIG. 5–1.   Chain reaction; five stages in a reaction which doubles at each stage.

this atom releases two neutrons, it would appear that these might in turn enter other uranium atoms and give rise to further fissions, so that quickly there might be an enormous number of atoms undergoing fission, as indicated in Figure 5–1.

At first thought it would seem that if such a reaction ever got started in a piece of uranium it would proceed with terrific rapidity until the whole thing had been destroyed. This would be truly the case if all the uranium atoms were fissionable and if no neutrons were lost. And with the enormous energy release of 200 MeV per fission, the reaction would be violently explosive. However, in natural uranium it is almost entirely the ^{235}U isotope that undergoes fission.* This isotope forms only $\frac{1}{140}$ of natural uranium. The more abundant isotope, ^{238}U, usually simply captures the neutron in an (n,γ) reaction which will be discussed later. Thus a single fission, or even a considerable number starting in a lump of natural uranium would not be likely to initate a continuing chain reaction, although there might be several successive fissions before it died out.

It is, however, possible, by various physical procedures, to separate the isotopes, at least partially, so that "enriched" ^{235}U may be produced, with a relatively high percentage of fissionable atoms. In this case, the likeli-

* ^{238}U nuclei can be fissioned only by neutrons of a few definite energies, likely to be available only in very small numbers in this haphazard process.

hood of a self-sustaining chain reaction becomes greater. Now, the concept of "critical size" enters the picture. In a mass in which a chain reaction is going on, some of the neutrons will be released near the periphery, and may escape. These are then lost, as far as propagation of the chain is concerned. If the volume is small, so many will be lost that the reaction will stop; if it is sufficiently large, the reaction may just proceed without building up to an explosive level, because just enough neutrons will be kept within the volume to produce one new fission for each one that has occurred. In a still larger volume the chain will spread, at a speed determined by the ratio of neutrons kept in the volume to the number of atoms undergoing fission.

As soon as the possibility of a sustained chain reaction became apparent, physicists saw its potentialities both for power and for wartime explosives. It will be recalled that fission was discovered in 1939. War was sweeping through Europe; the United States was not yet involved, but many people thought her entrance into the fighting was only a matter of rather brief time. Accordingly, a project was set up to study possibilities of exploiting this new source of energy, the "Manhattan Project."

The Atomic Pile or Nuclear Reactor. The first objective was to see whether a self-sustaining chain reaction could be established. Fermi, having earlier left Axis-dominated Italy, was in charge of this phase of the study. Details are fascinating, but would be out of place here. As is well known, he was successful and the first chain-reacting apparatus was put into action on December 2, 1942.

The principle is to capture enough of the neutrons released in fission: if they escape from one lump of uranium without producing a second fission, provision is made for their arrival at other lumps. For this purpose the space between lumps of uranium must be filled with material that will not absorb neutrons, but will slow them down by mechanical collisions, until they have too little energy to interact with the ^{238}U in the mass. Even at slowest speeds they will cause fission in the ^{235}U. Pure carbon was the first substance used as a "moderator," and the first "reactor" was a pile of blocks of very pure graphite with chunks of natural uranium at regular intervals. Stray neutrons from cosmic rays, or those deliberately introduced, served to start the reaction, and when the "pile" was large enough, it proceeded spontaneously. That is, for every neutron used to produce a fission, more than one was made available. If such a "pile" should be left alone, it would get hotter and hotter until it "blew up," not as a bomb, but simply separating into fragments too small to carry on the reaction. This can be prevented by inserting into the pile a rod of some material such as cadmium, that absorbs neutrons very strongly. If too much of the absorber is introduced, the chain will slow down and finally stop. It is possible to find the point of balance at which the chain will continue at a constant rate. This is the basic principle for all nuclear reactors, the so-called *atomic piles*, although other fuels may be used besides natural uranium, and other moderators besides carbon. A diagram of a working nuclear reactor is shown in Figure 5–2.

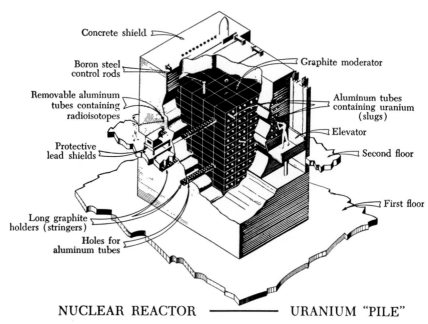

Concrete shield

Boron steel control rods

Graphite moderator

Removable aluminum tubes containing radioisotopes

Aluminum tubes containing uranium (slugs)

Elevator

Protective lead shields

Second floor

First floor

Long graphite holders (stringers)

Holes for aluminum tubes

NUCLEAR REACTOR ———————— URANIUM "PILE"

FIG. 5–2.   Diagram of working nuclear reactor.   (Courtesy of Atomic Energy Commission.)

Transuranic Elements.   As has been stated, it is possible to separate the isotopes of uranium by various physical processes.   Then, instead of natural uranium the fuel elements may contain material rich in ^{235}U; in this case, the whole unit can be more compact.   The smaller the amount of ^{238}U, the less the need for slowing down the neutrons to avoid their capture by this isotope.

However, this very capture leads to the production of a new element, which is also fissionable.

$$^{238}_{92}U\ (n,\gamma)\ ^{239}_{92}U$$

$$^{239}_{92}U \rightarrow\ ^{239}_{93}Np + \beta^- \ (T = 23 \text{ minutes})$$

$$^{239}_{93}Np \rightarrow\ ^{239}_{94}Pu + \beta^- \ (T = 2.3 \text{ days})$$

$$^{239}_{94}Pu \rightarrow\ ^{235}_{92}U + \alpha \ (T = 24,360 \text{ years})$$

Here are actually transuranic elements, neptunium and plutonium.* Plutonium has a very long half period for natural decay, but it is fissionable with fast or slow neutrons.   Since it is a different element, it may be separated chemically from the uranium in which it was created.   It can, therefore, be used as "fuel" in a reactor, although its more important use is in weapons, which will be briefly discussed below.

* Further transuranic elements have now been produced, up to atomic number 2-104. They are of little or no interest in the context of this book.

Production of Radionuclides in the Pile. In radionuclide production the nuclear reactor or pile, has two important roles. First, it supplies a copious source of slow neutrons, of much higher intensity than any cyclotron can produce. Target material to be bombarded by these slow neutrons can be introduced into channels in the pile, in suitable containers, and removed after the required time of bombardment. The most common reaction is simple capture:

$$^{23}_{11}\text{Na} \ (n,\gamma) \ ^{24}_{11}\text{Na}$$

$$^{59}_{27}\text{Co} \ (n,\gamma) \ ^{60}_{27}\text{Co}.$$

However, in some important cases the (n,p) reaction also proceeds:

$$^{32}_{16}\text{S} \ (n,p) \ ^{32}_{15}\text{P},$$

$$^{35}_{17}\text{Cl} \ (n,p) \ ^{35}_{16}\text{S}.$$

The second radionuclide source is fission products from spent fuel elements. Within the lump of uranium, the fission products are formed and in general do not escape, but decay there, eventually to stable end products as described above. However, the presence of this extraneous material in the fuel slug results in undue consumption of neutrons in interactions with the fission products. Eventually the uranium is so highly contaminated with these other substances as to become useless. It must then be removed from the reactor and replaced with a fresh fuel element. The uranium in the old one would be reusable if it could be separated from the contaminants; and some of these might also be valuable. The handling of these intensely radioactive chunks of material presents many problems, and a whole new field of "hot" radiochemistry has been developed. Certain radionuclides are now regularly separated from these old fuel elements. $^{131}_{53}\text{I}$, $^{140}_{56}\text{Ba}$, $^{137}_{56}\text{Cs}$, $^{89}_{38}\text{Sr} + ^{90}_{39}\text{Y}$, and many of the rare earths are supplied by the Atomic Energy Commission as fission products.

Nuclear Weapons. The "atomic bomb" has little to contribute to the program of uses of radionuclides, except for problems concerned with the possible radioactive debris. However, it should be discussed briefly.

Nuclear weapons can be made with ^{235}U, but the man-made element plutonium is usually employed. Most information about them is secret, and in any case irrelevant here, but certain basic principles may be mentioned.

The first concept is that of "critical size," which has been discussed above. If the volume of fissionable material is smaller than this, the reaction cannot build up. Even in a larger volume, an explosion would not necessarily develop. It will be recalled that 200 MeV of energy is released at each fission, most of this being expended as kinetic energy of the fission fragments. If the material is not constrained in any way, the result of a few generations in the fission chain would be that the mass would "push itself apart" and be reduced to a number of fragments of sub-critical size, in each of which the reaction would cease; a real "atomic explosion" would not occur. For this, a much larger number of fissions would have to occur in a very short time, and the mass would have to be prevented from splitting up prematurely.

This is brought about by confining two or more sub-critical masses of practically pure fissionable material inside a case of heavy material (called a tamper). At the instant of the desired explosion these sub-critical masses are shot into each other to form a mass greater than the critical value, while the tamper keeps the material from flying apart until a large number of fissions occur and a tremendous energy is released. The unit then blows apart with a terrific detonation, producing a blast wave with tremendous destructive force. During the brief instant of energy build-up the heat is such as to convert the metallic center to gas at a high temperature. When this gas is released, it expands to form a "ball of fire" emitting a tremendous flash of heat. Furthermore, the last generation of fission neutrons, released as the bomb flies apart, together with gamma rays released in the process, produce a highly lethal radiation.

If the explosion occurs at or near the earth's surface, a large amount of debris will be carried up with the cloud of fission products; much of this will have been made radioactive by the released neutrons. The larger particles will fall back fairly promptly, but the smaller ones will remain suspended for some time, and eventually be deposited over an appreciable part of the earth's surface. Explosions of low energy yield (so-called kiloton range) result in suspension mainly in the troposphere, to an altitude of possibly 50,000 feet. Most of this will have returned to the earth within a few weeks, in a fairly narrow band encircling the world at the latitude of the detonation.

For explosions of high energy yield (megaton range) most of the bomb debris will be propelled higher, into the stratosphere, from which it dribbles back to earth more slowly, over a period of years, during which some of it will reach all parts of the earth's surface. Of course during this period a great deal of the radioactivity will have decayed away, but there may still be enough to cause concern. This "fall-out" hazard will be considered in a later chapter.

Fusion (Thermonuclear) Reactions. The Hydrogen Bomb. It will be recalled (page 40) that when nucleons unite to form more complex nuclei, mass is lost. Part of this goes into the binding energy of the new nucleus, the rest is emitted as gamma radiation. If many nuclear fusions could be made to take place simultaneously, considerable energy could be released. However, it requires a good deal of energy to start such a reaction. This energy can be attained by raising the temperature to very high levels (of the order of a million degrees Centigrade). Under these circumstances the fusion processes are referred to as *thermonuclear reactions*.

Four such reactions apparently can be produced in practical abundance at this temperature level. They are:

$$^2H + {}^2H = {}^3He + n + 3.2 \text{ MeV.}$$
$$^2H + {}^2H = {}^3H + {}^1H + 4 \text{ MeV.}$$
$$^3H + {}^2H = {}^4He + n + 17 \text{ MeV.}$$
$$^3H + {}^3H = {}^4He + 2n + 11 \text{ MeV.}$$

The most practical way that sufficiently high temperatures can be obtained on earth, to initiate a large amount of such reactions, is by means of a fission explosion. Consequently by combining a quantity of deuterium or tritium or both with a fission bomb, one or more of the above reactions should be initiated, and if the energy can at first be constrained, a thermonuclear explosion may be produced. Since the essential elements are isotopes of hydrogen, these are frequently called hydrogen bombs.

"Dirty Bombs" and "Clean Bombs." Following the explosion of a fission bomb, even though it is so far above ground that there is no incidental dirt, as noted above there will be a large production of radioactive fission products, which will eventually reach the earth as fall-out. If a purely fusion bomb could be achieved, and exploded far enough above ground to prevent the released neutrons from activating the surroundings, this would be a truly "clean" bomb from the point of view of radioactive fall-out contamination. However, a small fission bomb is necessary to initiate the fusion reaction, so complete cleanness cannot apparently be achieved. Nevertheless, by adjusting the relative components of the fission-fusion system, some control may be had of the "dirty" radioactive residual.

REFERENCE

UNITED STATES ATOMIC ENERGY COMMISSION: *The Effects of Nuclear Weapons,* Washington, D. C., United States Government Printing Office, 1957.

6

Sources of the Radiations; Modes of Radioactive Decay

In decay of either naturally or artificially radioactive nuclides, only a very limited number of types of transformation has been observed. The only particles emitted are alphas and negative and positive electrons; any of these may be accompanied by gamma rays, or the gammas may be the only radiation.

Structure of the Nucleus. Much less is known about the actual structure of the nucleus than of the extra-nuclear part of the atom. Bohr, who developed the accepted concept of atomic structure, has proposed a nuclear model. Basing his ideas on assumed characteristics of nuclear forces, and on the fact that only certain ratios of neutrons to protons can exist in stable nuclei, he suggested a "liquid-drop" model. The nucleus may be compared to a small sphere of liquid; as the atoms are uniformly distributed in the drop, so the nucleons are distributed in the nuclear spherical volume. They are in a constant state of motion, but restricted within a very small radius. Thus they make many collisions per second, and all have the same average energy; in a stable nucleus no nucleon will ever accumulate enough energy to escape from the nuclear binding. However, radioactive nuclei have a certain excess of energy, and if a nucleon or group of nucleons can succeed in capturing a sufficient amount of this, it can and will escape. If not all the extra energy is utilized by the escaping particle, the new nucleus may be left in an "excited state," from which it will later recover by emission of a gamma ray, returning to the "ground" or most stable condition of the new nucleus. This may itself, of course, be radioactive.

This liquid-drop model is successful in accounting for many properties of nuclei. However strong evidence has been accumulating for some sort of shell structure in nuclei, analogous to the electron-shell structure in atoms. Nuclei with neutron numbers 2, 8, 20, 28, 50, 82, and 126 appear to be especially stable; this may correspond to the electron situation when the outermost orbit is completely filled. Similarly nuclei with Z equal to these numbers possess special properties. Certain decay schemes, and particularly some instances of isomerism (see page 66) may be partly explained by this hypothesis. However much more evidence needs to be collected along these lines. Meantime neither theory (nor any other) is essential to the considerations in this book.

Alpha Decay. Alpha particles, as has been shown, are helium nuclei, or aggregates of two protons and two neutrons each. Disintegration by alpha emission occurs only among the heavy naturally radioactive nuclides (Z > 83), a few artificially produced ones with either very long or very short periods, of atomic numbers between 60 and 85, and with $^8_4$Be and $^8_5$B. These two have very short half lives; each atom of the first decays into two alpha particles and of the second into two alphas and a positron. Alpha decay results in a daughter nucleus having atomic number two less and mass number four less than the parent.

Alpha particles from a particular nuclide either all have the same energy or are emitted in a few mono-energetic groups. In the first case it is assumed that every transition takes place directly to the ground state; there will then be no accompanying gamma rays. Alpha particles of several different energies are emitted when the nucleus can be left in different states of excitation, which will then return to the ground state by gamma emission. Each gamma ray then represents the difference between the disintegration energies associated with two alpha particle groups. A cloud chamber photograph of two groups of alpha particles from Th C and Th C′ was shown in Figure 3–2, page 34.

Since particular groups of alpha particles are mono-energetic, members of one group will all travel the same distance, or have the same *range* in any medium. Alpha particles from different radionuclides are emitted at velocities between 8000 and 15,000 miles per second, corresponding to ranges in air between 2.6 and 8.6 cm. The more rapid the disintegration rate, the greater is the alpha particle energy, there being an almost linear relation between the logarithm of the decay constant and the energy in MeV.

Alpha particles have little or no importance in clinical uses of radioactive nuclides, and will not be studied further at this time.

Beta Decay. Beta decay differs in several basic respects from alpha decay. The alpha particle is recognized as a group of nucleons, which may be part of a stable nuclear configuration, but electrons are not tolerated within the nucleus. Therefore it must be assumed that the electron is created and ejected. Negative and positive beta particles are believed to be created by the transformations

$$n \rightarrow p^+ + \beta^-,$$
$$p^+ \rightarrow n + \beta^+.$$

Accordingly, β^- decay would be expected when the neutron-proton ratio is too high for stability, (see Stability Curve, Fig. 1–5, p. 15) and β^+ decay when this ratio is too low. Thus β^- emitters would generally be expected to result from neutron bombardment, and β^+ from proton, although this is not rigidly adhered to. In general, the farther away from stability, the

Table 6–1. Isotopes of Iodine

Mass Number	n/p Ratio	Half Period	Radiation
119	66/53	18 min	β^+, EC*
120	67/53	30 min	β^+, EC
121	68/53	1.5 hr	β^+, EC, γ
122	69/53	3.5 min	β^+, EC
123	70/53	13.0 hr	EC, γ
124	71/53	4.5 days	β^+, EC, γ
125	72/53	60 days	EC, γ
126	73/53	13 days	β^-, β^+, EC, γ
127	74/53	STABLE	
128	75/53	25 min	β^-, γ
129	76/53	1.72×10^7 years	β^-, γ
130	77/53	12.6 hr	β^-, γ
131	78/53	8.1 days	β^-, γ
132	79/53	2.33 hr	β^-, γ
133	80/53	20.8 hr	β^-, γ
134	81/53	53 min	β^-, γ
135	82/53	6.7 hr	β^-, γ
136	83/53	86 sec	β^-, γ
137	84/53	22 sec	β^-, γ
138	85/53	5.9 sec	β^-
139	86/53	2.7 sec	β^-

* EC—electron capture, see page 64.

more rapid is the disintegration rate. These points may be illustrated by the radioactive isotopes of iodine, as shown in Table 6–1.

Positron emission is not as common as negatron; it occurs mainly in elements of low atomic weight, is not found above atomic number 79, and only rarely above atomic number 55.

Some nuclei which are close to the stability line may decay in both ways; in this case the percentage going by each route is constant. For example, $^{64}_{29}$Cu lies between the two stable isotopes $^{63}_{29}$Cu and $^{65}_{29}$Cu. In 39 per cent of its disintegrations, β^- particles are emitted, in 19 per cent, β^+. The remaining 42 per cent decay by the process of electron capture to be described below.

Product nuclei from either β^- or β^+ decay have the same mass numbers as their parents; the β^- daughter has an atomic number one greater, and the β^+ daughter one less than the parent.

Beta particles from a particular radionuclide are never emitted as a mono-energetic group, as in the case of alphas, nor even in a number of specific energy groups, but always have a continuous energy spectrum, as shown in Figure 6–1. For each beta-emitting nuclide there is a definite *maximum* energy, and all values below this may be observed; the actual shape of the curve varies somewhat from one radionuclide to another.

The Neutrino. It is not possible to explain this energy distribution on the same sort of decay phenomenon as for the alpha particle, even taking into account the neutron or proton transformation mentioned above. If each beta-decay process releases energy equal to E_{max}, but all values of

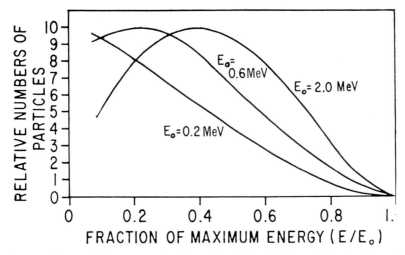

FIG. 6–1. Shapes of beta ray spectra for radionuclides of intermediate atomic number. (Courtesy of G. J. Hine, G. L. Brownell, and the Academic Press.)

lower energies are observed, which may be denoted by E_A, there has been a disappearance of energy $E_{max} - E_A$ that is unexplained. Difficulties also arise regarding conservation of momentum. In order to get away from these, Pauli suggested that a new type of particle, the *neutrino*, is involved in beta-decay. This is a fundamental particle of very small mass and electrically neutral. Then the above equation becomes

$$n \rightarrow p^+ + \beta^- + \bar{\nu}$$
$$p^+ \rightarrow n + \beta^+ + \nu$$

where $\bar{\nu}$ represents an anti-neutrino and ν a neutrino. There is no fundamental difference in their behavior and both are commonly spoken of as neutrinos. The neutrino carries away the energy indicated by $E_{max} - E_A$, and this may have any value from zero to almost E_{max}. Recent experimental evidence confirms the existence of the neutrino, with rest mass essentially zero.

The emission of beta particles may or may not be accompanied by emission of gamma rays. If the electron and the neutrino together utilize all the disintegration energy, there will be no gammas. If the nucleus retains some excess energy, this will be emitted as a gamma ray. The interval between beta and gamma emission is usually so short that they appear simultaneous. However, the delay is sometimes long enough so that the isomeric state is recognized. (See p. 66.)

Average and Maximum Beta Energy. In dosage calculations it is the average energy of the beta particles that must be used, rather than the maximum, ($\bar{E}_\beta$ rather than E_β max). There is no simple relation between the two.

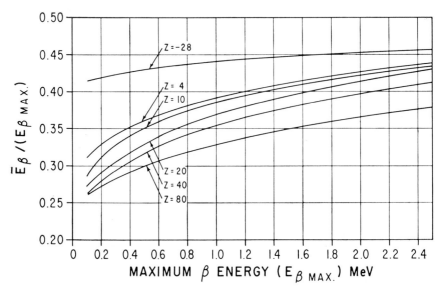

FIG. 6–2. Ratio of average to maximum β-ray energy for various values of Z. Positive values of Z refer to negative β-ray emission, negative values to positron emission. (After Hine and Brownell.)

$\overline{E}_\beta$ can be computed from the β-ray spectrum, but this is a tedious procedure. Figure 6–2, adapted from Hine and Brownell (Chapter 16)* gives the ratio $\overline{E}_\beta/E_\beta(\text{max})$, for a wide range of values of Z, for β^- emitters. The curve for $Z = -28$ is for positron emitters. A frequently used approximation is that $\overline{E}_\beta$ is about 1/3 $E_\beta(\text{max})$, but from this figure it is seen that the ratio varies from 0.25 to 0.45. Values for $\overline{E}_\beta$ for a number of nuclides are given in the appendix to this book. When accurate data are not available, satisfactory values may be obtained from the figure, interpolating for actual Z's if necessary. For instance, for the 2.25 MeV β of $^{90}_{39}$Y, $\overline{E}_\beta$ would be $0.408 \times 2.25 = 0.92$ MeV, instead of 0.75 MeV as given by the 1/3 rule.

K-electron Capture. An alternative transformation to positron emission is K-electron capture. It will be remembered that the positron results from the transformation of a proton into a neutron, with ejection of a positron and a neutrino. Another way in which a proton can be transformed into a neutron is by nuclear capture of an electron from the inner (K) electron orbit of the atom, and its amalgamation with a nuclear proton; here also the nuclear charge is decreased by unity. Since the atomic number is one less than that of the parent, the new atom will have the correct number of orbital electrons, but there will be one missing in the K-orbit and an extra one in an outer orbit. Readjustment will occur by an outer electron filling the vacancy in the K-orbit, with emission of K-characteristic x rays of the new atom.

* Note that in the Hine and Brownell book the energy is plotted on a semi-logarithmic scale, while in Figure 6–2 a linear scale is used. This causes the two to look quite different.

Gamma Decay. As already mentioned, radioactive decay involves not only the emission of particles, but sometimes also of energy in the form of radiation. This results from a decrease in nuclear mass greater than the mass of the ejected particles. This lost mass is transformed into energy according to the Einstein equation; part of it is used to accelerate the particles. However, after these have been ejected, there may be residual extra energy in the nucleus, which is then said to be in an excited state. The nucleus returns to normal by emitting this energy in the form of one or a series of gamma rays.

In general, the emission of gamma rays follows that of the particle in an extremely short time (less than 10^{-9} seconds), so that they appear to be simultaneous. However, in a considerable number of instances there is an appreciable interval before the gamma rays are emitted. This situation is discussed under *isomeric transition*, page 66. Gamma ray energies for a specific transformation occur always in the form of one or a few mono-energetic lines, not as a wide spectral range. In various nuclides, gamma energies have been observed between about 10 keV and 6 MeV. Typical beta and gamma decay schemes may be indicated as in Figure. 6–3.

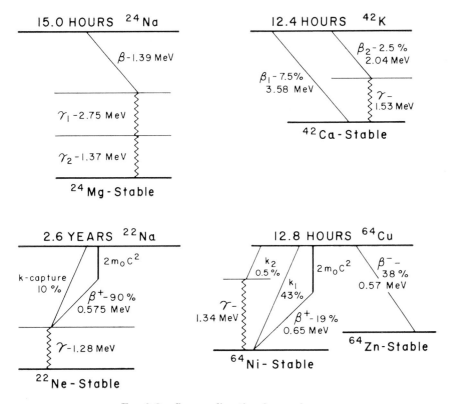

Fig. 6–3. Some radioactive decay schemes.

^{24}Na emits a β^- particle followed by two γ rays in cascade. There is only one mode of decay; every atom follows the same pattern. In ^{22}Na 10 per cent of the disintegrations are by electron capture and 90 per cent by positron emission. In considering the total positron energy, the annihilation radiation, $2\ m_oc^2 = 2 \times 0.511$ MeV must be included. That is, for every 0.575 MeV positron there are two 0.511 MeV new gamma rays to be added.

^{42}K also has two types of disintegration. In 75 per cent of the cases, a 3.58 MeV β^- particle is released. In the other 25 per cent the β^- has only 2.04 MeV and is followed by a 1.53 MeV γ ray, for the same total energy per atom disintegrating.

^{64}Cu has a very complicated pattern. It lies almost on the stability line, and can become a stable isobar by either β^- or β^+ decay. Thirty-nine per cent of the atoms go to stable ^{64}Zn by β^- decay, 19 per cent to ^{64}Ni by β^+ decay, and 42 per cent to ^{64}Ni by K-electron capture (which will be recalled as an alternative to β^+ decay). In 42.5 per cent of these last disintegrations, the entire disintegration energy (or essentially all) must be carried out by the ejected neutrino. However in 0.5 per cent, the nucleus is left in an excited state and must emit a 1.34 MeV gamma ray to come to stability.

Internal Conversion. When gamma ray energies are relatively low, this type of decay may be accompanied or replaced by *internal conversion*. This is a sort of intra-atomic photoelectric reaction, where the emitted gamma ray ejects a photoelectron from an orbit of its own atom. The photoelectron is ejected with an energy which is the difference between the gamma ray energy and the binding energy of the electron. For a given disintegration, these will be monoenergetic electrons. If there is also beta-particle emission, the continuous beta spectrum will have superimposed on it the lines of the conversion electrons. There will also, of course, be emission of the characteristic radiation of the daughter atom when the ejected photo-electron is replaced.

Isomeric Transition. Sometimes the excited state of a nucleus persists for an appreciable time; it is then said to be *metastable*. It is denoted by the letter m following the mass number in the superscript. The atom in this condition is an *isomer* of the final product nucleus, having the same atomic and mass numbers and only a difference in internal energy. Since in this case the gamma radiation is emitted some time later than the particle, the isomer may appear as a pure gamma-ray emitting nuclide. Such atoms are known with half periods from a fraction of a second to several months. The energy may all appear as gamma rays, or part of it may undergo internal conversion, with emission of conversion electrons.

In recent years several isomers have become important. An example of one which cannot be separated from its parent is ^{137m}barium, the daughter of ^{137}cesium. The cesium has a half life of 33 years, and emits only beta rays. The barium, with a half life of 2.6 minutes, emits the gamma ray which is attributed to the cesium as it is used in teletherapy sources.

Of more interest are the isomers of sufficiently long life so that they can be separated from their parents and used as essentially pure gamma-emitters. ^{99m}technecium, the 6-hour daughter of 67-hour ^{99}molybdenum, is now widely used in various scanning procedures. Other possibilities are ^{113m}indium, the 1.7-hour daughter of ^{113}tin; ^{87m}strontium, the 2.8-hour daughter of ^{87}yttrium; ^{140}lanthanum, the 1.7-day daughter of ^{140}barium. Various devices, called "cows," with a reservoir of the parent, and a means for separating the daughter, are available. These will be further discussed on page 76.

Although the great advantage of these isomers is that they emit no beta rays, and are often said to have a "pure" gamma emission, it must not be forgotten that there is usually also an emission of photoelectrons. These are generally of low energy, and do not complicate the diagnostic picture. However their possible significance in radiation dosage must not be overlooked (see page 118).

Other Modes of Decay. Proton emission has never been observed, although it has been carefully looked for. There appear to be strong theoretical reasons for its non-existence.

Neutron emission with appreciable lifetimes has not been observed and is not expected. "Delayed" neutrons are emitted from some highly excited fission products following beta-decay. Half lives are from a fraction of a second to about one minute; they are usually the same as that of the preceding beta-decay. The phenomenon is of no clinical importance, and is only mentioned for completeness of the picture.

Spontaneous fission sometimes occurs in some of the heaviest natural and artificial nuclides; it is very much less common than the normal alpha or beta reaction. For instance, ^{235}U emits alpha particles and has a half life of 7.1×10^8 years. It also occasionally undergoes spontaneous fission, but at such a rate that if this were the only mode of decay, the half life would be 1.9×10^{17} years.

Isotope Charts. Various charts have been developed for giving information about stable and radioactive isotopes of the elements. A popular type is in a sense an amplification of the stability curve shown in Figure 1–5. A sketch of a portion of such a chart is given in Figure 6–4. Z, the number of protons, is plotted along the vertical axis, and N, the number of neutrons, along the horizontal.* Stable nuclei are indicated as open squares, bearing the chemical symbol of the element; radioactive nuclei are indicated by shaded squares. Isotopes (nuclides with the same Z) obviously must appear along horizontal lines, and isobars (same Z + N) will be found on the diagonals. In general nuclides to the left of stable ones decay with β^+ emission or electron capture, since they have too few neutrons and must make one out of a proton. Those to the right of stable ones decay with β^- emission, since they have too few protons, and must make one out of a neutron.

---

* The coordinates are reversed from those of Figure 1–5 because available commercial charts use the scheme of Figure 6–4. These commercial charts carry in each square decay data, abundances, etc., for the particular nuclide.

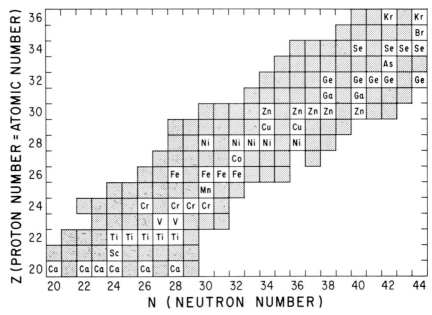

FIG. 6–4.   Diagram illustrating part of one type of isotope chart.

Radioactive Series.   Many of the alpha-emitting heavy nuclides occurring in nature, and of those which have been artificially produced, fall into four decay series, headed respectively by uranium, thorium, actinium, and neptunium. The uranium series is shown in Figure 6–5, with the beta and gamma transformations and half periods indicated. The final product, indicated as Ra G, is an isotope of lead, $^{206}_{81}$Pb. The parent element of each series must have a very long half life, otherwise there would be none remaining on earth; it would all have decayed since its creation, and its shorter-lived descendants would have also. It is probably because neptunium has a half life of only two million years that it is not found in nature. (The age of the earth is at least 1000 times this, so that if there had originally been any created, the amount left now would be undetectable.) Any members later than a long-lived first ancestor will always exist, no matter how short their half lives, because the supply will be continually replenished.

With the discovery of nuclear fission a large number of beta-decay series were observed among the fission products, as mentioned in Chapter 5. Since here the half periods of the parents are very short, continued existence of the daughters is not assured.

Radioactive Equilibrium.   In Chapter 2, disintegration rules for radioactive nuclei were outlined. There the only radioactivity corresponded to the transformation of a single radionuclide. However, the daughter substance may in turn be radioactive, and so on. Relations among quantities present of different members of the series depend on the various decay constants.

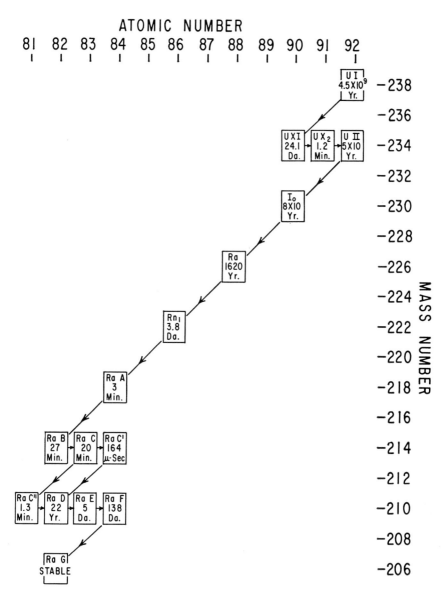

FIG. 6-5. The uranium series.

Consider a radioactive parent, which decays into a radioactive daughter. Let N_p and λ_p represent the number of atoms of the parent and its decay constant, and N_d and λ_d those of the daughter. According to the law of radioactive decay (page 21) if there are present N_p atoms of a particular nuclide, whose decay constant is λ_p,

$$- dN_p = \lambda_p N_p,$$

and
$$N_p = N_p^o e^{-\lambda_p t}, \qquad\qquad 6-(2)$$

where N_p^o represents the original number of atoms of this nuclide at time $t = 0$. Every atom of N_p which decays becomes an atom of N_d, and this in turn decays with its own rate. Therefore

$$\frac{dN_d}{dt} = \lambda_p N_p - \lambda_d N_d, \qquad\qquad 6-(3)$$

the first term representing the growth from the parent and the second the decay of the daughter. Mathematical development of this equation leads to*

$$N_d = \frac{\lambda_p}{\lambda_d - \lambda_p} N_p^o (e^{-\lambda_p t} - e^{-\lambda_d t}) + N_d^o e^{-\lambda_d t} \qquad 6-(4)$$

Here again the first term shows net growth of the daughter from the parent, and the second the contribution from any daughter atoms initially present. For products resulting from an initially pure parent fraction, the second term is zero.

In considering special parent daughter relationships, three cases are evident, depending on whether the parent or the daughter is longer-lived or whether their lives are the same. In the first case λ_p is less than λ_d, and after a sufficiently long time $e^{-\lambda_p t}$ is so much larger then $e^{-\lambda_d t}$ that the latter can be neglected. Then

$$\frac{N_p}{N_d} = \frac{N_p^o e^{-\lambda_p t}}{\dfrac{\lambda_p}{\lambda_d - \lambda_p} N_p^o e^{-\lambda_p t}} = \frac{\lambda_d - \lambda_p}{\lambda_p} \qquad 6-(5)$$

or the ratio of the amounts of the two nuclides becomes constant. They are then said to be in a state of equilibrium.

---

* This development involves the solution of differential equations, which is beyond the mathematical training expected of readers of this text.

Equations 6—(4) and 6—(5) can easily be transformed to give the relations in terms of half lives instead of decay constants. Since

$$\lambda = \frac{0.693}{T},$$

$$N_d = \frac{T_d}{T_p - T_d} N_p^o \left(e^{-0.693\ t/T_p} - e^{-0.693\ t/T_d} + N_d^o\ e^{-0.693\ t/T_d} \right) \qquad 6\text{—}(6)$$

and at equilibrium

$$\frac{N_p}{N_d} = \frac{T_p - T_d}{T_d} \qquad\qquad\qquad 6\text{—}(7)$$

The time required for equilibrium to be attained depends on the relative values of T_p and T_d.

As mentioned above three cases may be considered:

a. Parent longer-lived than daughter   —$(T_p > T_d)$
b. Parent and daugher having equal lives—$(T_p = T_d)$
c. Parent shorter-lived than daughter   —$(T_p < T_d)$

As an example of (a), consider the pair ^{99}Mo — ^{99m}Tc.

$$T_p = 66\ hr;\ T_d = 6\ hr.\quad \frac{T_p - T_d}{T_d} = \frac{60}{6} = 10.$$

Start with 100 mCi of ^{99}Mo; this contains $4.6 \times 10^{12} \times \dfrac{66}{24} \times 100 =$ 12.65×10^{14} atoms, which is N_p^o. N_p and N_d for subsequent times can be calculated from the above equations, considering that the parent was initially free of any of the daughter. In Figure 6-6 the lower curves show the number of atoms of parent and daughter over a period of two weeks. After an initial increase N_d (N_2) reaches a maximum and then decreases at the same rate as N_p (N_1); the two are in equilibrium. The ratio of the two,

$$\frac{N_p}{N_d} = \frac{T_p - T_d}{T_d} = \frac{66 - 6}{6} = 10.$$

When both parent and daughter have relatively short lives, the equilibrium is said to be transient.

Equilibrium curves are frequently plotted to show the *activities* or numbers of atoms disintegrating per unit time, rather than the number of atoms present. The activity is in each case, of course the number of atoms present multiplied by the decay constant, so $A_p = N_p\lambda_p$ and $A_d = N_d\lambda_d$. If the data of the above example are treated in this way, the upper curves of Figure 6–6 are obtained.   For the 100 mCi of the parent originally present, the curves show the atoms of each nuclide decaying at any instant. Decrease in activity of each nuclide is at the rate of λ_p, characteristic of the parent.

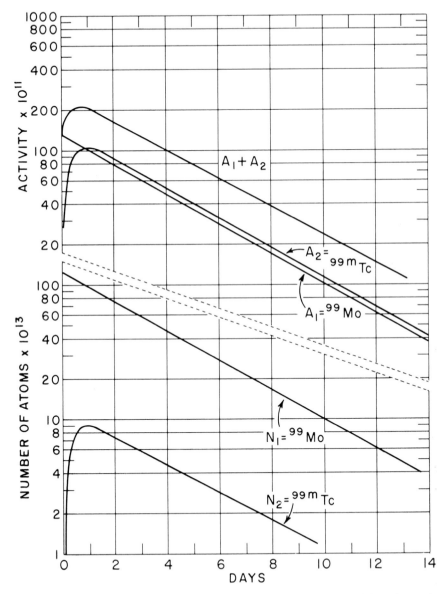

FIG. 6–6.   Transient radioactive equilibrium. Upper curves, A_1, activity of parent; A_2, activity of daughter; $A_1 + A_2$, total activity in preparation.   Lower curves, N_1, decay of parent; N_2, growth and decay of daughter.

Since the number of millicuries present is determined by the number of atoms disintegrating rather than by the number present, it appears from Figure 6-6 that at transient equilibrium the number of millicuries of the daughter is greater than that of the parent. It is seen from formulas 6—(1), 6—(4) and 6—(5) that this should be so.

$$A_p = N_p \lambda_p \text{ and } A_d = N_d \lambda_d$$

$$= \lambda_d \frac{\lambda_p}{\lambda_d - \lambda_p} = \frac{\lambda_d}{\lambda_d - \lambda_p} \lambda_p N_p = \frac{\lambda_d}{\lambda_d - \lambda_p} A_p = \frac{T_p}{T_p - T_d} A_p$$

Since $\dfrac{T_p}{T_p - T_d}$ is greater than unity, A_d is always greater than A_p, or the daughter millicuries are greater than those of the parent.

If the half life of the parent is very much longer than that of the daughter, so that it does not decay appreciably over the period of study, the situation is that shown in Figure 6-7; the equilibrium is called *secular*. In this

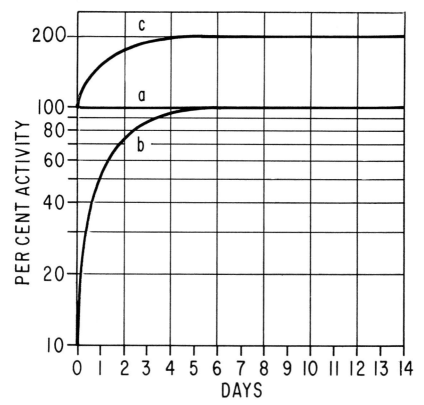

FIG. 6–7. Secular radioactive equilibrium. *a*, decay of parent (not demonstrable in period of observation); *b*, growth and decay of daughter; *c*, total activity in preparation of initially pure parent.

case λ_d is very much greater than λ_p, so that $\lambda_d - \lambda_p$ is essentially equal

to λ_d. Then $A_p = \lambda_p N_p$ and $A_d = \lambda_d N_d = \dfrac{\lambda_d \lambda_p}{\lambda_d - \lambda_p} N_p = \lambda_p N_p$.

Thus the two activities are equal; the same number of atoms of each decays per unit time after equilibrium has been reached, or the same number of millicuries of each is present. This may be illustrated by the growth of radon ($T_d = 3.8$ days) in an initially pure preparation of radium. ($T_p = 1620$ years $= 267000$ days.)

$$\lambda_p = 2.6 \times 10^{-6}. \ \lambda_d = 0.18. \ \lambda_d - \lambda_p \text{ is essentially } = \lambda_d,$$

whence $\dfrac{\lambda_d - \lambda_p}{\lambda_d} = 1$, and $A_d = A_p$.

$b.$ Parent and daughter having same half lives. No such case is known. Mathematically it can be treated by making $T_p = T_d + \delta$, where δ is a very small quantity; the equations become lengthy and are of no practical significance.

$c.$ Parent shorter-lived than daughter. In this case $\lambda_p > \lambda_d$. At all times $\lambda_p t$ is greater than $\lambda_d t$, so $e^{-\lambda_p t}$ is less than $e^{-\lambda_d t}$ and the expression in parentheses in 7—(4) is negative. However $\dfrac{\lambda_p}{\lambda_d - \lambda_p}$ is also negative, giving a positive value for N_d. This increases and then decreases at the rate of λ_d. There is no equilibrium.

In Figure 6–8 are given values for the N's and the A's for the reaction $^{131}\text{Te} \rightarrow {}^{131}\text{I}$. $T_p = 1.25$ days; $T_d = 8$ days. $\lambda_p = 0.555/\text{day}$. $\lambda_d = 0.0865/\text{day}$. N_p for 100 mCi of $^{131}\text{Te} = 5.5 \times 10^{14}$ atoms. N_d rises to a maximum and then decays at the rate λ_d. There is no equilibrium.

Growth of Radionuclide in Neutron Flux. The production of a radionuclide by steady bombardment of a stable source may be considered analogous to the growth of a short-lived daughter in an infinitely long-lived parent. Thus the time necessary for a target to be bombarded in a pile or cyclotron to produce a desired activity can be determined. In this case $-\lambda_p N_p$, the rate of destruction of the parent, is the rate of production of the radioactive daughter, and may therefore be replaced by R. Since $\lambda_p N_p$ is an extremely small fraction of the stable atoms of the target, $e^{-\lambda_p t}$ is essentially unity. Furthermore λ_p is very much smaller than λ_d, the decay rate of the product, whence $\lambda_d - \lambda_p$ is essentially equal to λ_d. Then equation 6—(4) becomes

$$N_d = \frac{R}{\lambda_d} (1 - e^{-\lambda_d t}) \qquad\qquad 6\text{—}(8)$$

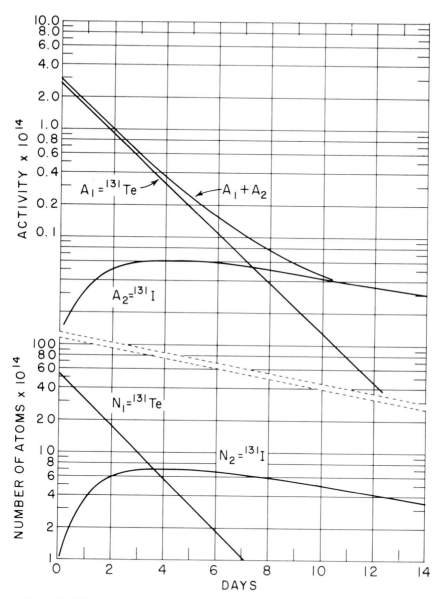

Fɪɢ. 6–8. The case of no equilibrium. Upper curves, A_1, activity of parent; A_2, activity of daughter, $A_1 + A_2$, total activity in preparation. Lower curves, N_2 decay of parent; N_1, growth and decay of daughter.

If t becomes very long, $e^{-\lambda_d t}$ becomes very small and N_d approaches $\dfrac{R}{\lambda_d}$ as a limiting value, the maximum amount of the daughter isotope that could ever be produced. The ratio of N_d at any time to its value at the maximum is

$$\frac{N_d}{N_d \text{ (max)}} = \frac{\dfrac{R}{\lambda_d}(1 - e^{-\lambda_d t})}{\dfrac{R}{\lambda_d}} = 1 - e^{-\lambda_d t} \qquad 7-(9)$$

Thus if t is one half period, $1 - e^{-\lambda_d t} = 0.5$ or half the maximum amount can be produced in a bombardment of one half period. Similarly three-fourths of the maximum are produced in two half periods, and so on. In practice it is seldom economical to irradiate for more than two half lives of the product.

In Chapter 4, page 47, an example was given of the production of ^{198}Au by slow neutron bombardment of ^{197}Au. The above formulae were used in the calculation of the quantity of ^{198}Au produced. Of course the process may be complicated by neutron bombardment of the first daughter radionuclide to form a second. Details of calculations in such cases are outside the scope of this book.

Radioactive "Cows." When a radioactive nuclide has a daughter of shorter life, it is often possible to separate the two, mechanically or chemically. The supply of the parent can be maintained, and the daughter periodically removed or "milked" from it. Several such systems are in use, being familiarly known as "cows." The earliest was the radium-radon installation. The radium salt was in solution: the radon gas could be pumped off and used without disturbing the parent. Here N_p remained practically constant, as illustrated in Figure 6–9.

A popular "cow" in current use is the ^{99}Mo $-$ ^{99m}Tc combination, where the separation is effected by means of a chemical solution poured over the "cow," dissolving the Tc but not affecting the Mo. The growth of ^{99m}Tc in ^{99}Mo was illustrated in Figure 6–6. Here, however, no "milking" had taken place; the curves represent the situation of the daughter left with the parent. If the separation takes place daily, the effect is as shown in Figure 6–9. In practice the total amount of the daughter cannot be obtained, but often up to 90 per cent can be removed.

Other available systems are ^{90}Sr $-$ ^{90}Y; ^{87}Y $-$ ^{87m}Sr; ^{132}Te $-$ ^{132}I; ^{140}Ba $-$ ^{140}La; ^{113}Sn $-$ ^{113m}In. Doubtless in the near future there will be many more, since this is a practical way of making many short-lived nuclides available.

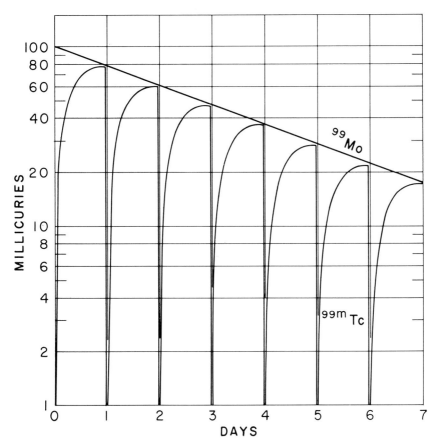

FIG. 6–9.   Radioactive "Cow": ^{99}Mo-^{99m}Tc.   The technecium grows to equilibrium in 24 hours, regrows in another day and is again removed, and the procedure is repeated daily.

REFERENCES

BRUCER, MARSHALL: *Trilinear Chart of the Nuclides.*   St. Louis, Mallincrodt Nuclear, 1968.

HINE, G. J. and BROWNELL, G. L.:   *Radiation Dosimetry*, Chapters 2 and 16, New York Academic Press, Inc., 1956.

General Electric Chart of the Nuclides, Knolls Atomic Power Laboratory, Schenectady, New York, 1956.

GLASSER, O., QUIMBY, E. H., TAYLOR, L. S., WEATHERWAX, J. L. and MORGAN, R. H.: *Physical Foundations of Radiology*, 3rd Ed., Chapter 4, New York, Paul B. Hoeber, Inc., 1961.

MORGAN, R. H. and CORRIGAN, K. E.:   *Handbook of Radiology*, Section 4, Chicago, Yearbook Publishers, Inc., 1955.

Nuclear Research Center, Karlsruhe, Chart of the Nuclides, revised to 1961.   Gersbach und Sohn Verlag, Munich, Germany.

POLLARD, E. C. and DAVIDSON, W. L.:   *Applied Nuclear Physics*, 2nd Ed., Chapters 5 and 6, New York, John Wiley & Sons, Inc., 1951.

RUTHERFORD, E., CHADWICK, J. and ELLIS, C. D.:   *Radiations from Radioactive Substances.*   Chapters 3, 7, 8, 9, 14, 15, Cambridge, England. University Press, 1951.

7

Interaction of Radiation and Matter

RADIATION can be detected only by its action on matter. The uses of radiation depend on effects produced in living or non-living material. Any such effect must necessarily be the result of a transfer of energy from the radiation to the matter. This means that a beam of radiation will have its energy diminished as it traverses a material medium. The interactions by which such energy transfer can be brought about, and the results of the interactions on the matter and on the radiation form the subject of this chapter.

Characteristics of the Radiations. The radiations to be considered are charged and uncharged particles, and photons, or electromagnetic rays; all may have considerable energy. The charged particles are alphas, deuterons, protons, and positive and negative electrons; the uncharged one are neutrons. The electromagnetic rays are gamma or x rays. Alpha particles, $^4_2\alpha$, have a mass number 4 and two positive charges; those from radioactive substances travel at velocities up to about 15,000 miles per second. Protons, ^1_1H, and deuterons, ^2_1H, have mass numbers 1 and 2 respectively and a single positive charge. They are not emitted in radioactive disintegrations, but are accelerated in such instruments as the cyclotron, and for the same energies as the alpha particles, have considerably greater velocities. Negative and positive electrons have masses only of the order of $\frac{1}{1800}$ of a mass unit, and single charges of the indicated sign. Both types are emitted in radioactive disintegrations, the negative ones can be accelerated to high velocities artificially; some may travel with speeds up to 99 per cent of that of light. Neutrons, ^1_0n, have unit mass and no charge. They may have velocities ranging from thermal to many thousands of miles per second. Electromagnetic rays or photons have neither charge nor mass, and travel with the speed of light.

Energies of the Radiations. The energy of *particle radiation* is kinetic;

$$KE = \tfrac{1}{2} m v^2, \qquad\qquad 7-(1)$$

or energy in ergs equals $\frac{1}{2}$ mass in grams multiplied by square of velocity in cm per second. For the alpha particle, m is 6.643×10^{-24} gm, v at 12,000 miles per second is 2×10^9 cm per second.

$$KE = \tfrac{1}{2} \times 6.643 \times 10^{-24} \times (2 \times 10^9)^2 = 1.3 \times 10^{-5} \text{ erg.}$$

Since 1 erg $= 6.24 \times 10^5$ MeV the kinetic energy of the alpha particle traveling with this speed is 8 MeV. Similar calculations can be made for other particles of appreciable mass, namely deuterons, protons, and neutrons.

For beta particles a new phenomenon has to be considered; the increase of mass as velocity attains high values.

Einstein postulated that no particle can travel faster than the speed of light in a vacuum. If the above formula for kinetic energy is applied to a million-volt electron it becomes

$$1 \text{ MeV} = 1.602 \times 10^{-6} \text{ ergs} = 1/2 \times 9.108 \times 10^{-28} \text{ gm} \times v^2 \text{ cm/sec.}$$

Whence $v = 6 \times 10^{10}$ cm/sec. But this is twice the speed of light, and hence inadmissible.

One of the predictions of Einstein's special relativity theory is that the mass of a particle must increase as its velocity increases. If the particle velocity is denoted by v, the speed of light by c, and the ratio v/c by β, the formula for mass at velocity v, in terms of the "rest mass" is

$$m_v = \frac{m_o}{\sqrt{1-\beta^2}}. \qquad\qquad 7-(2)$$

This formula will be accepted without derivation; its validity has been thoroughly demonstrated.

In Chapter 4, the equivalence of mass and energy was discussed, and the energy equivalence of an electron at rest was given as $m_o c^2 = 0.511006$ MeV. Obviously if the electron gets heavier by virtue of its motion, its equivalent energy will increase. The total energy will then be $m_v c^2$. This energy may be considered as having two components, one the rest mass energy, the other the kinetic energy. Then

$$m_v c^2 = m_o c^2 + \text{KE, or}$$

$$\text{KE} = (m_v - m_o)c^2. \qquad\qquad 7-(3)$$

An electron going at 0.9 the speed of light will have mass m $= \dfrac{m_o}{\sqrt{1-0.81}}$

$= 2.3\ m_o$. The total energy then is $2.3\ m_o c^2$ or 1.175 MeV. Of this $m_o c^2 = 0.511$ MeV is rest energy, and the remainder, 0.664 MeV is, kinetic. Kinetic energies of electrons or beta particles in general practice range from about 0.1 to 3.0 MeV.

The energy of the *photons* is determined in a different manner. These have no associated mass, but are electromagnetic waves traveling with the speed of light.

The wave pattern may be indicated as in Figure 7–1. The *wave length*, or distance from crest to crest, is usually denoted by the Greek lower case lambda (λ). The velocity, which is the velocity of light, 2.998×10^{10} cm per second, is denoted by c. The frequency, or number of waves passing a given point per second, is indicated by the Greek lower case nu (ν).

$$\nu = \frac{c}{\lambda} \text{ or } \lambda = \frac{c}{\nu}. \qquad\qquad 7\text{--}(4)$$

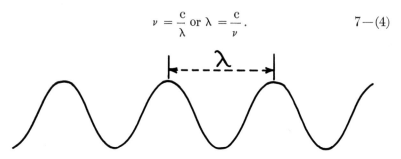

Fig. 7–1.   Diagram to illustrate wave motion.   Wave length, λ, = distance from crest to crest.

The range of wave lengths to be considered is of the order of 1.0 to 0.01 Angstrom units or 10^{-8} to 10^{-10} cm., which means frequencies of the order of 10^{18} to 10^{20} per second. The shorter the wave length or the higher the frequency, the greater is the energy of the radiation.

However, in describing the interaction of photons with matter, it is difficult to deal with waves, so they are to be considered in a second aspect, as *particles of pure energy*. This is not a contradiction. Neither particle nor wave picture describes the radiation fully, just as neither floor plan nor elevation describes a building completely, but both are true as far as they go. In this sense the energy of the particle is given by

$$E = h\nu \text{ ergs}, \qquad\qquad 7\text{--}(5)$$

where h is a number known as Planck's constant, and equal to 6.625×10^{-27} erg-seconds. Thus, for a photon of wave length 0.1 Å, or frequency

$$\frac{3 \times 10^{10*}}{0.1 \times 10^{-8}} = 3 \times 10^{19} \text{ per second, E} = 6.625 \times 10^{-27} \times 3 \times 10^{19} = 2 \times 10^{-7}$$

ergs $= 0.125$ MeV. Photon energies in practice range from a few keV to a few MeV.

There are convenient relations among wave length, voltage and energy:

$$E = h\nu \text{ ergs}, \; = \frac{hc}{\lambda} \text{ ergs} = \frac{hc}{\lambda} \times 6.24 \times 10^5 \text{ MeV}. \qquad 7\text{--}(6)$$

* This value is used for c, instead of 2.998×10^{10} as given above, for simplification of the computations.

In these formulas λ is expressed in cm. If it is expressed in Angstrom units

$$E \text{ (keV)} = \frac{6.625 \times 10^{-27} \times 3 \times 10^{10} \times 6.24 \times 10^8}{\lambda \times 10^{-8}} = \frac{12.40}{\lambda} \text{ Angstrom.}$$

$$7-(7)$$

Possible Types of Interactions of Radiation and Matter. The nature of matter has been discussed in Chapter 1. It is composed of atoms, consisting of nuclei, orbital electrons, and a great deal of empty space. Any of the kinds of radiation just discussed, in traversing atoms, may do one of three things:

 a. Pass through without encountering any opposition;
 b. Interact with an orbital electron;
 c. Interact with the nucleus.

That which passes through with no interaction is not detected, and is of no interest in this discussion. By far the greatest amount of energy interchange results from interactions with orbital electrons.

Interaction of Alpha Particles with Matter. Consider first an alpha particle with a velocity of some thousands of miles per second, or an energy of a few million electron volts, a mass about 7000 times that of an electron and a double positive charge. If it passes close to an orbital electron, it will exert a powerful attraction on it, and may pull it entirely out of its orbit and give it a considerable velocity. The atom will then be left lacking an electron, and therefore with a net positive charge; it is a *positive ion*. The electron flying off by itself is a *negative ion;* it may temporarily attach itself to another atom, in which case the whole thing is the negative ion. It may, however, continue on as a fast-moving electron, when it is essentially equivalent to a beta particle. It will not attach itself to the disrupting alpha particle, because this has been moving so fast that the electron cannot catch it. However, the alpha particle did lose some energy in the encounter, possibly several hundred electron volts, and after many interactions it will be slowed down sufficiently so that it can pick up two electrons to take their places in orbits around the now slowed-down alpha particle which is essentially a helium nucleus. The final state of the alpha particle, then, is as the nucleus of a helium atom. Alpha particles, being much heavier than electrons, will not be deflected from their straight paths by the encounters with orbital electrons, and since all those from a particular alpha-emitter have the same energy, they will travel the same distance in a particular medium, or have a definite *range*. The cloud chamber photograph in Figure 3–2, page 34, was made by a mixture of alphas from thorium C and thorium C′, with energies of about 8.8 and 5.6 MeV respectively. The two ranges are clearly shown.

Even the most energetic alpha particles lose their energy fairly rapidly in traversing matter, so that their ranges are not more than a few cm in air, or a small fraction of a mm in solid substances. The range increases rapidly with the energy or velocity of the alpha particle. The 5.3 MeV alphas from $^{210}_{84}$Po have a range of 3.6 cm in air, while the 7.6 MeV particles from $^{214}_{84}$RaC' travel 6.6 cm in this medium.

A positive ion and a negative ion are always produced simultaneously; it is not possible to obtain one without the other. The two together constitute an *ion pair*. The *specific ionization* is defined as the number of ion pairs produced per millimeter of path of the ionizing particle, and is approximately inversely proportional to the particle velocity. Thus an alpha particle ionizes more and more strongly as it slows down, until it reaches a maximum just before it is stopped. The 7.6 MeV alphas just mentioned would have an initial specific ionization of about 2000 ion pairs per millimeter of air, and just before the end of their range, of about 7000.

The energy lost by the particle per ion pair formed varies in different substances, and, to a certain extent, with different ionizing particles. On the average, about 34 electron volts are lost by the particle for every ion pair formed in air. Thus a 5 MeV alpha particle, when its energy is eventually used up, will have produced approximately $\dfrac{5,000,000}{34} = 15 \times 10^4$ ion pairs. Most of these will not have resulted from direct action by the alpha particle, but from action of the secondary electrons which the alpha particle has set in motion as it tore them from their atoms. Their behavior is essentially the same as that of beta particles, which will be discussed in the next section.

If the alpha particle makes a direct collision with a nucleus, the result may be nuclear disintegration, as described in Chapter 4. This is an extremely rare event, and of little importance in the discussion of the interaction of radiation and matter.

The behavior of deuterons and protons is essentially the same as that of alpha particles, and need not be considered separately.

Interactions of Beta Particles with Matter. In the interactions of beta particles of either sign with orbital electrons, mutal attraction of unlike charges and repulsion of like ones is the operative agency, as with alpha particles, and ionization is again the result of the "collision." However, in these cases the interacting particles are of essentially the same mass, and hence the impinging particle may be widely deflected by the encounter, moreover it may lose most of its energy in a single interaction. Thus the beta particles will pursue very tortuous paths, and even if all started with the same energy they would not have the same range, as do the alphas. The particles are finally slowed down to thermal velocities, the negative ones attach themselves to atoms needing electrons. The positrons disappear by combining with negative electrons to form *annihilation radiation*. This is a process similar to that described in Chapter 4 where the loss of matter resulted in the production of radiation. The same law is followed:

$$E \text{ (ergs)} = m \text{ (gm)} \times C^2 \text{ (cm/sec)}^2$$

In this case the masses are essentially equal and about 9.1×10^{-28} gm each. Whence

$$E = 2 \times 9.1 \times 10^{-28} \times (3 \times 10^{10})^2 \text{ ergs} = 2 \times 0.51 \text{ MeV.} \qquad 7-(8)$$

or two photons, each of about one-half million electron volts, are produced, There must usually be two, to comply with the laws of conservation of momentum. Rare specific cases resulting in production of one or three photons may be neglected.

If a beta particle of either sign passes near an atomic nucleus, its path will be bent somewhat toward the nucleus if it is a negative electron, away from it if it is positive. This change in direction is considered a negative acceleration of the charged particle, and according to classical electromagnetic theory, in such circumstances electromagnetic energy must be radiated. This is, in fact, the phenomenon leading to the production of the continuous spectrum of x rays in x-ray tubes, as the electrons from the hot cathode are slowed (negatively accelerated) by the target atoms. This radiation, particularly as it is produced in the passage of beta particles through matter, is called *bremsstrahlung* (from the German meaning "braking radiation") and represents an energy loss for the electron. This type of interaction becomes more important as the energy of the beta particle increases, and as the atomic number of the material traversed increases. It can be shown that the *fraction* of the beta energy which appears as external bremsstrahlung is approximately equal to $\dfrac{ZE}{3000}$ where E is the maximum energy of the particle in MeV and Z is the atomic number of the absorber. Thus, for 2 MeV beta particles passing through ^{29}Cu, the external bremsstrahlung is $\dfrac{29 \times 2}{3000} = 2$ per cent of the total energy. In ^{82}Pb it would be $\dfrac{82}{29}$ times as much, or about 6 per cent.

Interaction of Neutrons with Matter. Neutrons, having no charge, do not interact with electrons; their only interaction is with nuclei, in the form of actual collisions. In such an encounter the neutron may be scattered, absorbed with emission of a photon, absorbed with emission of a heavy particle such as a proton, absorbed with production of fission of the target nucleus. A particular case of nuclear scattering interaction occurs when neutrons and hydrogen atoms are involved. Since neutrons and protons (hydrogen nuclei) have essentially the same mass, an energetic neutron striking a hydrogen nucleus can drive it away from its orbital electron, thus making it a positive ion. This can then ionize in the same manner as a positively charged "heavy" particle. (See alpha particle, above.) In absorption processes new stable or radioactive nuclei may be formed. Some of these processes have been described in Chapter 4. Nuclides may thus exhibit very different reactions on collision with neutrons, and the characteristics may change with neutron energy in a complicated way. There are few generalizations which can be made with regard to the variations with atomic number or mass number. Since clinical users of radionuclides are mainly interested in neutron interactions only for the production of such substances they will not be further discussed in this chapter.

Interaction of Photons with Matter. The interaction of photons with orbital electrons takes place in different ways depending on whether the electron is essentially free in an outer orbit or tightly bound in an inner one. In the first case the picture may be imagined as similar to the interaction of beta particles with orbital electrons, although the force is not now due to the interaction of electric charges. The photon "collides" with an electron and knocks it from its position, giving up some of its energy and being deflected from its path. Thus it proceeds in a new direction as a photon of less energy or longer wave length. This is called a *Compton collision*; the electron is a Compton or recoil electron. The difference in wave length between the incident and scattered photon depends only on the angle of scatter. Regardless of the initial energy of the photon, the change in wave length is given by

$$\Delta\lambda = 0.024 \ (1 - \cos \theta) \ \text{Angstrom}, \qquad\qquad 7\text{—}(9)$$

where θ is the angle of deflection or scatter, as indicated in Figure 7–2. Thus for a 90° deflection, since cos 90° = 0, any photon has its wave length increased by 0.024 Å. For a 100 keV photon, $\lambda = \dfrac{12.40}{100} = 0.124$ Å, and the 90° scattered ray has a wave length of 0.124 + 0.024 = 0.148 Å, corresponding to 84 keV. However for a 1 MeV photon, with a wave length of 0.0124Å, 90° scattered wave length is 0.036 Å, corresponding to 350 keV, a much more drastic reduction in energy. A photon cannot give up all its energy in a Compton collision. If it is scattered directly backward $\theta = 180°$, cos $\theta = -1$ and the wave length is increased by 0.048 Å. If the initial wave length were vanishingly small, the final one would still be equivalent to 260 keV. If the original photon were only 10 keV, with $\lambda = 1.24$ Å, the final wave length of 1.288 Å would correspond to 9.6 keV.

If the electron is tightly bound in an inner orbit, the photon in removing it may give up all of its energy and cease to exist. Part of the energy goes to overcoming the binding energy* of the electron in its orbit, and the rest

---

* This binding energy of orbital electrons must not be confused with nuclear building energy (p. 40).

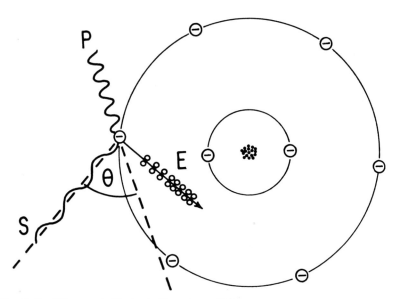

FIG. 7–2.   Diagram to illustrate Compton collision.
  P, primary photon; S, scattered photon; θ, angle of scatter; E, Compton electron producing ion pairs. (Note the change of scale in the ion track. Each ion pair in E should
be as large as the initial atom. It is not practicable to make the illustration completely
to this scale.)

to accelerating this electron. This is a *photoelectric collision*, the electron is
a *photoelectron*. In order to be capable of a photoelectric interaction, a
photon must have sufficient energy to overcome the binding energy of the
electron in its orbit, but not so much more that the electron is incapable of
taking all that remains. The binding energies of electrons in the K and L
orbits of certain elements are listed in Appendix F. From this it is seen that
the binding energy for a K electron in nickle is 8.34 keV. Hence a 10 keV
photon could eject this electron and have 1.66 keV additional to accelerate
it. The ejected electron is then effectively a 1.66 keV beta particle (though
never called this). However a 10 keV photon could not eject a K electron
from tin (binding energy = 25.5 keV), but it could remove an L electron
from this atom, since this requires only 3.53 keV. A 1 MeV photon would
not readily undergo photoelectric interaction with a tin K electron; this
would result in the production of essentially a 1 MeV electron. Such an
interaction is not impossible, but it is unlikely. (See Appendix F for
binding energies.)

  The ejected electrons, in either Compton or photoelectric encounters,
proceed as ionizing particles in exactly the same manner as primary beta
particles.

  A photon interacting with a nucleus *may* disintegrate it, but this is
improbable except for photons of several MeV of energy. The usual re-
  7

action of a high energy photon passing close to the field of a nucleus is its complete transformation into a *positron-negatron pair*.* Again according to the Einstein equation

$$E = m \ c^2.$$

For such a pair the mass is $2 \times 9.1 \times 10^{-28}$ gm, and the necessary energy to produce it is

$$E = 2 \times 9.1 \times 10^{-28} \times 9 \times 10^{20} \text{ ergs} = 1.02 \text{ MeV.}$$

Photons of less energy than this cannot undergo pair formation. If the energy is greater, the excess goes to accelerating the particles. These then traverse matter in exactly the same manner as primary beta particles, ionizing as they go. They are eventually slowed down to thermal velocities; the positron unites with a free electron to produce two 0.51 MeV photons of annihilation radiation, as described above, and the negatron is annexed by something that needs an extra electron.

Recombination and Production of Characteristic Radiation. The net result of the passage of any charged particle or photon through matter is the production of *ions;* for this reason these are called *ionizing radiations*. In producing ionization, the radiation must impart energy to the matter. The ionized state is extremely temporary. In a very small fraction of a second the ionized atom finds another electron, *recombines* with it, and returns to normal. When the vacancy left in a photoelectric interaction is filled, the atom gives up the energy that the photon left with it when it removed the electron. This energy is emitted in the form of one or a few photons, the sum of whose energies is exactly the energy which bound the electron there in the first place. For this reason it is called *characteristic radiation*; its energy is characteristic of the particular orbit in the particular atom from which it arose.

For an atom of any element, the characteristic radiation arising from replacement of an electron in the K orbit (K-characteristic) is more energetic than from the L orbit, and so on, as indicated by the binding energies in Appendix F. Characteristic radiation from any orbit increases in energy as the atomic number of the element increases.

The characteristic radiation is not truly mono-energetic, but exhibits a group of slightly different values depending on whether the replacing electron came from the L, M, etc. orbits, or from completely outside the atom. The K_α radiation, resulting from replacement from the L orbit, has slightly less energy than the K_β from the M, and so on.

Recombination after a Compton interaction results in general in the production of much less energetic photons. The radiation is usually in the visible or ultra violet region.

---

* The term *negatron* is used for the negative electron at any time, but especially when it is paired or contrasted with a positron.

Wilson Cloud Chamber. The paths of ionizing particles in a gas may be made visible by an apparatus called a Wilson Cloud Chamber. An enclosed volume of very clean gas saturated with water vapor is suddenly cooled by expansion, to produce supersaturation. In air containing dust particles, under this condition a fog would be formed, but if the gas is dust-free there is no fog. However, if a beam of radiation is passed through the air in the chamber, the ions will serve as condensation centers for the fog droplets; thus the paths of the ionizing particles can be followed. Figure 3–2, page 34, showed cloud chamber photographs of alpha particles. In Figure 7–3 are shown tracks of slow and fast beta particles; it will be re-

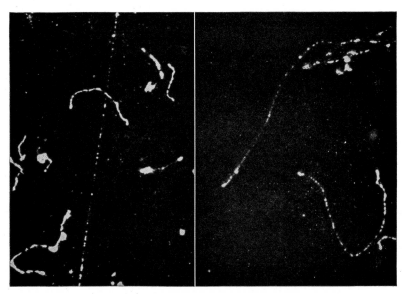

Fig. 7–3.   Cloud tracks of slow (curved path) and fast (straight path) beta particles. (Courtesy of C. T. R. Wilson and the Royal Society of London.)

called that specifiic ionization increases as the particle is slowed down. The cloud tracks due to a beam of photons are actually the tracks of the secondary electrons ejected in Compton and photoelectric interactions. Neutrons, not being themselves ionizing particles, do not leave tracks, but when a neutron interacts with a nucleus, tracks start at the point of interaction and by their characteristics the nature of the interaction may be inferred.

Bubble Chamber. For the study of energetic particles, cloud chambers must be very large to show the entire track. The bubble chamber, invented by D. A. Glaser in 1952, overcomes this difficulty by having the particles traverse a liquid instead of a gas. Thus the track lengths are much shorter. Liquids can, for brief periods, be heated above their boiling points without actually boiling. Charged particles traversing such a superheated liquid cause bubbles to form along their tracks, by a phenomenon which may be considered as local boiling spots. These bubble paths can be photographed in a manner analogous to the cloud tracks in a cloud chamber. These bubble chambers are very important tools in the study of products of high energy accelerators.

Absorption and Scatter of Radiation. Up to this point in this chapter the discussion has concerned *individual* interactions of specific particles or photons with individual atoms. In general, the interest is in the *gross* effect on the matter which receives energy, and on the radiation beam which loses it.

The beam, in traversing matter, tends to become more and more heterogeneous. This is particularly true with photons, where an initially homogeneous beam is quickly "contaminated" by Compton and photoelectrons, characteristic x rays, lower energy scattered x rays, and (if the original energy was high enough) annihilation radiation. The final result on matter of the absorption of energy is a very slight rise in temperature, although part of the energy may have gone to producing chemical changes, etc.

In addition to absorption of the radiation with utilization of its energy for ionization, part of the rays may be removed from the beam by *scatter*, and so be lost to the detector or to absorbers lying farther along its path. This effect is more marked the larger the beam of radiation impinging on the scattering material, and the smaller the detector . Both absorption and scatter must be considered in studying the interactions of radiation and matter.

Absorption of Beta Radiation. Absorption is usually studied by measuring the radiation transmitted by increasingly thick layers of material, or "filters," and plotting the data as an "absorption curve," as in Figure 7–4. Semi-logarithmic paper is usually employed, as the decrease is likely to be so rapid at the beginning that a linear plot may be difficult to read. Such curves are usually nearly linear on semi-logarithmic paper. This does not arise from a simple absorption function of mono-energetic particles, but is due to a fortuitous combination of a continuous beta-ray spectrum (see p. 63) and the contribution of scattered radiation to the total activity. The exact shape of the absorption curve depends on the geometrical arrangements of sample, absorbers, and detector, as well as on the nuclide. The linear part of such an absorption curve as the one in the figure can be represented by the equation

$$A_t = A_o e^{-\mu t}, \qquad\qquad 7-(10)$$

where A_o is the initial activity and A_t that after passage through a thickness of filter t; μ is the linear absorption coefficient, the rate of absorption per unit thickness of the material.* A half thickness or half value layer bears the same relation to the absorption coefficient as does the half period to the decay constant for a radioactive nuclide;

---

* The similarity to the isotope decay equation is obvious.

$$t(\tfrac{1}{2}) = \frac{0.693}{\mu}. \qquad 7-(11)$$

Frequently, instead of the *linear* absorption coefficient (absorption per unit thickness), the mass absorption coefficient is used (absorption per unit mass). This is μ/ρ, the linear absorption coefficient divided by the density. Filter thickness may be expressed in terms of grams per square centimeter, as shown in the lower legend for abscissa in Figure 7–4. The filter thickness is given in cm and the density in gm/cm³. Then thickness (cm) × density (gm/cm³) = filter (gm/cm²). For example, the range of 0.5 MeV beta particles in Al is 0.59 mm or 0.059 cm. The density of Al is 2.7 gm/cm³. Then the range of these betas is 0.059 cm × 2.7 gm/cm³ = 0.159 gm/cm².

In practice the value of the filter in gm/cm² is usually determined directly by measuring the area of the filter and weighing it; for thin filters of soft

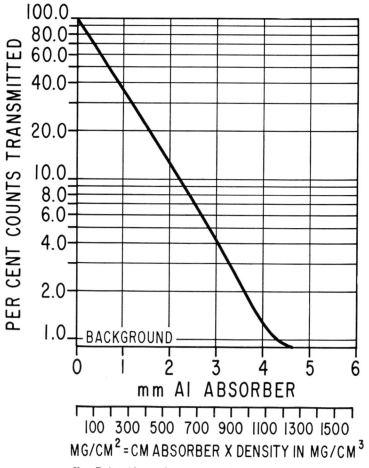

FIG. 7–4.   Absorption curve for beta radiation.

Table 7–1. *Ranges of Beta Particles of Various Energies in Various Materials*

Maximum Energy MeV	Range mg/cm²	Water 1.0	Lucite 1.2	Aluminum* 2.7	Lead 11.3
		Density—Gm/Cm³			
		Range—Mm			
0.05	4.0	0.04	0.03	0.02	0.004
0.1	13.5	0.14	0.12	0.05	0.012
0.2	40	0.40	0.33	0.15	0.035
0.3	80	0.80	0.67	0.30	0.071
0.5	160	1.6	1.3	0.59	0.14
0.7	210	2.1	1.8	0.78	0.19
1.0	400	4.0	3.3	1.5	0.35
1.5	650	6.5	5.4	2.4	0.58
2.0	950	9.5	7.9	3.5	0.83
2.5	1200	12	10.0	4.4	1.06
3.0	1500	15	12.5	5.5	1.33

* Pyrex glass essentially the same.

and dense metals such as lead the results are likely to be more accurate than those given by direct measurement. Linear absorption coefficients are usually given in terms of cm⁻¹ (absorption per cm); mass absorption coefficients are specified by cm² gm⁻¹ (cm squared per gram.)*

It must be remembered that, unlike the curve for radioactive decay, which has no cut-off, these curves come to a definite termination when all the beta particles have been absorbed. Absorption coefficients and half value layers apply only to the region of partial absorption, during which the plot is a straight line on semi-logarithmic paper.

Range of Beta Rays. A value usually desired for beta radiation is the *range*, or the thickness of filter necessary to stop all the particles. In the practical determination of the range, correction must be made for the background (see Chapter 15) and the curve may be complicated by a bremsstrahlung component as in Figure 7–5. Extrapolation of the linear part of the curve to the background axis gives the range with sufficient accuracy for practical purposes. There is an empiric formula for range of relatively energetic beta rays in gm/cm² of aluminum,

$$R = 0.543 \ E - 0.160, \qquad\qquad 7-(12)$$

where E is maximum beta-particle energy. This is approximately correct for energies greater than 0.5 MeV. On this basis the range of the 1.7 MeV beta particles of ³²P would be 0.763 gm/cm² or 2.8 mm Al. In the lower

* $\dfrac{\mu \ \text{cm}^{-1}}{\text{gm/cm}^2} = \dfrac{\mu}{\rho} \ \text{cm}^2\text{gm}^{-1}.$

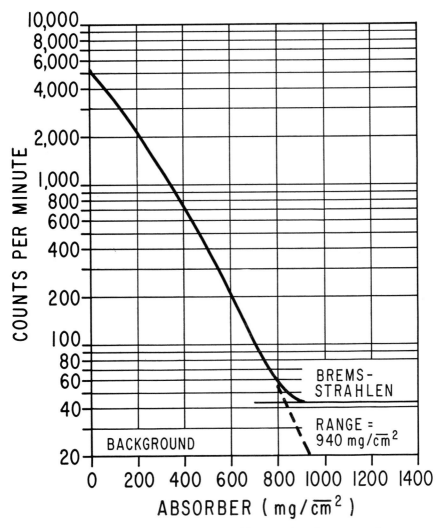

FIG. 7–5. Determination of range of beta particles in presence of
bremsstrahlung component.

energy region there is no good formula. Measurements have been made
for various energies. Some published data, especially that of Friedlander
and Kennedy, have been used to develop Table 7–1.

Scattering of Beta Particles. As a narrow beam of beta particles penetrates matter, some of the particles will be scattered away from the original
path. Some of them may undergo very wide angular deflections, so that
the path is essentially reversed; this is called *back-scatter*, and introduces
complications into many measurements with radionuclides. For instance,
consider three identical very thin beta sources, mounted under identical

detectors. The first is on a thin film of cellophane, the second on a relatively thin piece of solid material, and the third on a thick piece (Fig. 7–6). Practically no beta particles will be scattered back from the first source, an appreciable number from the second, and the maximum quantity from the third; thus the three detectors will give different results for the three identical sources.

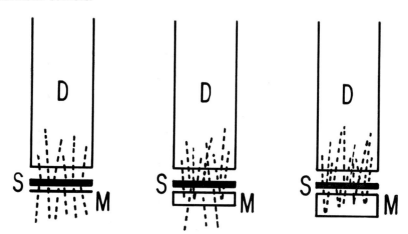

FIG. 7–6.   Back-scattering of beta particles. Identical sources and identical detectors; successively thicker mounts.

Back scatter increases with the thickness of the mount, up to about one-third of the maximum range of the particles. After this, most of the scattered radiation will be absorbed before it returns to the detector, since the particles seldom travel in straight paths perpendicular to the face of the mount. Back scatter increases relatively rapidly with Z for low atomic numbers, and then more slowly. The effect may be masked by more rapid absorption of the scattered particles within the mount.

Practical aspects of this subject will be discussed in Chapter 16.

Self-Scattering and Self-Absorption of Beta Particles. When a beta-emitting source to be measured has an appreciable thickness, particles emitted from lower layers may be absorbed in upper ones, and particles may be scattered at any level. If sample thicknesses are more than 1 or 2 per cent of the range of the particles, a correction must be made for these effects. Practical methods for carrying this out are also discussed in Chapter 16.

When thicker and thicker samples are prepared from an active material, the counting rate at first increases because of greater total activity, and then becomes constant. This constant or "saturation" value is obviously not a measure of the total activity, but usually is related to that in the upper layer whose thickness is the range of the beta particles in question. It is sometimes easier to prepare all samples of a fixed thickness greater than this range, and make no correction for self-absorption. Thin and thick samples containing the same amounts of radioactive material will of course give different counting rates. Comparison of values for "thin" samples is usually impossible unless each reading is corrected for self-absorption and selfscatter. If "thick" samples are all the same thickness, comparisons based on counting rates are valid.

Absorption (Attenuation)* of Photon Beams. A homogeneous or mono-energetic beam of x or gamma rays in passing through matter loses energy at a rate which can be described by the exponential equation

$$I_t = I_o \, e^{-\mu t}, \qquad\qquad 7-(13)$$

where t is the thickness of the sheet of matter and μ the linear absorption coefficient for the particular photon energy in the particular matter. An absorption curve can be obtained in the same manner as for beta rays; it will not exhibit a "range" but will continue indefinitely, as in Figure 7–7. Half value layer and linear absorption coefficient can be determined from such a curve. As in the case of the beta particle coefficients, the mass absorption coefficient, μ/ρ is frequently employed. In fact, most tabulated data are in terms of mass absorption coefficients, because values for different absorbers for a particular photon energy are more nearly alike. This is demonstrated in Table 7–2 which gives linear and mass absorption coefficients for a limited number of photon energies for water (or tissue), aluminum and lead. Tabular values are frequently in terms of photon wave length rather than energy; one is readily obtained from the other by the formula $\lambda = \dfrac{12.40}{\text{keV}}$, obtained earlier in this chapter. It is also an advantage

Table 7–2. Linear and Mass Absorption Coefficients

KeV	λ	Water, $\rho = 1.0$			Aluminum, $\rho = 2.7$			Lead, $\rho = 11.3$		
	A	μ cm^{-1}	μ/ρ cm^2gm^{-1}	% Transmitted by 1 cm	μ cm^{-1}	μ/ρ cm^2gm^{-1}	% Transmitted by 1 cm	μ cm^{-1}	μ/ρ cm^2gm^{-1}	% Transmitted by 1 cm
20	0.620	0.786	0.786	45	97.8	32.5	—	635	56	–
40	0.310	0.264	0.264	77	12.95	4.80	—	158	14	—
100	0.124	0.168	0.168	84	1.255	0.465	29	63.5	5.62	—
200	0.062	0.137	0.137	87	0.411	0.152	66	11.0	0.97	—
400	0.031	0.106	0.106	90	0.248	0.092	77	2.14	0.19	12
1000	0.012	0.071	0.071	93	0.160	0.059	85	0.68	0.06	51
2000	0.006	0.049	0.049	95	0.113	0.042	88	0.51	0.045	60

* *Attenuation* is generally preferable to *absorption*, because the indicated decrease in the beam includes that due to scatter as well as that due to absorption. However, since "absorption" curves and coefficients are more commonly referred to, the custom it followed here.

that when mass absorption coefficients are used, physical or chemical state, temperature, etc. do not exert important effects.

The absorption coefficient μ/ρ is made up of three parts; the photo-electric (τ/ρ), Compton (σ/ρ), and pair (κ/ρ) (if the energy is sufficiently great).

$$\mu/\rho = \tau/\rho + \sigma/\rho + \kappa/\rho. \qquad\qquad 7\text{—}(14)$$

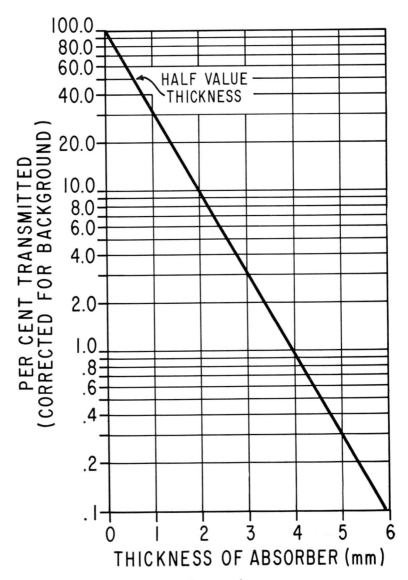

FIG. 7–7.   Absorption curve for gamma rays.

Photoelectric absorption increases rapidly with increase in atomic number of the absorber, and decreases rapidly with increasing energy of the photon. Approximately $\tau/\rho = k_1 Z^3/E^3$, where k_1 is a constant of proportionality. Compton absorption for any particular energy depends only on the number of electrons present, and therefore is independent of Z since there are essentially the same number of electrons per gram for all substances. It decreases with increasing photon energy. Approximately $\sigma/\rho = k_2/E$. σ/ρ,

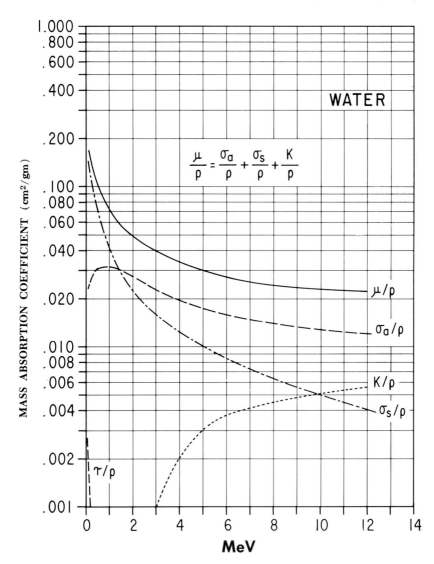

$$\frac{\mu}{\rho} = \frac{\sigma_a}{\rho} + \frac{\sigma_s}{\rho} + \frac{K}{\rho}$$

WATER

FIG. 7–8. Mass absorption coefficients for photons in water.
See text for detailed discussion.

referring to energy loss by the Compton process, has two components, $(\sigma/\rho)_a$ and $(\sigma/\rho)_s$. The first one is true energy absorption; the second is energy loss from a particular beam by scatter. Only the part defined by $(\sigma/\rho)_a$ is used in producing ionization, although the entire σ/ρ is lost from the beam. Pair formation increases both with increased energy and increased atomic number, so that approximately $\kappa/\rho = k_3 Z E$.

Thus, the total absorption coefficient is an extremely complicated function of the photon energy and the atomic number of the absorber. There

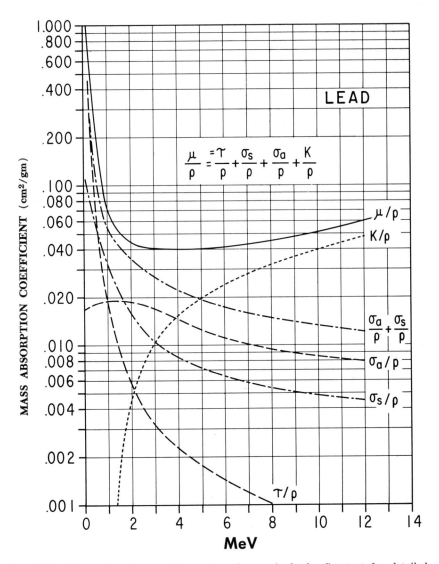

Fig. 7-9. Mass absorption coefficients for photons in lead. See text for detailed discussion.

are formulas for calculation of the different components, and these or the total coefficients are tabulated in various places.

The curves of Figures 7–8 and 7–9 have been constructed from these tabulated coefficients. For water, the photoelectric component vanishes at about 200 kv; pair formation is not significant before 3 MeV. Hence the total attenuation coefficient at any voltage between these two is simply the sum of Compton absorption and Compton scatter coefficients. For lead, on the other hand, photoelectric absorption is appreciable to several MeV; pair formation sets in just above 1 MeV and rapidly becomes important. The total attenuation coefficient is made up of these two plus the two Compton contributions. It is to be noted that μ/ρ goes through a minimum at about 4 MeV and then increases with increasing voltage. This is, of course, due to the increasing amount of 0.511 MeV annihilation radiation added to the beam as the result of pair production.

The relative importance of the different processes, for various energies and absorbers, is indicated in Table 7–3.

Table 7–3. Relative Importance of Different Types of Absorption

Photon Energy	Type of Absorption	
	Water	Lead
Up to 10 keV	τ	τ
10 — 50 keV	$\tau = \sigma$	τ
50 — 100 keV	$\sigma > \tau$	τ
100 — 500 keV	mostly σ	$\tau \stackrel{=}{>} \sigma$
500 —1000 keV	σ	$\sigma > \tau$
1000 —10,000 keV	$\sigma > > \kappa$	$\sigma > \kappa$
Higher than 10,000 keV	$\sigma \stackrel{=}{<} \kappa$	$\kappa \stackrel{=}{>} > \sigma$

REFERENCES

FRIEDLANDER, G., KENNEDY, J. W. and MILLER, J. M.: *Nuclear and Radiochemistry,* 2nd Ed., Chapter 4. New York, John Wiley & Sons, Inc., 1964.

GLASSER, O.: *Medical Physics,* Vol. 2. Roentgen Ray Quality (Absorption coefficients, p. 892) Chicago, Year Book Publishers, 1950.

GLASSER, O., QUIMBY, E. H., TAYLOR, L. S., WEATHERWAX, J. L. and MORGAN, R. H.: *Physical Foundations of Radiology,* 3rd Ed., Chapter 4, New York, Paul B. Hoeber, Inc., 1961.

JOHNS, HAROLD E.: *The Physics of Radiology,* 2nd Ed., Chapters 5 and 6, Springfield, Charles C Thomas, 1961.

LAPP, R. E. and ANDREWS, H. L.: *Nuclear Radiation Physics,* 3rd Ed., New York, Prentice-Hall, Inc., 1963.

MORGAN, R. H. and CORRIGAN, K. E.: *Handbook of Radiology,* Sections 2 and 4, Chicago, Yearbook Publishers, Inc., 1955.

RUTHERFORD, E., CHADWICK, J. and ELLIS, C. D.: *Radiations from Radioactive Substances,* Chapter 1, Cambridge, England, University Press, 1951.

8

Basic Considerations Regarding Medical Uses of Radioactive Nuclides

THE subject of medical and other biological uses of radioactive nuclides is treated in detail in the other two volumes of this series. Nevertheless certain general considerations should be outlined here before specific matters of radiation dosage are discussed.

Medical uses of radioactive substances fall into two broad categories, tracer (or "diagnostic") studies and therapy. In the first, the aim is to obtain some information about the condition or function of an organ or system, without in any way affecting its state at the time. In the second, as in all radiotherapy, the aim is to alter the system by the action of radiation, usually to kill or inactivate certain tissues or groups of cells.

The tracer field is much the broader and has more ramifications than therapy. It always involves the detection of relatively small quantities of radioactive material. In general the sensitivity of such methods greatly exceeds that of chemical or other physical procedures. It will be remembered that 1 μCi of any radioactive nuclide represents a disintegration rate of 37000 per second. With good detection apparatus a few disintegrations per minute are readily counted. (Details are given in Part II of this volume.) A popular example is to consider the introduction of 1 mCi of a radioactive nuclide (^{131}I for example) into a swimming pool 50 $\times$ 20 feet, with an average depth of 5 feet, giving a volume of approximately 5000 cubic feet or 135 $\times$ 10^6 cubic centimeters. After thorough mixing, 5 cu cm of the mixture is taken and its radioactivity measured with a carefully calibrated instrument. It is found to contain about 4 $\times$ 10^{-5} uCi (100 disintegrations per minute). True this is a small quantity, and needs very careful measuring procedures, but it is not at the limit of detectability. The actual volume of the swimming pool can be found by dividing the total amount of radionuclide introduced by that found in one cu cm.

$$\frac{1000 \ \mu\text{Ci}}{1/5 \times 4 \times 10^{-5} \ \mu\text{Ci/cm}^3} = 1.2 \times 10^8 \text{ cu cm or } 4500 \text{ cu ft.}$$

The weight of the tracer radionuclide used is (page 26) less than 0.01 μgm, and less than one-millionth of this is in the measured sample. It is apparent that quantities of material too small to be detected otherwise, toxic or otherwise dangerous drugs, etc. may be adapted to these procedures if the radioactive material can be obtained carrier-free, or in very high specific activity.

There are of course limitations, some of which are immediately obvious. The period during which useful observations can be made depends on the half life of the nuclide; if this is very short, possibilities are curtailed. It is unfortunate that all radioactive isotopes of nitrogen and oxygen have half lives of a few minutes or a few seconds. Again, if external measurements are to be made on material within the body, it is almost essential that the nuclide be a gamma-emitter. (True, some powerful beta-emitters can be detected by their bremsstrahlung, but the doses necessary are too large to be considered tracers.) Unfortunately isotopes of hydrogen and carbon which have usable half lives emit no gamma rays.

Three other limitations must be considered. The first is a possible chemical effect of the drug administered (not necessarily the radioactive part) which might alter the metabolism or bring about other changes in the subject. An example of this is toxicity. If the radionuclide can be obtained in high specific activity, the problem is never serious. Consider for instance arsenic. The maximal clinical dose is 5 μgm of arsenic trioxide, which would contain about 4 μgm of arsenic. Four μgm of ^{74}As would be 500 mCi. Obviously any imaginable tracer dose would be far below this. A specific activity of 1 mCi per μgm, which is very low, would be on the borderline of acceptability.

A different sort of chemical effect occurs in the use of iodine isotopes in thyroid study. The normal daily intake of iodine is of the order of 150 μgm. A test dose containing appreciably more than this amount would upset normal thyroid metabolism, that is, an abnormally small per cent would be deposited in the gland, and an abnormally high per cent excreted by the kidneys. Tracer studies based on either of these phenomena would give erroneous results. The administration of the radioactive iodine tracer should not alter the daily intake of the element by more than 10 or 15 μgm. Fifteen μgm of I-131 would be many millicuries of carrier-free material, and even a small amount of carrier could be tolerated. However if the radioactive dose were given with 100 μgm of carrier, the tests could be meaningless. (Some of the early uptake studies were of little value because of the relatively high amounts of stable iodine included.)

Another limitation which must at least be considered is a possible radiation effect. It is now known that some blood components are very sensitive to radiation, that a dose of even one rad may produce observable effects. (Doses and dose determinations will be discussed in the next chapter.) An administered 100 μCi of ^{32}P to a human being may deliver a dose of 1 rad to the blood, and if blood studies are the object of the test, the results may be wrong. Tracer doses of this magnitude are used in attempts at tumor localization, where any such small change as that mentioned would be insignificant. They have also been used in red cell survival studies, and here it would seem desirable to find a label that would deliver a smaller radiation dose.

A third possible complication is the so-called "isotope effect." It is usually assumed that all isotopes of an element are chemically and biologically indistinguishable, and this is usually the case. However when the isotopes differ considerably in mass, as in ^1H and ^2H, or even ^{12}C and ^{14}C, differences may exist in certain chemical reaction rates. This is seldom of any significance in medical tracer studies, but must not be overlooked by the basic research worker.

Tracer procedures may be employed to follow the behavior of a certain element or compound in the body, or to follow the path of any molecule to which a radioactive atom has been attached, when the latter takes no part in the metabolism. The first would be typified by iodine uptake and excretion by the thyroid gland, the second by the measurement of blood volume by dilution of any labeled compound. Many examples of these will be found in the other two volumes of this series.

Conditions are more rigid for the first type of study mentioned above. If a certain compound is to be followed, its metabolic behavior must be thoroughly known, and the binding of the radionuclide in the molecule must be firm. For instance if a particular iodine-labeled substance is to be followed, and the eventual breakdown products detected, it is essential that the iodine stay with its molecule or known part of molecule, and not become free and attach itself to something else. This, of course, is true for all labeled substances, but frequently only the behavior in the first brief period is of interest. Afterward the only concern with the radioactivity is the radiation dose delivered; what happens to the breakdown products is of little or no concern. Such would be the case when a radioactive substance is used to measure circulation time.

Tracer studies may be divided into basic research and diagnostic aids,— though the dividing line is sometimes difficult to identify. Physiologic determination of uptake, absorption and excretion of an element or compound may be straightforward. Formerly such studies were generally possible only by administering an overload of the material under consideration, and seeing when and where excess quantities appeared.

Turnover studies may be readily carried out. The rate of disappearance after a steady state is reached is typified by the disappearance of radioactive iodine from the thyroid gland after the administration of a tracer dose. Since the radioactive material is an isotope of the element iodine, all iodine in the gland will behave in the same manner as the tracer, and the total disappearance rate can be determined.

Reutilization of metabolic products can be observed. If erythrocytes labeled with radioactive iron are obtained from a donor and injected into the blood stream of the recipient, it would be expected that the number of labeled cells would decrease with time, as some of the cells died and became hemolized. This does happen at first, but then the number of labeled cells increases again. It is apparent that the hemoglobin from the destroyed cells is being incorporated into new ones.

Other metabolic products can be traced, particularly in urine and feces after a labeled compound has been administered. The permeability of phase boundaries can be measured,—gastrointestinal tract to blood, blood to cerebrospinal fluid, etc.,—by the time and rate of appearance of the label in one compartment after its administration into another.

Diagnostic studies may be based on isotope dilution, or radionuclide transport, radionuclide localization and practically any other phenomenon in which radioactive material is introduced into the body. Detailed discussion of these will be found in the other two volumes of this series; there is no need to go into them here.

As for therapy, the main problem is to get enough radioactive material into a suitable location so that the diseased tissues will receive an adequate radiation dosage, while normal structures are not irreparably damaged. This can usually best be accomplished when the radionuclides can be encapsulated and kept as sealed sources, to be placed outside or inside the body as the radiotherapist decides in a particular case. They may be in large quantities, as "telecurie" sources, when all procedures are similar to those with high voltage x-ray machines. They may also be in the form of small tubes or needles, which can be introduced into body cavities, or directly into diseased tissues and removed after the desired dose has been administered. This is analogous to radium therapy and is carried out in the same manner. For either of these types of procedure it is essential to have a relatively long-lived radionuclide. On the other hand, permanent implants such as radon seeds should be made with relatively short-lived nuclides.

It is sometimes possible to utilize a short-lived substance for therapy by some sort of physiological localization. This may be by confinement in a body cavity by the cavity wall, as in use of radioactive colloids in chest or abdominal cavities, or of radioactive solutions in the bladder. Or it may be by a true differential uptake in the tissues, as is the case of radioactive iodine in the thyroid gland, or in certain thyroid cancers. Here the degree of differential becomes very significant. This question is discussed in detail on page 138.

In all clinical uses of radioactive nuclides a knowledge of radiation dosage is necessary. For tracer studies it must be assured that there is not enough dose to produce a radiation effect which might vitiate the results of the study. Furthermore, as will be seen in later chapters, when therapy is not the object, the permissible dose to the individual and to the specific organs is defined and should not be exceeded. It must then be possible to determine this dose with reasonable accuracy. In the case of therapy the doses to diseased and normal tissues must be known to see whether an adequate differential can be maintained and the desired clinical dose delivered. All these aspects of the dosage problem will be considered in the next chapter.

8

9

Dosage Calculations for Radioactive Nuclides

RADIOACTIVE nuclides may be employed as sources for external irradiation, in which case they are encapsulated or in some way controlled as to position, or they may be administered to an individual for internal irradiation, when, in general, control is lost; the material is distributed more or less uniformly throughout the organism. Sources may be used primarily for beta or for gamma irradiation. It must be remembered that every positron emitter has also two 0.51 MeV photons per disintegration, which must be considered in any dosage problem.

External (Controlled) Sources. External sources may be employed for α-, β-, or γ-irradiation. In these cases the radioactive material is confined either on a plaque or in a container, in a known distribution.

For photon radiation the exposure unit is the *roentgen* which is based on the production of ionization in air. No similar unit exists for particles. For all radiation the absorbed dose unit is the *rad* which is 100 ergs absorbed per gram of any absorber. These units and the relation between them will be discussed in detail in following sections. Dose rates from radioactive sources can be determined with suitable instruments, or can be calculated, when certain basic data about the nuclides are available.

External Alpha-Particle Sources. Since α particles have ranges in tissue of the order of 0.1 mm or less, such sources would have very limited biological or chemical applications. Loevinger[1] has measured surface emission from polonium plaques with an ionization chamber, and has studied the effects of these radiations on human skin. His source, a 1-cm disc of nickel on which 15 mCi of polonium had been deposited, was covered with a gold plating approximately 1 micron thick, to reduce "creeping" of polonium from the nickel, and was further covered with a Mylar film of 0.9 mg/cm². The dose rate at the surface of the Mylar, measured with a suitable ionization chamber, was approximately 20,000 rads per minute per mCi. The range of the polonium α particles was about 3.5 mg/cm², or about 35 microns. The more penetrating α particles of thorium X have a range about twice as great, but they are always contaminated by the β and γ radiation from later members of the thorium series. Alpha irradiation from external sources is of little clinical importance and dosage considerations will not be carried further.

External Beta Particle Sources. Controlled beta sources are usually either flat plaques for surface irradiation, or tiny seeds or grains for implantation. In the case of the flat applicator, its face is placed in contact either with the lesion itself, or with the tissues immediately over it. The dose delivered at a particular level below the source depends on the nuclide, the thickness of the source, and the thickness of the tissue layer.

There is no simple and general method of calculating beta ray dose from such external applicators. Rossi and Ellis[2] have developed some charts which can be used without the necessity of extensive mathematical calculation, and these will be presented here. Their basic assumption is that the average absorption coefficient for beta rays in tissue is a function of the *maximum* beta energy; the relation is given in Figure 9–1. From this the absorption coefficient may be read for any beta energy. Now for flat sources, a general set of curves is prepared, shown in Figure 9–2, in which

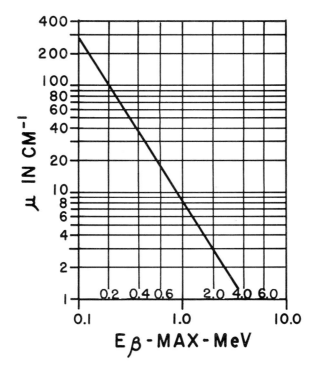

FIG. 9–1. Average absorption coefficient in tissue, for beta rays from an infinite plane source, as a function of maximum beta energy. (Courtesy of H. H. Rossi, R. H. Ellis, Jr., and the American Roentgen Ray Society.)*

* This curve does not agree with Figure 7, Chapter 16, of Radiation Dosimetry, by Hine and Brownell, since this is based on infinite plane sources and theirs on point sources. Using Hine and Brownell figures and formulas, the same results will be obtained as using Rossi's, but it is not possible to use charts or formulas interchangeably.

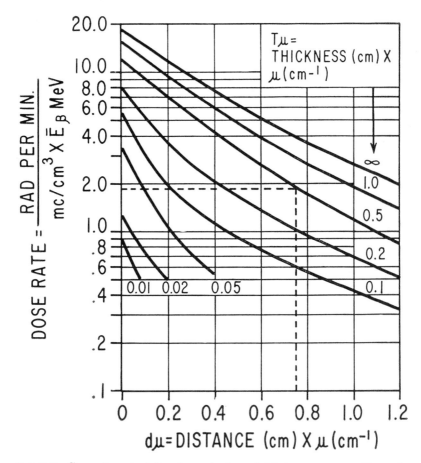

FIG. 9–2. Curves for calculating dose rates from flat beta ray sources. For explanation, see text. (Courtesy of H. H. Rossi, R. H. Ellis, Jr., and the American Roentgen Ray Society.)

one coordinate is the distance in tissue from the beta source, multiplied by the absorption coefficient, and the other is the rads* per minute divided by the product of the *average* energy of the radiation, $\overline{E}_\beta$, (see p. 64) and the concentration of the nuclide in millicuries per cubic centimeter of applicator. The parameter of the set of curves is the thickness of the source multiplied by the absorption coefficient. This complicated-sounding chart makes dosage determination relatively simple, once the relevant constants have been established.

For example, consider a flat applicator of 1.25 mm thickness which contains ^{32}P at a concentration of 2 mCi per cu cm in a plastic medium of

* Rossi's published curves are based on dosage in "equivalent roentgens." This unit is now obsolete, and his data have been re-calculated to give doses in rads in accordance with present conventions as used throughout this chapter.

approximately unit density. It is desired to find the dose rate at a depth of 2 mm in tissue. For ^{32}P, E_β (max) is 1.7 MeV, and $\overline{E}_\beta$ is 0.70 MeV. (See Appendix C.) From Figure 9–1, for energy 1.7 MeV, μ is 3.8* per cm. The thickness, t, of the applicator is 0.125 cm and the depth d is 0.2 cm. Therefore $t\mu = 0.5$ and $d\mu = 0.76$. The curve for $t\mu = 0.5$ will therefore give the dose rate. For an abscissa of 0.75, the ordinate for this curve is 1.85. This number, multiplied by the concentration and by $\overline{E}_\beta$ gives $1.85 \times 2 \times 0.70 = 2.6$ rads per minute at this depth. One millimeter closer to the surface the value is 6.1 rads per minute, and at the surface it is 17. These curves are adequate for determining dose rate in tissue beneath radioactive slabs, as long as the diameter of the slab is a few times the tissue depth under consideration.

For small implants, an approximation may be made on the basis of spheres. The curves of Figure 9–3, plotted in the same coordinates as Figure 9–2, give the dose rates. For example, find the dose rate 3 mm from the center of an yttrium-90 pellet 1 mm in diameter and containing 250 μCi of the nuclide. The volume of the pellet is 5.25×10^{-4} cubic centimeters, and the concentration is $\dfrac{250 \times 10^{-3}}{525 \times 10^{-6}} = 475$ mCi per cu cm.

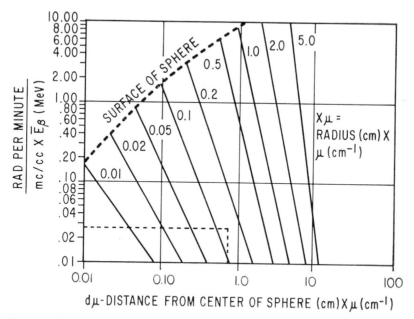

Fig. 9–3. Curves for calculating beta dose rates from small spheres. For explanation, see text. (Courtesy of H. H. Rossi, R. H. Ellis, Jr., and the American Roentgen Ray Society.)

---

* From the curve it is not possible to read μ so accurately; $\mu = 4$ would be obtained. The value 3.8 is used because this is the value used for Figure 9–2. Using $\mu = 4$, the rads per minute are 2.8.

For ^{90}Y, E_β(max) is 2.24 MeV and $\bar{E}_\beta$ is 0.93 MeV. From Figure 9–1, $\mu = 2.4$ cm^{-1}. The radius of the pellet is 0.05 cm and the distance d is 0.3 cm. Therefore $x\mu = 0.12$ and $d\mu = 0.72$. The dose rate will be found for the abscissa 0.72, one-fifth of the way between the $x\mu$ curves 0.1 and 0.2. The reading for the 0.1 curve is 0.012, and for the 0.2 curve, 0.084. Therefore for 0.12 it would be 0.026. This, multiplied by the concentration and by $\bar{E}_\beta$ gives $0.026 \times 475 \times 0.93 = 11.5$ rads per minute. The rads delivered at this distance in the total life of the pellet will be 11.5 times the average life of the isotope in minutes. The half life of ^{90}Y is 65 hours. Therefore the total D_β at the distance in question is $11.5 \times 65 \times 60 \times 1.443 = 65000$ rads. One millimeter farther out the dose would be 8 rads per minute.

The dosage problem for external beta ray sources is not a very important one in practice, and more detailed consideration does not seem warranted here.

External Gamma Ray Sources.   Gamma ray exposures are specified in roentgens. One roentgen is defined as "that quantity of x- or gamma radiation such that the associated corpuscular emission per 0.001293 grams of air, produces, in air, ions carrying 1 esu of quantity of electricity of either sign." The associated corpuscular emission consists of the Compton and photoelectrons liberated by the photons in their passage through matter. The passage of one roentgen of radiation will result in the production of 2.083×10^9 ion pairs per cubic centimeter of air under standard conditions. The energy absorption in tissue for one roentgen of fairly high energy photons is essentially equivalent to one rad. This relation will be discussed later in connection with addition of beta and gamma ray doses.

The basic value for calculation of gamma ray dosage from any encapsulated source is the exposure rate in roentgens per hour at a distance of one centimeter in air from a point source of one millicurie. This is called the specific gamma constant, and is variously designated by I_γ, Γ, and K. However, I_γ might be expected to have a connotation of intensity, and K is already used for other purposes in physics. Accordingly, the symbol Γ (capital Greek gamma) is becoming generally accepted, and will be used here. The value of this constant may be determined experimentally if the disintegration *rate* is known. If the disintegration *scheme* is known, Γ may be calculated from known physical constants.[3,4]

Consider a nuclide which emits one gamma ray of energy E_γ MeV per disintegration. In one hour the energy emitted by 1 mCi is $3.7 \times 10^7 \times 3600 \times E_\gamma$ MeV, and the flux per sq cm at a distance of 1 cm from the point source of 1 mCi is

$$F = \frac{3.7 \times 10^7 \times 3600 \times E_\gamma \times 10^6}{4\pi} \text{ eV per sq cm per hr.} \qquad 9\text{—}(1)$$

This energy will be absorbed in air according to the true linear absorption coefficient μ_a. That absorbed in a unit area of a thin shell (thickness dr) at

1 cm from the point is $F\mu_a$ dr. This absorbed energy produces ions. W, the energy required to produce an ion pair, is approximately 34 electron volts, and N, the number of ion pairs per roentgen is 2.083×10^9 per cubic centimeter of air.   Whence

$$\Gamma = \frac{F\,\mu_a dr}{NW \times dr} = \frac{3.7 \times 10^7 \times 3600 \times E_\gamma \times 10^6 \times \mu_a \times dr}{4 \times 3.1416\ 34 \times 2.083 \times 10^9 \times dr}$$

$$= 1.5 \times 10^5\ E_\gamma\mu_a \text{ roentgens per mCi-hr at 1 cm.}$$

$$9\text{---}(2)$$

For the calculation of Γ it is necessary to know the *true* absorption coefficient.   Coefficients usually tabulated are for $\mu = \tau + \sigma_a + \sigma_s + \kappa$; for these calculations σ_s must be eliminated.   Radiation corresponding to this factor is removed from the beam by scatter but is not utilized for the production of ions.   Values for the true mass absorption coefficients for photons of various energies in air are shown in Figure 9–4.   The true linear absorption coefficient can be obtained by multiplying values from this curve by the density of air, 0.001293 gm per cu cm.

The true mass absorption coefficient in air, for gamma rays of energies from 0.06 to 2.0 MeV is about 0.028 cm²/gm, and hence the linear coefficient

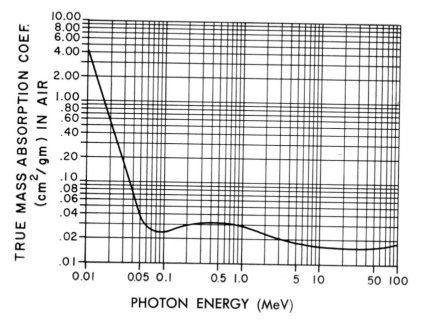

Fig. 9–4.   True mass absorption coefficients for gamma rays in air. (Density of air = 0.001293 gm per cu cm.) (Courtesy of G. J. Hine, G. L. Brownell, and the Academic Press.)

is 0.028 cm²/gm $\times$ 0.001293 gm/cm³ = 3.62 $\times$ 10⁻⁵/cm. Then within this energy range, approximately

$$\Gamma = 1.5 \times 10^5 \times 3.6 \times 10^{-5}\ E_\gamma = 5.4\ E_\gamma. \qquad 9\text{—}(3)$$

It must be remembered that in the above calculations the radionuclides are assumed to have half lives long enough so that no appreciable decay takes place during the first hour. For short-lived nuclides a correction is necessary. The procedure adopted is to find the energy flux per second, and then find the total for the lifetime of the material, by multiplying the flux per second by the average life in seconds. Then the part of this which is used up in the first hour (see equation 2—(7)) gives the correct value of Γ. Values for this constant in Appendix C have been obtained in this manner for all nuclides with half lives less than 6 hours.

If a nuclide emits more than one gamma ray, a similar calculation can be made for each one, and the sum taken. If gamma rays are emitted only in a fraction of the disintegrations, this can be allowed for. For example, ⁶⁰Co emits two gamma rays per disintegration, of energies 1.173 and 1.332 MeV. The values of μ are essentially the same for the two, 0.34 $\times$ 10⁻⁴ per cm. Then $\Gamma = 1.5 \times 10^5 \times (1.173 + 1.333) \times 0.34 \times 10^{-4} = 12.8$ r* per mCi-hr at 1 cm. Using the approximate formula of 9—(3), the value would be 5.4 (1.173 + 1.132) = 13.5, which would be a reasonable approximation if absorption coefficients were not available. Values of Γ are tabulated in Appendix C for most nuclides used at present in medicine. A curve to facilitate determination of other Γ's is given in Figure 9–5.[3] Here are plotted values of Γ for one gamma ray of the indicated energy per disintegration. If several gammas are emitted, the partial values can be obtained from the curve and added. Thus for the two gammas of ⁶⁰Co the contributions are 6.1 and 6.7 or a total of 12.8 R per mCi-hr at 1 cm. If gammas are emitted in only part of the disintegrations, the value from the curve must be multiplied by the appropriate fraction.

It must be remembered that for every positron emission, two photons of 0.51 MeV result. These must be included in the calculation of Γ for all positron emitters. From Figure 9–5, Γ for 0.51 MeV is 3.1 R/mCi-hr at 1 cm. Hence if every atom disintegrated by positron emission only, Γ would be 2 $\times$ 3.1 = 6.2 R/mCi-hr at 1 cm. If gammas are also emitted, their contribution to Γ must be added.

The exposure rate at any practical distance from a gamma-emitting point source in air can be obtained by means of the inverse square law. For a source of N mCi at a distance of d cm, the exposure rate is $\dfrac{N\ \Gamma}{d^2}$ R per hour.

For extended sources the inverse square law will not be followed. Furthermore, if the source contains a considerable quantity of radioactive material,

---

* The value 12.9 given in Appendix C, results from using three significant figures in the value for μ; 12.8 however is generally used at present.

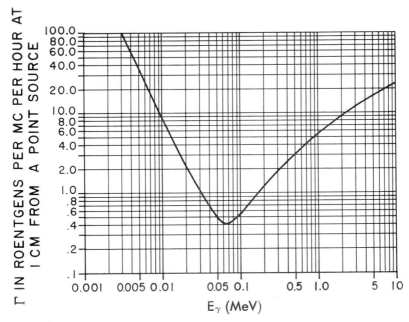

FIG. 9–5.   Gamma ray dose rate in roentgens per millicurie-hour
at 1 cm from a point source.

such as the large ^{60}Co units used in therapy, there will be appreciable self-absorption and each individual installation must be calibrated by means of suitable instruments. For smaller sources (tubes or plaques) exposure rates at various places can be found by considering the source as a close array of point sources of small activity, and integrating to obtain the total exposure at the point in question. Due allowance must be made for filtration by container walls, which varies with the obliquity of the path of the rays through them. This procedure has been carried out for a wide range of radium sources and the results are available in various texts. It does not seem desirable to reproduce them here.

Besides radium, at the present time radioactive cobalt, cesium, gold, and iridium are being employed in small sources used in body cavities or implanted directly into tissues. The radiations from ^{60}Co and ^{137}Cs have nearly enough the same average energy as radium so that the same dosage tables can be used, with the correction factor in the ratio of the Γ's, $\left(\dfrac{12.8}{8.25} \text{ for } ^{60}\text{Co}\right)$ for the dose delivered per mCi-hr. Radiations from ^{198}Au and ^{192}Ir are less penetrating, but still within the energy range in which this type of approximation should be satisfactory.

Radioactive Nuclides Administered Internally (Out of Control). Nuclides may be ingested or injected intravenously in soluble form; they may also be instilled into cavities in the form of colloidal suspensions. These colloidal suspensions may also be injected directly into solid tissues, with the hope that they will not diffuse away, and into vascular or lymphatic systems in the hope that they will drain into a particular organ or region. In any of these cases, they will be deposited with a degree of non-uniformity; measurements by means of external instruments are usually impracticable or unsatisfactory and calculations of the types used for fixed sources are not applicable. However, when the physical factors of half life and radiation energy, and some physiological factors of uptake and excretion are known, it is frequently possible to make satisfactory estimates of tissue dosage. The approach is different for particle and photon emitters.[4]

Alpha-Emitting Nuclides in the Body. Since the range of the α particles from available nuclides does not exceed about 70 microns in tissue, for uniform irradiation within a mass the radioactive atoms would have to be distributed uniformly with spacings of this magnitude. All of the energy carried by the α-particles would be absorbed almost exactly where it is emitted.

One μCi emits 3.7×10^4 particles per second. For a concentration of C μCi per gram, of an α-emitter whose particles have an energy of E MeV, the total energy released and absorbed per second per gram is $3.7 \times 10^4 \times E \times C$ MeV, and since 1 rad is equal to 6.24×10^7 MeV absorbed

$$d_\alpha/\text{sec} = \frac{3.7 \times 10^4 \text{ E C}}{6.24 \times 10^7} = 5.92 \times 10^{-4} \text{ E C rad.} \qquad 9\text{—}(4)$$

For doses in longer periods the same line of reasoning will be followed as for β-doses in the next section.

However, in the case of α-doses another factor must be taken into account, the relative biological effect. It has been found that the biological effectiveness of a particular radiation may depend not only on the energy absorbed from it, but on the distribution of the ions in the material. For many biological reactions, heavy charged particles are more efficient than electrons or photons. In order to take this into account, a special dose unit has been developed, the *rem*. The dose in rems is the dose in rads multiplied by the relative biological effectiveness (RBE). For certain reactions α particles are about four times as effective as β's, whence the dose in rems, *for these reactions*, would be four times the dose in rads. The whole concept of RBE is rather inexact, and doses in rems are accordingly approximate. In actual fact, the rem was devised for use in protection problems, where it might be necessary to consider additive effects of various types of radiation. It was never meant to be used as a dose unit in biological or clinical practice. (Further discussion of this subject will be found in Chapter 10.)

The greatest interest in internal α-dosimetry lies not in masses of appreciable size, but rather in the fact that most α-emitters (radium, plutonium) are bone-seekers, and that soft tissue immediately adjacent to, or enclosed in the bone may receive a considerable dose. The problem has been considered in some detail by Hoecker[5] and by Spiers.[6] Spiers bases his calculations on the experimental observation that when radium is deposited in the bone, about half the radon escapes via the blood. He can then determine the number of α particles per cubic micron deposited by the radium and its decay products, and hence the dosage in bone, based on uniform distribution of the radioactive material in the bone. He extends his calculations to very small cavities of various sizes in the bone, and develops the formula

$$\text{Dose rate} = 34 \times 10^3 \text{ N F rads/day*} \qquad 9—(5)$$

where N is the number of α particles per cubic micron per day, and F is a factor depending on cavity size, which he tabulates.

When it is possible to obtain a bone section and make autoradiographs, as in the work of Hoecker and Roofe, the actual distribution of the α-tracks in the medium can be studied. They found numerous microscopic localizations of about the same radium density, but the frequency of the localizations varied greatly from one bone to another. Obviously the assumption of uniform distribution of the radioactive material is useful only as a first approximation.

Beta-Emitting Nuclide in the Body. When a radionuclide emits only beta rays, the dose is essentially confined to the region containing the material, at least in most human organs. The range of these particles in tissue is generally only a few millimeters, and most human organs are large in comparison. This, however, is not true for organs in small animals used in experiments with nuclides emitting high energy beta particles. Proper estimate of correction factors in these cases is difficult, but some discussion of the problem will be given later.

Consider a beta-emitting nuclide uniformly distributed throughout a volume large in relation to the range of the beta particles, with a concentration of C μCi per gram. Then, since 1 μCi produces 3.7×10^4 disintegrations per second, the energy released and absorbed per gram of tissue per second (except for a rim close to the boundary), is $3.7 \times 10^4 \bar{E}_\beta$ C MeV, where $\bar{E}_\beta$ is the *average* beta ray energy per disintegration in MeV. Now it will be remembered that one rad is equivalent to 6.24×10^7 MeV absorbed per gram, whence

$$d_\beta \text{ (sec)} = \frac{3.7 \times 10^4 \times \bar{E}_\beta \text{ C}}{6.24 \times 10^7} = 5.92 \times 10^{-4} \text{ C } \bar{E}_\beta \text{ rad}, \qquad 9—(6)$$

and $$d_\beta \text{ (min)} = 3.55 \times 10^{-2} \text{ C } \bar{E}_\beta \text{ rad.} \qquad 9—(7)$$

* In the published paper dose rates are given in "reps," one rep being 83×10^{-12} ergs per cubic micron. A rad is 100×10^{-12} ergs per cubic micron of unit density material, and a suitable correction has been applied to Spiers' published formula.

If decay is very rapid (half lives of a few hours), it is not satisfactory to multiply d_β/min by 60 to obtain d_β/hr. At the end of the hour the amount of nuclide is appreciably less than at the beginning. The decision as to the half life level at which this multiplication is valid is made on a basis of the degree of accuracy desired. For instance, if a difference of 3 per cent from the beginning to the end of the hour is acceptable, $\lambda = 0.03$/hr. The corresponding half life T (in hours) $= \dfrac{0.693}{0.03} = 23$ hours. Thus for half lives greater than 23 hours, the formula could be used, but for shorter ones the method leading to equation 9—(11) below must be employed. Thus for half lives longer than about 20 hours, decay is slow enough so that

$$d_\beta \text{ (hr)} = 60 \times d_\beta \text{ (min)} = 2.13 \text{ C } \overline{E}_\beta \text{ rads,} \qquad 9—(8)$$

and for half lives longer than about 20 days

$$d_\beta \text{ (day)} = 51.2 \text{ C } \overline{E}_\beta \text{ rads.} \qquad 9—(9)$$

For complete decay of the nuclide, the total dose is given by the dose per minute multiplied by the average life in minutes. The average life is 1.443 times the half life; the latter is usually tabulated in days. Therefore

$$\mathbf{D}_\beta = d_\beta \text{ (min)} \times T \text{ (days)} \times 1440 \text{ (min per day)} \times 1.443$$
$$= 73.8 \text{ C } \overline{E}_\beta \text{ T rads.} \qquad 9—(10)$$

The part of the dose delivered in any time can be found by use of the decay equations of Chapter 2. If the amount of the nuclide remaining at any time t is $Q_t = Q_o e^{-\lambda t}$, the amount used up is $Q_o - Q_t = Q_o(1 - e^{-\lambda t})$, and the part of the dose delivered in time t is

$$\mathbf{D}_\beta \text{ (t)} = \mathbf{D}_\beta \text{ } (1 - e^{-\lambda t}). \qquad 9—(11)$$

Thus one-half the total dose will have been delivered by the end of one-half period, three-quarters by the end of the second half-period, and so on.

As an example of dosage from an internal beta-emitter, consider a patient who has received 5 mCi of ^{32}P as treatment for polycythemia vera. Assuming uniform distribution and no excretion of phosphorus, the concentration in a 70-kg man is $\dfrac{5000}{70,000} = 0.07$ μCi per gram. $\overline{E}_\beta = 0.694$ MeV and T 14.3 days. $D_\beta = 73.8 \times 0.07 \times 0.694 \times 14.3 = 51$ rad. Half of this will be delivered during the first two weeks.

In practice, elimination and non-uniform concentration will make the dose somewhat different from that calculated by these formulas; these topics will be discussed later in this chapter. (See page 127.)

Dose in Regions Small in Comparison to Range of Beta Particles. The general solution of dosage problems for organs small in comparison to the range of the beta particles has not been developed. Rossi and Ellis have given data for spheres, which may be used as an approximation for other shapes. Their curves are shown in Figure 9–6, the coordinates being in terms of the same units as Figure 9–3. For example, consider one lobe of a thyroid of a 2-day-old chick to be represented as a sphere 1.5 mm in diameter. Assume that 20 μCi of ^{131}I have been deposited in this lobe,*

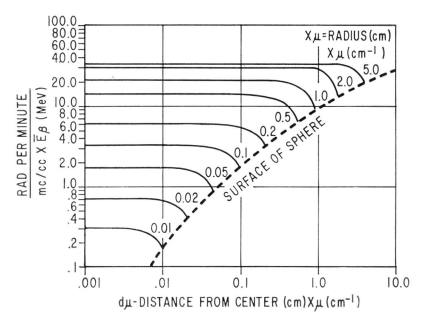

FIG. 9–6. Curves for calculating dose rate from beta-emitters deposited inside sphere small in relation to range of beta particles. (Courtesy of H. H. Rossi, R. H. Ellis, Jr. and the American Roentgen Ray Society.)

and it is desired to find the dose rate at its center and at its surface. For ^{131}I there are several beta rays; the most important is 0.608 MeV, and this may be used as E_β(max), whence $\mu = 18$ cm^{-1}. $\bar{E}_\beta = 0.180$ MeV. The radius is 0.075 cm so for the surface $\mu x = 1.35$. The distance for the center may be considered 0.01 cm, since the curve is flat at that point and the reading will not increase toward the center. The concentration is 11.4 mc per cu cm. Data will be obtained by interpolation between the $x\mu$ curves for 1.0 and 2.0. For the center the reading is $\frac{1}{3}$ of the way between 21 and 30, or 24; this multiplied by 0.180 $\times$ 11.4 gives 49 rads per minute. For the surface $x\mu = d\mu = 1.35$, and the dose rate is 10.3 $\times$ 0.180 $\times$ 11.4 = 21

---

* The separation of the two lobes is such that each may be considered independently of the other.

rads per minute. The dose rate in an extended medium with the same concentration would be [from formula 9—(7)] $3.55 \times 10^{-2} \times 11.4 \times 1000 \times 0.180 = 72.5$ rads per minute.

Application to Treatment of Very Small Masses. According to the above section, the dose in a spherical mass, from a given concentration of radioactive material deposited uniformly within it, decreases with the radius of the mass. Since there is a limit to the amount of radionuclide which can be administered to a human being, there is a limit to the concentration which can be obtained. Thus, in practice, doses to very small isolated masses are strictly limited. The problem may be considered particularly with regard to the desire to treat small metastatic deposits of thyroid cancer with radioactive iodine. By following the above procedure, the doses at the center and the surface of spheres of various radii are found, relative to the dose in an extended mass containing radioactive material in the same concentration. From these can be found the relative concentrations in small masses necessary to give the same dose as unit concentration in the large one. Data for iodine and for phosphorus are presented in Table 9–1.

Table 9–1. Doses in Small Spheres, Relative to Doses in an Extended Volume, for the Same Concentration of Iodine or Phosphorus

	Sphere Diameter—Mm								
	0.1	0.3	0.5	0.7	1.0	2.0	3.0	5.0	10.0
	Iodine-131								
Ratio Average D in Sphere to D_β	0.077	0.27	0.33	0.42	0.50	0.67	0.77	0.9	0.9
μCi/gm in Sphere to give dose $= D_\beta/\mu$Ci	13	3.7	3	2.4	2	1.5	1.3	1.1	1.1
	Phosphorus-32								
Ratio as above	0.012	0.033	0.06	0.084	0.11	0.25	0.33	0.50	0.72
μCi/gm as above	81	30	17	12	9	4	3	2	1.4

Dose in Objects Floating in Radioactive Solutions. The same curves of Figure 9–6 can be used to find the dose in a small spherical organism immersed in a solution of radioactive material. If the sphere contained radioactivity at the same concentration as the medium, the entire system would receive radiation at the same rate, which would be that of the large volume with uniform distribution of radionuclide. But if the organism contains no activity, the dose at its center would be that in an extended medium, minus that at the center due to the sphere itself.

Consider a frog's egg, stripped of its jelly, floating in a medium containing ^{32}P in a concentration of 1 mCi per cu cm, with none permeating the egg.

The diameter of the egg is 3 mm; the dose rate at a point 0.5 mm inside the surface is to be determined. For ^{32}P, E_β(max) is 1.7 MeV and $\bar{E}_\beta$ is 0.694 MeV; μ is 4 cm^{-1}. The distance from the center, d, is 0.1 cm (radius is 1.5 mm). Therefore $\mu d = 0.4$ and $\mu x = 0.6$. The reading at $\mu d = 0.4$ for $\mu x = 0.6$ is 12, hence the dose rate at this point due to the sphere itself is $12 \times 1 \times 0.694 = 8.32$ rads per minute. The dose rate in the extended medium is $3.55 \times 10^{-2} \times 1 \times 1000 \times 0.694 = 24.6$ rads per minute. Hence the dose rate at the point in question, with no radioactive material in the egg, is $24.6 - 8.3 = 16.3$ rads per minute.

Gamma Ray Emitting Nuclides in the Body. In the case of gamma rays emitted within an organ or anywhere within the body, absorption is rarely complete within the tissue of interest. The approach to the dosage problem must therefore be different from that for beta rays.

When the nuclide is distributed throughout a volume of tissue such as V (Figure 9–7), with a concentration of C μCi per gram, the exposure rate per hour at any point P due to the quantity of radionuclide CdV present in a small volume dV at a distance r from P will be

$$d(\exp_\gamma) = \frac{10^{-3}\ \Gamma\ C\ e^{-\mu r}}{r^2} \quad \text{roentgens per hour,} \qquad 9\text{--}(12)$$

where μ is the *effective* absorption coefficient of the radiation per centimeter of tissue. The value of this absorption coefficient depends on the fraction of the scattered radiation which is absorbed within the tissue. Its evaluation is very complicated, but fortunately, for absorption in unit density material, it is essentially constant, and less than 0.03 cm^{-1} for gamma ray energies in the range from 0.1 to 2.0 MeV. (The exposure rate for 1 μCi at 1 cm is $10^{-3}\ \Gamma$.)

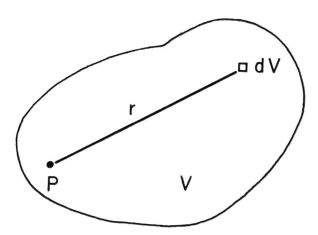

FIG. 9–7.   Basis for calculation of exposure rate from gamma-emitter distributed through large volume of tissue.

The total exposure rate at point P then is

$$\exp_\gamma/hr = 10^{-3}\ \Gamma\ C\ \int_v \frac{e^{-\mu r}}{r^2}\ dV \text{ roentgens per hour.} \qquad 9-(13)$$

This expression is not readily integrated except when the volume is a sphere, but it can be evaluated for some other shapes. It may be called the *geometrical factor* and represented by g. In any volume the value of g will depend on the position of the point of reference, being a maximum at the center and a minimum at the surface. Usually what is desired is an *average* gamma dose rate, and for this purpose it is desirable to define an *average* geometrical factor, $\bar{g}$. For a sphere of unit density material, of radius R,

$$\bar{g} = 3\pi R, \text{ for radii up to 10 cm.} \qquad 9-(14)$$

For the average human body, Hine and Brownell have developed values for $\bar{g}$, based on data published by Bush.[7] These are given in Table 9–2.

Table 9–2. ***Average Values of Geometrical Factor for the Human Body for Gamma Ray Dosage Calculations***

Gamma Ray Emitter Uniformly Distributed in Average Human Body
(*Courtesy of G. J. Hine, G. L. Brownell, and Academic Press*)

Weight of Individual Kg	Height of Individual—Cm						
	200	190	180	170	160	150	140
	Values of $\bar{g}$						
100	138	139	142	145	147	150	154
90	134	136	138	140	143	146	148
80	129	130	131	134	136	139	141
70	123	124	125	126	129	131	135
60	117	118	119	120	122	125	128
50	112	113	114	116	117	119	122
40	102	104	105	106	108	109	110

For cylinders of a wide range of sizes, values obtained by Focht, Quimby, and Gershowitz[8] are given in Table 9–3. These are for an "average point" as determined by the method of Bush.*

The exposure rate per hour is then $10^{-3}\ \Gamma\ C\ \bar{g}$ roentgens per μCi per gram. Corresponding rates per minute and per day are $1.7 \times 10^{-5}\ \Gamma\ C\ \bar{g}$

---

* Previously published tables, in earlier editions of this book, and in other texts, were erroneously stated to be for the average point. It was recently discovered that the values were wrongly labeled in the original publication; they were actually for a point at end of the axis, and hence were much too low for an average.

Table 9–3. Average Geometrical Factor, ḡ, for Cylinders Containing a Uniformly Distributed Gamma-Ray Emitter ($\mu = 0.028/cm$); Applicable to Gamma Energies from 0.06 to 2.0 MeV

Length of Cylinder (cm)	Radius of Cylinder (cm)										
---	1	2	3	5	7	10	15	20	25	30	35
1	3.8	7.5	10.2	13.0	13.5	13.8	15.1	16.0	17.5	18.0	19.0
2	6.5	11.7	15.7	21.6	23.2	25.2	28.1	30.5	32.8	35.4	37.3
3	8.4	14.7	19.8	27.7	31.0	34.5	39.2	42.9	46.5	49.5	52.5
5	10.6	18.8	25.6	36.0	42.4	48.5	56.1	62.6	68.2	73.0	77.2
7	11.6	21.4	29.3	41.4	50.0	59.0	68.7	77.8	84.7	90.2	93.8
10	12.7	23.6	33.0	47.1	57.8	70.2	83.2	94.0	103	109	113
15	13.7	25.6	36.4	53.2	66.1	81.4	99.7	113	123	130	135
20	14.2	26.7	38.0	56.3	72.2	89.6	111	127	139	147	152
30	14.5	27.6	39.7	59.9	76.8	98.8	124	144	159	172	179
40	14.8	28.2	40.7	62.4	80.0	103	133	156	175	187	197
50	14.8	28.4	41.3	64.1	82.2	106	139	165	185	199	208
60	14.8	28.7	41.7	65.5	84.0	109	143	171	193	206	216
70	14.8	28.8	41.9	65.6	85.3	111	146	174	196	212	222
80	14.8	28.8	42.1	65.8	86.0	112	148	176	198	214	226
90	14.8	28.9	42.3	66.0	86.5	113	149	177	199	216	228
100	14.8	29.2	42.5	66.2	86.8	114	150	179	201	218	230

For photons of less energy than 0.06 MeV, the absorption coefficient μ increases and these values of ḡ are no longer applicable. A discussion of values of ḡ for lower energy photons will be found on page 126.

9

and $2.4 \times 10^{-2} \Gamma C \bar{g}$. The total gamma exposure Exp_γ is of course exp_γ/hr multiplied by the average life in hours:

$$exp_\gamma/min = 1.7 \times 10^{-5} \Gamma C \bar{g} \text{ roentgen}$$
$$exp_\gamma/hr = 10^{-3} \Gamma C \bar{g}, \text{ for half lives greater than 20 hours} \qquad 9\text{—}(15)$$
$$exp_\gamma/day = 2.4 \times 10^{-2} \Gamma C \bar{g} \text{ for half lives greater than 20 days}$$
$$Exp_\gamma = 10^{-3} \Gamma C \bar{g} \times 1.443 \times 24 T = 0.0346 \Gamma C T \bar{g} \text{ roentgens}$$

where T is the half life in days.

To obtain the absorbed dose in rads from the exposure in roentgens, it is necessary to have the conversion factor f rads per roentgen, for the γ energy and the tissue in question. For muscle tissue and for photon energies from 0.2 to 3.0 MeV this factor varies between 0.95 and 0.98. Obviously no appreciable error will be introduced within this range by using rads instead of roentgens in the above formulae, without any change of value. Equations (15) then become:—

$$d_\gamma/min = 1.7 \times 10^{-5} \Gamma C \bar{g} \text{ rads}$$
$$d_\gamma/hr = 10^{-3} \Gamma C \bar{g} \text{ rads, } T > 20 \text{ hr} \qquad 9\text{—}(15a)$$
$$d_\gamma/day = 2.4 \times 10^{-2} \Gamma C \bar{g} \text{ rads, } T > 20 \text{ days}$$
$$D_\gamma = 0.0346 \Gamma C \bar{g} \text{ rads}$$

The sum of the β and γ doses then are given by adding equations 9—(6-11) and 9—(15a):

$$d_{\beta+\gamma}/hr = C(2.13 \bar{E}_\beta + 10^{-3} \Gamma \bar{g}) \text{ rads} \qquad T > 20 \text{ hr} \qquad 9\text{—}(16)$$
$$d_{\beta+\gamma}/day = C(51.2 \bar{E}_\beta + 0.024 \Gamma \bar{g} \text{ rads} \qquad T > 20 \text{ d}$$
$$D_{\beta+\gamma} = C T(73.8 \bar{E}_\beta + 0.0346 \Gamma \bar{g}) \text{ rads}$$

For partial decay the formula is analogous to that for partial beta dosage:

$$D_\gamma(t) = D_\gamma (1 - e^{-\lambda t}).$$

Very Low Energy Gamma Rays. When a nuclide decays by electron capture or internal conversion, radiation is emitted in the form of characteristic x rays, whose energy depends on the atomic number of the element concerned. Some of these have such low energy that they are absorbed in a centimeter or less of tissue. These may be considered as behaving like beta radiation, and their energy included with $\bar{E}_\beta$. This is true for characteristic x rays below about 0.015 MeV. For those of higher energy the procedure is less simple. Detailed analyses have been published by Smith and Harris.[9] A somewhat simplified version of their work follows:

When an atom decays by electron capture, a vacancy is created in the electron shell from which the capture was made—usually the K shell.

This vacancy is filled by an electron from an outer orbit, and a K-character-istic x ray of the daughter nuclide is emitted. This may escape from the atom, or it may in turn eject electrons from outer orbits. The K-radiation which leaves the atom (if its energy is greater than 0.015 MeV) contributes to the total photon dose, of which Γ is the statement. That which interacts with outer electrons in its own atom will eventually be deposited as β-like radiation.

The fraction of disintegrations that occur by K-capture may be denoted by k_K. (For L and other captures there would be similar coefficients, but in general these are not significant.) If a nuclide decays entirely by K-capture, k_K is unity; with a branching disintegration it is the appropriate fraction.

The *K fluorescent yield* is the fraction of the K-shell vacancies that result in x rays escaping from the atom; it is usually denoted by ω_K (see Appendix F). The energy of this K-characteristic radiation is denoted by E_K. Then the radiation escaping from the atom as photons which contribute to Γ is $k_K \omega_K E_K$.

The remaining energy $k_K (1 - \omega_K) E_K$ is used in releasing electrons and very low energy photons by interactions in outer orbits. Accordingly it will form part of the "average beta" factor. Furthermore, for every K- x ray a vacancy will have been created in an L or M orbit, and when they are filled, characteristic radiation from these orbits will be emitted. This is all so low in energy that it can be included with $\overline{E}_\beta$. As a first (and usually satisfactory) approximation, consider that all this comes from the L orbit. Then the number of L-characteristic photons, of energy E_L will also be $k_K \omega_K$ and the total energy will be $k_K \omega_K E_L$. Therefore the total contribution to the "average β energy" will be $k_K(1 - \omega_K) E_K + k_K \omega_K E_L$. Some radionuclides can decay by electron capture to more than one energy state. These must be considered separately. Sometimes an appreciable part of the capture is from the L-orbit; this is specified in the decay scheme. In this case k_L will be the fraction involved, and since all L-characteristic radiation is in the readily absorbable range, an additional factor for the "β-like" radiation will be $k_L E_L$.

In the case of internal conversion, the γ ray emitted by the nucleus under-goes a photoelectric interaction with one of its own orbital electrons. The energy of the ejected electron will be the energy of the γ ray, E_γ, less the binding energy of the shell from which the electron was ejected, B_K for the K-shell. The ratio of the number of conversion electrons to the number of unconverted photons is called the γ-ray conversion coefficient, it is denoted by α_K for the K-orbit. There may be conversion factors for other orbits; they are seldom significant. Vacancies in any shell caused by removal of electrons will be filled as discussed above for electron capture. The fraction of disintegrations resulting in a photon of energy E_γ is denoted by f. If all photons are of this energy, f = 1.

If N_K denotes the number of escaping photons, and N_{eK} the number of K-electrons per disintegration, then the sum of these two is unity, and their ratio is α_K.

$$\frac{N_{eK}}{N_K} = \alpha_K \text{ and } N_{eK} + N_K = 1$$

$$\text{Whence } N_{eK} = \frac{\alpha_K}{1 + \alpha_K} \quad \text{and } N_K = \frac{1}{1 + \alpha_K}.$$

The part of the radiation which has been converted (captured) gives rise to K-characteristic rays. These will follow the same procedure as after electron capture, that is a fraction ω_K will escape as photons, and $(1 - \omega_K)$ will be degraded as discussed before, to contribute to "β". Furthermore, all the first ejected electrons must be included in this factor. For a particular E_γ there are then $\dfrac{f\ \alpha_K}{1 + \alpha_K}$ electrons of energy $(E_\gamma - B_K)$, and $\dfrac{f}{1 + d_K}$ escaping photons of energy E_γ.

To summarize: Let

E_β = total local energy deposited per disintegration, MeV/dis
$\overline{E}_\beta$ = average energy of β-disintegration, MeV/dis
E_ϵ = energy due to electron capture and subsequent low energy products, MeV/dis
E_e = energy due to conversion electrons and subsequent products, MeV/dis
E_p = local energy deposited by γ-rays of energy less than about 0.015 MeV, MeV/dis
$E_\beta = \overline{E}_\beta + E_\epsilon + E_e + E_p$.
B_K, B_L = binding energies in K and L electron shells, MeV
E_K, E_L = energies of K and L characteristic x rays, MeV
ω_K = K fluorescent yield
f = fraction of disintegrations giving rise to a photon of energy E_γ
k_K, k_L = fractions of disintegrations that occur by L and K capture respectively.
N_{eK}, N_{eL} = numbers of K and L conversion electrons respectively arising from a photon of energy E_γ.
α = internal conversion coefficient

The contributions to E_β are

From electron capture, $E_\epsilon = k_K(1 - \omega_K)\ E_K + k_K\ \omega_K\ E_L$ 9—(17)
From internal conversion $E_\epsilon = f\ N_{eK}(E_\gamma - B_K) + f\ N_{eK}\ (1 - \omega_K)\ E_K + f\ N_{eK}\ \omega_K\ E_L$ MeV.

The contribution to gamma energy, which will enter into Γ are

From electron capture $k_K \, \omega E_K$ MeV
From internal conversion $f(1-N_{eK}) \, E_\gamma + f N_{eK} \, \omega E_K$ MeV.   9—(18)

These contributions must be evaluated as described on page 106, using the true absorption coefficients in air for the various energy levels.

If there is a branching type of disintegration, with part of the nuclei decaying by electron capture and the rest by β^- or β^+, the contribution to E_β from the electron capture is likely to be unimportant. But in the evaluation of Γ, the characteristic x rays must not be neglected.

As an example, consider [113]tin in equilibrium with [113m]indium. The decay scheme, which is simple, is shown in Figure 9–8. The tin has a half life of 119 days; the indium of 104 minutes. If the tin is to be used, it will almost certainly be accompanied by the indium. It is, however, possible to separate the daughter and use it alone.

Consider first the tin:

$\omega = 0.84 \quad k = 1 \quad E_K = 0.024$ MeV $\quad E_L = 0.003$ MeV.
$E_\epsilon = (1 - 0.84) \times 0.024 + 0.84 \times 0.003 = 0.006 = E_\beta$ for the tin.

The gamma contribution is 0.84×0.024 MeV; for this $\Gamma = 0.84 \times 1.4 = 1.3$, for the tin.

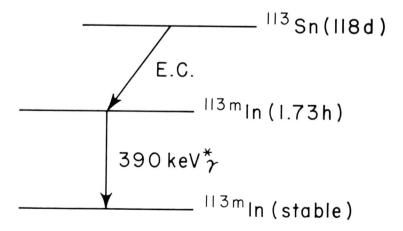

DECAY SCHEME [113]Sn – [113m]In

[113]Sn (118d)

E.C.

[113m]In (1.73h)

390 keV *γ

[113m]In (stable)

*~35% internal conversion

Fig. 9–8.   Decay scheme for [113]tin with [113m]indium.

Now consider the indium

$f = 1 \quad \omega = 0.84 \quad E_\gamma = 0.392 \text{ MeV} \quad B_K = 0.028 \text{ MeV} \quad \alpha = 0.44$

$N_{eK} = \dfrac{0.44}{1.44} = 0.30 \qquad N_K = 0.70 \qquad E_e = 0.30\ (0.392 - 0.028) +$

$(1 - 0.84)\ 0.024 + (0.84 \times 0.003) = 0.11$ for the indium.

The gamma contribution is 0.70 of 0.392 MeV photons plus 0.30×0.84 of 0.024 MeV. For these $\Gamma = 0.7 \times 2.4 + 0.25 \times 1.4 = 2.03$ for the indium. However because of the short half life, this will have to be corrected as discussed on p. 108. The true value is 1.75.

Thus for the two nuclides in equilibrium

$E_\beta = 0.006 + 0.11 = 0.12$

$\Gamma = 1.3 + 1.75 = 3.05$

The Absorbed Fraction. A different approach to the dosimetry of internal emitters has been developed by Brownell, Ellet, and Reddy, and by Loevinger and Berman[10,10a,11] on a basis of the so-called "absorbed fraction," that is, the part of the total emitted gamma energy which is absorbed in a volume of specified mass and geometry. They have made extensive computations using the Monte Carlo method of following many theoretical photons through many assumed interactions. They have published data for spheres, ellipsoids, and elliptical cylinders of various sizes for a range of gamma energies. None of their figures is exactly comparable to the cylinders of Table 9–2. All spheres are comparable, and their elliptical cylinders are roughly the shape of the human body, so those values may be compared with data of Table 9–1. From their data certain useful generalizations may be drawn. For energies from 0.08 to 1.46 MeV, the absorbed fractions in any particular ellipsoid or sphere do not vary by more than ± 10 per cent; for the most part the variations are less. Below 0.08 MeV they increase slowly to 0.06 MeV and then much more rapidly. It would seem therefore that for practical clinical dosimetry a set of average values within this range would be satisfactory, as it was in calculating the $\bar{g}$'s.

In order to determine the dose in rads from the absorbed fraction, it is necessary to know the concentration in μCi/gm, the mass in gm and the emitted gamma energy per disintegration. The energy emitted in the mass per minute is then:

$3.7 \times 10^4 \text{d/sec} \times 60 \text{ sec/min} \times C\mu\text{Ci/gm} \times$ mass in gm $\times E\gamma \text{ MeV/d} =$
$2.22 \times 10^6 \text{ C } E_\gamma \text{ MeV/min/gm} \times \text{gm}$

The part absorbed in the A.F. The dose in rads per minute is then

$$d_\gamma/min = \frac{2.22 \times 10^6 \, C \, E_\gamma \, MeV/min/gm \times gm \times A.F.}{6.24 \times 10^7 \, MeV/gm/rad \times gm}$$

$$= 0.355 \, C \, E_\gamma(A.F.) \quad \text{and} \qquad\qquad 9\text{—}(19)$$

$d_\gamma/hr = 2.1 \, C \, E_\gamma(A.F.)$ $T > 20 \, hr$

$d_\gamma/day = 504 \, C \, E_\gamma(A.F.)$ $T > 20 \, days$

$D_\gamma = 72.8 \, C \, T \, E_\gamma(A.F.).$

These formulas hold for all energies; they are not subject to the limitations imposed on $\bar{g}$ because of changes in absorption coefficients. Absorbed fractions for uniform distribution of energy in small spheres are given in Table 9–4.

Determination of dose by the two methods may be compared by considering the gamma dose in a 1 kg sphere from 1 mCi of ^{131}I deposited therein. By formula 9—(15), since radius = 6.2 cm, making $\bar{g} = 58$,

$$D_\gamma = 0.0346 \times 2.2 \times \frac{1000}{1000} \times 58 \times 8.05 = 34.4 \, \text{rads (neglecting elimina-}$$

tion). In determining dose by absorbed fractions, each gamma ray component and its particular absorbed fraction must be considered. For ^{131}I the principal components and their contributions are listed below:

MeV	Percent	Absorbed Fraction	$E_\gamma A.F.$	Contribution to D_γ
0.080	2.2	0.135	0.0108	
0.284	5.3	0.137	0.039	1.2
0.364	82.0	0.142	0.052	25.0
0.638	9.0	0.144	0.090	4.8
0.724	3.0	0.144	0.104	1.8
TOTAL				32.8

The two results are within 4 per cent of each other, which is good agreement. It appears that, while more approximations may be involved in the use of the Γ and $\bar{g}$ factors, the method is much simpler, particularly when there are a number of different photon energies.

A relationship between $\bar{g}$ and A.F. can be obtained from equations 9—(15a) and 9—(19):

$D_\gamma = 0.0346 \, \Gamma \, T \, C \, \bar{g} \, \text{rads} = 72.8 \, C \, T \, E_\gamma(A.F.) \, \text{rads.}$
and from 9—(3) $\Gamma = 5.4 \, E_\gamma$ between 0.06 and 2.0 MeV. Thus within this range

$$0.0346 \times 5.4 \, E_\gamma \, \bar{g} \, T \, C = 72.8 \, E_\gamma(A.F.) \, T \, C \qquad\qquad 9\text{—}(20)$$

or

$$\bar{g} = \frac{72.8(A.F.)}{0.187} = 390 \, A.F. \qquad\qquad 9\text{—}(21)$$

Values of $\bar{g}$ obtained in this way and by the standard formula for spheres are compared in Table 9–5.

Table 9-4.   Absorbed Fractions for Uniform Distribution of Activity in Small Spheres* and Thick Ellipsoids*

Mass (kg)	A.F.										
	0.020 MeV	0.030 MeV	0.040 MeV	0.060 MeV	0.080 MeV	0.100 MeV	0.160 MeV	0.364 MeV	0.662 MeV	1.460 MeV	2.750 MeV
0.3	0.684	0.357	0.191	0.109	0.086	0.085	0.087	0.099	0.096	0.092	0.077
0.4	0.712	0.388	0.212	0.121	0.096	0.093	0.097	0.108	0.108	0.099	0.083
0.5	0.731	0.412	0.229	0.131	0.104	0.099	0.104	0.116	0.117	0.104	0.089
0.6	0.745	0.431	0.244	0.140	0.111	0.105	0.111	0.122	0.124	0.109	0.093
1.0	0.780	0.486	0.289	0.167	0.135	0.125	0.130	0.142	0.144	0.125	0.106
2.0	0.818	0.559	0.360	0.212	0.173	0.160	0.162	0.174	0.173	0.153	0.127
3.0	0.840	0.600	0.405	0.245	0.201	0.188	0.186	0.197	0.195	0.174	0.143
4.0	0.856	0.629	0.438	0.271	0.222	0.209	0.205	0.216	0.213	0.190	0.156
5.0	0.868	0.652	0.464	0.294	0.241	0.277	0.222	0.231	0.228	0.204	0.167
6.0	0.876	0.671	0.485	0.312	0.258	0.241	0.236	0.245	0.240	0.216	0.177

* The principal axes of the small spheres and thick ellipsoids are in the ratios of 1/1/1 and 1/0.667/1.333.
Courtesy of G. L. Brownell, W. H. Elliott and A. R. Reddy.

Table 9-5. Comparison of ḡ for Spheres, by Two Methods

I	II	III	IV	V	VI	VII	VIII	IX	X	XI	XII
		ḡ = 3πr	ḡ = 390 A.F.								
			$E\gamma - MeV$								
Mass kg	Radius cm		0.06	0.08	0.10	0.16	0.36	0.66	1.46	Av	Ratio III/XII
0.3	4.2	40	42	34	33	34	34	39	37	36	1.05
0.5	4.9	46	51	41	39	40	45	46	41	43	1.07
1.0	6.2	58	65	53	49	51	55	56	49	54	1.07
2.0	7.8	73	83	68	63	64	68	67	60	68	1.07
5.0	10.6	100	115	94	88	87	91	89	79	93	1.07

Within this energy range values for $\bar{g} = 3\pi r$ average about 7 per cent higher than those obtained from A.F. This is acceptable for the sake of simplicity.

For lower energies equation 9—(21) does not hold. It will be remembered that $\Gamma = 1.5 \times 10^5 \, E_\gamma \, \mu_\alpha$. (See 9—2). The value $\Gamma = 5.4 \, E_\gamma$ is based on a constant μ_α of about 0.35×10^{-4} cm^{-1}. Below about $E_\gamma = 0.06$ MeV, μ_α increases rapidly and Γ must be determined for each energy. $\bar{g}$ will also change, since the μ in formula 9—(12), which refers to absorption in tissue, will also increase. Values for $\bar{g}$ have not been computed for these higher absorption coefficients.

Some approximate data can be obtained from the A.F. tables. Rewriting 9—(20), using $\Gamma = 1.5 \times 10^{-5} \, E_\gamma \, \mu_\alpha$, the following is obtained:

$$0.0346 \times 1.5 \times 10^{-5} \, E_\gamma \, \mu_\alpha \, \bar{g} \, T \, C = 72.8 \, E_\gamma \, T \, C \, A.F. \qquad 9—(22)$$

$$\text{or} \qquad \bar{g} = \frac{72.8 \, A.F.}{0.0346 \times 1.5 \times 10^{-5} \, \mu_\alpha} = 0.014 \, \frac{A.F.}{\mu_\alpha} \qquad 9—(23)$$

Using A.F. values from Table 9–3, and values of μ_α from appropriate physical tables (Johns, Physics of Radiology, page 700) it is found that $\bar{g}$ for 0.04 MeV decreases to about 80 per cent of the formula value, for 0.03 MeV to about 60 per cent. Here, however, the decrease is greater the larger the volume, and this variation becomes really severe at 0.02 MeV.

It is evident that the formulas developed in this book break down at about 0.04 MeV. As an approximation it may be concluded that tabulated values of $\bar{g}$ can be used down to about 0.06 MeV, then down to about 0.04 MeV values should be 0.8 of those listed. For lower energies the doses should be determined directly from the A.F.'s.

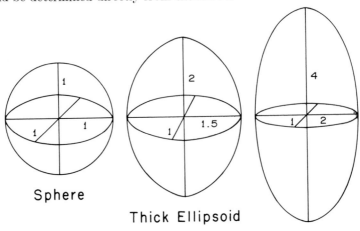

FIG. 9–9.   Diagrams of sphere and ellipsoids to be used as models for organs of various shapes.

Brownell and his associates have also studied "thick ellipsoids" and "flat ellipsoids." The axes of the former are in the ratios 1/1.5/2 and of the latter 1/2/4 (see Fig. 9–9). They find that for masses from 0.3 to 60 kg the differences between the "thick" ellipsoids and the spheres of the same volume are practically negligible. By extension, then, it can be assumed that $\bar{g}$ for a thick ellipsoid is the same as that for a sphere of equal volume. For "flat" ellipsoids, average values of the absorbed fraction are 85 per cent of those for spheres of the same volumes, with variations of less than ± 5 per cent from 0.08 MeV to 0.662 MeV. The $\bar{g}$'s should be in the same ratio.

To summarize:

Figure	Ratio of axes	$\bar{g}$
Sphere	1/1/1	$3\pi r$
Thick Ellipsoid	1/1.5/2	Same as for Sphere of same Volume
Flat Ellipsoid	1/2/4	0.85 of Sphere of same Volume

Hence for fairly compact organs whose shapes are better represented by ellipsoids than by spheres, the procedure would be to find the radius of the sphere of equivalent volume, from the formula $v = 4/3\,\pi\,r^3$. Thus a spleen of 150 gm might be assumed to be a flat ellipsoid. The radius is obtained from $150 = 4/3\,\pi\,r^3$, whence $r = 3$ cm. $\bar{g}$ for the equivalent sphere is $3\pi \times 3 = 28$, for the flat ellipsoid it is $0.85 \times 28 = 24$.

The absorbed fractions discussed above do not include a contribution from photons scattered into the target volume from surrounding tissues. When this volume is located more or less centrally in the trunk, this contribution will increase the absorbed fraction by about 20 per cent for energies between 0.04 and 0.16 MeV. For higher or lower energies the increase is unimportant. When an organ under study is thus situated, the correction should be used for photons within the stated energy range.

An analytical approach to the problem of absorbed fraction in cylinders has recently been published by Widman and Powsner.[11] Their results, published in the form of a family of curves involving the dimensions of the cylinder and the absorption coefficient, cover a wide range of factors. It is difficult to read their absorbed fractions to better than two significant figures,—but this is adequate for all practical purposes. Values of $\bar{g}$ obtained from their data agree with those in Table 9–5 to better than ± 10 per cent, over a wide range of lengths and radii of cylinders.

Effective and Biological Half Life. In the formulas developed above, the physical half life of the radionuclide has been employed. However, frequently physiological elimination removes some of the material, so that the decrease in quantity in any organ is due to both elimination and physical decay. In many cases elimination follows an exponential law, with a different rate from the physical decay. Then

$$Q_t = Q_o\, e^{-\lambda_p t}\, e^{-\lambda_b t} = Q_o\, e^{-(\lambda_p t + \lambda_b t)} \qquad 9-(24)$$

where λ_p and λ_b are the physical and biological decay coefficients respectively. These are equal to $\dfrac{0.693}{T_p}$ and $\dfrac{0.693}{T_b}$, where T_p and T_b are physical and biological half lives. The net result is

$$Q_t = Q_o\, e^{-\lambda_e t}. \qquad 9-(25)$$

where $\lambda_e = \lambda_p + \lambda_b$, and is the "effective" decay constant.

$$\text{Whence} \frac{0.693}{T_e} = \frac{0.693}{T_p} + \frac{0.693}{T_b}$$

$$\text{or} \quad \frac{1}{T_e} = \frac{1}{T_p} + \frac{1}{T_b}. \qquad 9-(26)$$

This expression is sometimes presented in one of the forms

$$T_e = \frac{T_p \times T_b}{T_p + T_b} \qquad T_b = \frac{T_p \times T_e}{T_p - T_e}. \qquad 9-(27)$$

In all these expressions, T_p is the tabulated physical half life, T_e the experimentally determined effective half life. T_e can never be greater than T_p. T_b, the biological half life, can be obtained by calculation from these two.

For example, a patient has been given a tracer dose of [131]I. Daily measurements over the thyroid gland reveal that the quantity therein is decreasing at such a rate that the effective half life is 6 days instead of the physically accepted value of 8.04 days. This effective half life is of course the value which should be used in dosage calculations when it is known. Use of the physical half life will give maximum dose, the actual one will be somewhat less. The effective half life is not always available. Average values for many nuclides are given in National Bureau of Standards Handbook 52, but in the individual case there may be considerable variation from the average. In the case of the ^{131}I patient just mentioned, if a therapeutic dose were administered, the substitution of 6 for 8.04 in the dosage formulae would result in an actual dose only 74 per cent of the maximum.

The biological half life represents the actual turnover of the *element*, not only of the radioactive isotope, in the tissues. For the iodine case just mentioned

$$\text{mentioned} \qquad T_b = \frac{8.04 \times 6}{8.04 - 6} = 23.6 \text{ days.}$$

If the factor 0.96 rads per roentgen is introduced into the formula, the factor 0.0346 becomes 0.0331. It must be realized that this applies strictly to muscle tissue. For bone, the rads per roentgen vary from 1.32 for 0.1

MeV to 0.87 for 1.0 MeV photons. Correct values for various anatomical sites are often difficult to obtain. Accordingly it must be remembered that these doses cannot be strictly accurate.

When the radioactive material is distributed uniformly throughout the entire body, every organ receives the same dose. The dose in a small organ is not a fraction of the entire body dose. $D_{\beta+\gamma}$ is the dose in rads to the whole body or to any part thereof,—that is, every gram absorbs the same number of ergs of energy.

While for single organs, the β dose is the same for all regions large in relation to the range of the particles, the gamma dose is strongly dependent on the volume. Thus the dose for a particular nuclide will be different if it is concentrated in a small region or dispersed through the body. For instance (see calculations below) 1 mCi of ^{131}I concentrated in the thyroid gland would give a thyroid dose of about 10 rads in the first hour. The same amount of the nuclide distributed throughout the body would give a whole body dose of only 0.035 rad in the first hour.

If the radionuclide is concentrated in one organ, then D for that organ will be calculated for the suitable volume, concentration, and $\bar{g}$ factor. However if the material is distributed throughout the skeleton, or the blood vessels, a special situation arises. The concentration for the β's is μCi/gm blood (or per gm bone). The concentration of the γ's, however, must be considered *as if* the nuclide were distributed throughout the whole body, since gamma rays from one part of the blood or skeleton will irradiate all the rest of it in almost the same manner as from uniform distribution. Therefore the γ concentration will be μCi/gm whole body. The dosage equation then becomes

$$D_{\beta+\gamma} = T_e \,(C_\beta \times 73.8 \, \bar{E}_\beta + C_\gamma \times 0.0346 \, \Gamma \, \bar{g}). \qquad 9-(28)$$

It is admitted that this is an approximation, but it is a better one than considering the gamma concentration to be only in the bones or blood vessels.

Examples of Dosage Problems. In any particular case the relative importance of beta and gamma dosage depends on the radiation energies and on the size and shape of the mass containing the radioactive material. Widely different cases may be illustrated by the dose to the thyroid gland from ^{131}I deposited therein, and dose to the entire body from ^{24}Na administered intravenously.

For the first case, consider a 40-gram thyroid gland containing 3 mCi of ^{131}I. Essentially all of the isotope not deposited in the gland by 24 hours after administration has been excreted and may be neglected. The following are the constants of the irradiation:

T_{eff} (measured) = 5.5 days,
$\bar{E}_\beta$ = 0.180 MeV,
Γ = 2.20 r per mCi at 1 cm,
$\bar{g}$ for 40 gm sphere = 19.

Whence $\qquad D_\beta = 73.8 \times 0.180 \times 5.5 \times \dfrac{3000}{40} = 5500$ rads,

$$D_\gamma = 0.0346 \times 2.20 \times 5.5 \times 19 \times \frac{3000}{40} = 600 \text{ rads*}$$

$D_{\beta+\gamma} = 6100$ rads, of which 90 per cent is due to the beta rays. The part of this dose delivered in the first week is

$$(1 - e^{-7 \times 0.693/5.5}) = (1 - 0.41) = 0.59.$$

Half would have been delivered in 5.5 days, and three fourths in 11 days.

In contrast, consider the dose to the entire body of a 60 kg man receiving an intravenous dose of 500 mCi of ^{24}Na.

$T_{eff} = T_{phys} = 0.625$ day,

$\bar{E}_\beta = 0.553$ MeV,

$\Gamma = 18.7$ r per mCi-hr at 1 cm,

$\bar{g}$ for a 60 kg man 170 cm tall is 120.

$$D_\beta = 73.8 \times 0.553 \times 0.625 \times \frac{500}{60,000} = 0.212 \text{ rad.}$$

$$D_\gamma = 0.0346 \times 18.7 \times 120 \times 0.625 \times \frac{500}{60,000} = 0.407 \text{ rad.}$$

$D_{\beta+\gamma} = 0.62$ rad, of which 66 per cent is due to the gamma rays.

Essentially all of this dose will be delivered in 4 days, which is 7 half lives.

On page 112 a calculation was done for dosage from ^{32}P uniformly distributed throughout the body. It was pointed out there that this did not represent the true situation; after an early uniform distribution, the nuclide becomes more concentrated in some tissues than in others. Accurate information on this is difficult to obtain, but John Lawrence[12] has presented data based on his extensive observation of patients undergoing therapy with this nuclide. For the 5 mCi dose in a 70 kg patient discussed on page 112, the dose for uniform distribution and no elimination was 51 rads to the whole body. According to Lawrence, this situation may be considered as prevailing for the first 3 days, during which 14 per cent of the nuclide has decayed. Therefore, up to this point, 3 days, the whole body dose is $51 \times 0.14 = 7$ rads.

From here on, concentration in a compartment consisting of bone, marrow, liver, and spleen (the "bone compartment" of Lawrence) is 10 times

---

* Gamma ray dose will now be stated in terms of rads instead of roentgens, in accordance with the discussion of the previous page.

that in the rest of the body, and the effective half life is 11 days. The "bone compartment" weighs about 12,000 grams and the "soft tissue compartment about 58,000 grams. Since 14 per cent of the material has decayed, there remain $0.86 \times 5000 = 4300$ μCi. Since the relative concentrations are 10 to 1,

$$\text{Concentration (bone)} = \frac{\mu\text{Ci bone}}{12,000}$$

$$\text{Concentration (soft tissue)} = \frac{\mu\text{Ci soft tissue}}{58,000}$$

and $\quad \dfrac{\mu\text{Ci bone}}{12,000} = 10 \times \dfrac{\mu\text{Ci soft tissue}}{58,000}$

whence $\dfrac{\mu\text{Ci bone}}{\mu\text{Ci soft tissue}} = \dfrac{10 \times 12,000}{58,000} = 2$ (approximately).

Therefore $\frac{2}{3}$ of the 4300 μCi are in the bone, and $\frac{1}{3}$ in the soft tissue, or approximately 2850 μCi in bone and 1450 μCi in soft tissue. The bone dose after the third day is then

$$\frac{2850}{12,000} \times 0.7 \times 11 \times 73.8 = 136 \text{ rads,}$$

and the soft tissue dose is 14 rads.

To each of these must be added the original 7 rads for the first 3 days, therefore the total bone dose is $136 + 7 = 143$ rads, and the total dose to the soft tissue compartment is 21 rads, from the 5 μCi of ^{32}P administered intravenously.

This analysis does not allow for early excretion of ^{32}P which may be important especially if the material is given by mouth.

Dosage with Iodine Isotopes Other than ^{131}I. Both longer-lived and shorter-lived iodine isotopes have been used for diagnostic purposes. ^{132}I with half life 2.26 hours, and ^{130}I, half life 12.3 hours, have been advocated for therapy, particularly in the very toxic hyperthyroids, where iodine turnover is very rapid. The thyroid dose resulting from 1 μCi per gram of each, deposited in a 30 gm gland, is shown in Table 9–6. It is assumed that T_{eff} with ^{131}I has been determined to be 6 days, whence T_{biol} is 23.6 days, and T_{eff} for the other isotopes can be calculated. $\bar{g}$ is taken as 17.

It is immediately apparent that the dose from ^{125}I is about 40 per cent of that from ^{131}I, in spite of its very much lower energy. Accordingly it would not be desirable to use several times as much of the longer-lived nuclide as of the shorter.

Table 9–6. Dose Delivered to Thyroid Gland by Various Isotopes of Iodine

Isotope Mass No.	T_{phys} Days	T_{eff} Days	$\overline{E}_\beta$ MeV	$\Gamma R / mCi\text{-}hr$ at 1 cm	$D_{\beta+\gamma}$ per μCi per gm Rads
123	0.54	0.53	0.028	2.2	1.77
124	4	3.4	1.62	7.2	420
125	60	17	0.021	1.23	38.6
126	13	8.3	0.16	2.5	110
130	0.51	0.51	0.285	12.1	14.3
131	8.04	6	0.180	2.20	87.5
132	0.094	0.094	0.483	9.4	3.9

Approximate Formula for Thyroid Dose with ^{131}I. If an average effective half life of 6 days is assumed, and an average $\bar{g}$ for the thyroid gland of 15, a formula may be developed for rapid calculation of thyroid dose, when the radioiodine content of the gland is known and the gland weight can be estimated. In formula 9—(16), C becomes $\dfrac{\text{I in gland}}{\text{gland weight}}$, and

$$D_{\beta+\gamma} = \frac{\text{I in gland}}{\text{gland weight}} \times 6\ (73.8 \times 0.180 + 0.0346 \times 15 \times 2.20)$$

$$= 90 \times \frac{\text{I in gland}}{\text{gland weight}}. \qquad\qquad 9\text{—}(29)$$

In using this formula it should be kept in mind that if the effective half life is appreciably greater or less than 6, the dose will be proportionately greater or less. Gland size will not make a significant difference unless the gland is really enormous, more than 100 grams.

Calculation of Quantity of Radio-Nuclide to Administer to Deliver a Specified Dose. Formula 9—(16) can be used to plan administration of a specified dose; it is only necessary to put in the known constants and the desired dose, and solve for C, the concentration per gram of the tissue in which the material will be deposited. If all of the material remains in the tissues, there will be no correction for elimination, but if there is excretion, this must be allowed for.

For example, it is desired to administer 8000 rads to a thyroid gland estimated to weigh 60 grams, using ^{131}I. On a tracer study the gland took up 65 per cent of the dose in 24 hours; this decreased with an effective half life of 5 days.

$\overline{E}_\beta = 0.180$ MeV; $\bar{g}$ (60 gm sphere) $= 23$; $\Gamma = 2.20$; $T = 5$; $D_{\beta+\gamma} = 8000$ rads; C = concentration to be found.

$8000 = 5\ C\ (73.8 \times 0.180 + 0.0346 \times 23 \times 2.20)$.

Solving this equation for C, the result is 106 μCi per gm.

This is the concentration to be *retained* in the gland; according to the up-take study this would be 65 per cent of that *administered*. Therefore the amount to be administered would be $\frac{100}{65} \times 106$ or 163 μCi per estimated gram of gland weight. $163 \times 60 = 9750$ μCi or 9.75 mc to be administered to deliver the desired dose in the gland specified.

Calculations for Administered Dose for a Short-Lived Iodine Isotope. In the above calculation the dose delivered during the first 24 hours, the period of accumulation of the radioactive isotope in the gland, was neglected; it would be very small compared to the total. This, however, cannot be the case for the short-lived isotopes, nor can their decay during the first hours be omitted.

Consider a very toxic patient, who has been studied with [131]I. Her thyroid content at 4 hours was 90 per cent of the administered dose, and at 24 hours, 80 per cent. The effective half life was 2.5 days, whence the biological half life was 3.6 days. The gland was estimated to weigh 60 gm, so $\bar{g} = 23$. It was decided to treat her with [130]I to a dose of 6000 rads.

By the use of the above formula it is found that there must be 27 mCi of this isotope in the gland at 4 hours, to give 6000 rads thereafter. Since the 4-hour uptake is 90 per cent, 30 mCi would have been the necessary initial dose. But in 4 hours the decay is to 80 per cent, whence to have 30 mCi available at 4 hours, $\frac{30}{0.80}$ or 37.5 mCi must have been injected. Now in the first 4 hours some of this will have been irradiating the gland. Uptakes were not determined for earlier periods, but as an approximation it may be assumed to have been linear. Then it was 22.5 per cent at one hour, 45 per cent at 2 hours, and 67.5 per cent at 3 hours. If 45 per cent be assumed as the average content of the gland for those first four hours, this would mean a gland content of $0.45 \times 37.5 = 17$ mCi. But the 2-hour decay must also be considered; it provides a reduction to $90 \times 17 = 15$ mCi. The dose delivered to the gland by this average 15 mCi content in 4 hours is 4 times the dose per hour.

$$4 \times \frac{15{,}000}{60} (2.13 \ \bar{E}_\beta + 10^{-3} \ \Gamma \ \bar{g}) = 880 \text{ rads.}$$ Then the total dose given by the 37.5 mCi administered would be 6880 rads. For a dose of 6000 rads, the administered quantity of [132]I should be $\frac{6000}{6880} \times 37.5 = 33$ mCi.

Non-uniformity of Irradiation. In reality the radionuclide distribution is never actually uniform, and sometimes it is decidedly patchy within such an organ as the thyroid gland. In these cases the calculated dose is an average, but local maxima and minima may vary widely from this dose. On a basis of radioautographs, Sinclair[13] estimates that in toxic diffuse goiter the maximum dose averages three times the mean and in non-toxic

10

nodular goiter ten times the mean. No data are given for the minimum doses. There is little that can be done about these variations at the present time.

However, there may be also a broader variation, a difference in uptake of the nuclide by different organs, as has already been noted in the case of the thyroid gland and radioiodine. In no other instance is the differential between uptake in a particular organ and the rest of the body as great, but significant variations do exist. Uptake, deposition, and elimination for a particular nuclide may vary with its chemical form, solubility, presence of carrier, and so on. The Report of Committee II of the International Commission on Radiological Protection, on Permissible Dose for Internal Radiation, lists critical organ, effective half life, fraction in critical organ of that in body, and so on, for a large number of radionuclides. These values furnish useful starting points for some dosage studies, but reservations as to the applicability of the table to the particular chemical compound under consideration must always be kept in mind.

An illustration of the use of this table can be made with a study of the behavior of some iron isotopes, which are used in the study of blood composition and behavior. According to the table the spleen is the critical organ, concentrating 2 per cent of an intravenous dose of either isotope; the weight of the spleen is 150 g. Physical and effective half lives for both nuclides are given, and the β and γ constants are obtained from Appendix C. When the calculations are made according to formula 9—(16) it is found that 100 μCi of ^{55}Fe results in a dose to the spleen of 1.1 rads, while the same amount of ^{59}Fe delivers 9.7 rads. The average dose to the whole body, assuming uniform distribution of 70 per cent of the material, is 0.2 rad for ^{55}Fe and 0.6 rad for ^{59}Fe. The liver, accumulating 15 per cent of the material, receives 1.5 rads from ^{55}Fe and 5.8 rad from ^{59}Fe.

Special Dosage Problems. 1. *Dose to blood and to entire body from ^{131}I for treatment of thyroid cancer.* A problem which is important in the treatment of thyroid cancer with radioiodine is the determination of the dose to the blood and to the entire body, from a therapeutic dose of radioactive iodine most of which either concentrates in thyroid tissue or is excreted. There have been several studies of this problem.[13-16] The treatment developed by Seidlin, Yalow, and Siegel will be reviewed here, with adjustment of their constants to conform with the use of rads instead of reps as the dose unit.

The dose in any tissue has been shown to be proportional to the concentration of the isotope within that tissue. For a concentration of C μc per gm, the beta dose rate is 2.12 $\overline{E}_\beta$ C rads per hour. Hence for a concentration of ^{131}I in the blood denoted by C_b, the dose rate to the blood, due to beta radiation is 2.12 $\times$ 0.180 $\times$ C_b = 0.38 C_b rads per hour. The gamma dose rate will depend not on the concentration in the blood, but on that in the whole body, since gamma rays released outside the blood vessels will still irradiate the entire organism. This will depend on a concentration

C_t, the average for the whole body, which the authors assume to be roughly equivalent to half the blood concentration; $C_t = \frac{1}{2}C_b$. The gamma ray dose rate is $10^{-3} \Gamma C_t \bar{g}$ rads per hour. For a 60 kg man this is $10^{-3} \times 2.20 \times 120 \times \frac{1}{2} \times C_b = 0.13 C_b$ rads per hour. Then the total dose rate to the blood is $0.51 C_b$ rads per hour.

The beta dose rate to the whole body would be half that to the blood if $C_t = \frac{1}{2} C_b$, but the gamma dose rate would be the same throughout. Hence the total dose rate to the body outside the blood vessels is $0.32 C_b$ rads per hour. The gamma dose to the rest of the body from the iodine concentrated in the thyroid can be shown to be negligible for calculations of the degree of accuracy possible here.

Table 9–7. Calculation of Blood Dose in a Thyroid Cancer Patient

Hours after Administration	C_b μCi per gm Blood	Hours for this Average Concentration	Average C_b during Interval	0.51 C_b × Hr. Rads
4	1.8	4	0.9	3.8
8	1.3	4	1.55	3.2
12	0.9	4	1.10	2.2
24	0.65	12	0.78	4.8
48	0.60	24	0.62	7.5
96	0.4	48	0.5	12.3
192	0.2	96	0.3	14.6
288	0.1	192	0.15	14.6
at 24 days	0.025			14.8*

Total D$_{blood}$ .... 77.8 rads

and total $D_{tissue} = \dfrac{0.33}{0.53} \times 77.8 = 48$ rads

* The dose from 24 days on is the dose per hour at that time multiplied by the average life in hours.

It now becomes a question of evaluating C_b, which of course changes constantly as the iodine is eliminated. This has to be done for the individual patient, by taking repeated blood samples and determining the average concentration during the period represented by each sample. Details for one patient are given in Table 9–7. This patient received 100 mCi of ^{131}I. Blood samples were taken at the indicated intervals; the average concentration during an interval was assumed to be the mean of the values at the start and the end of that interval.

The elimination pattern varies greatly among thyroid cancer patients. In the 82 cases reported by the authors of the above-mentioned report, the *average* blood dose per 100 mCi administered was 55 rads, but the extremes were from 18 to 200 rads per 100 mCi administered, depending on elimination and retention of the isotope. It must be emphasized that the ratio $C_t = \frac{1}{2} C_b$ does not necessarily hold for any other radionuclide in the blood stream. Values must be determined in any particular case.

2. *Dose to bladder mucosa from* ^{82}Br *in a rubber balloon.* For treatment of widespread but superficial cancer of the bladder mucosa, radiation may be administered by radioactive material introduced into a balloon in the bladder. Various radionuclides have been employed; ^{82}Br seems to be one of the most satisfactory. The balloon is introduced into the bladder and then filled with 100 cc of a solution of calcium bromide. Various techniques are used for introducing the material and maintaining it in place; description of these would be out of place here.[17]

For the calculation it will be assumed that 250 mCi of the nuclide are introduced and that the bag will be tolerated for 4 hours. T = 35.3 hours; $\overline{E}_\beta$ = 0.137 MeV; Γ = 14.6 r per mCi-hr at 1 cm; $\overline{g}$ = 31. The attenuation of the beta radiation by the stretched rubber balloon has been experimentally determined; about 30 per cent is transmitted. The dose per hour at the inner surface of the balloon is $\frac{1}{2}$ that at the center of the sphere, for both beta and gamma components; the beta component is further reduced by the bag before it gets to the bladder mucosa. Then

$$d(\text{mucosa}) \text{ per hour} = 0.5 \times \frac{250{,}000}{100} (2.13 \times 0.137 \times 0.3 + 14.6 \times$$

31×10^{-3}) rads per hour. In four hours the total dose at the surface of the mucosa is 2700 rads. The beta radiation would be mostly absorbed by any urine seeping between the bag and the mucosa, but the gamma radiation would not be affected. At a depth of 2 mm the beta radiation would be completely gone, but the gamma radiation would be very little less than at the surface.

3. *Dose from Constant Body Burden of Radioactive Nuclide.* All of the formulas developed up to this point are based on administration of a single dose of a nuclide, followed by its physical decay and physiological elimination. In a case where such material is continuously taken in and eliminated, as by drinking contaminated water or breathing contaminated air over a considerable period of time, a "body burden" is accumulated. If elimination just balances intake, a state of equilibrium exists; in other cases the burden may increase constantly. This depends on the manner in which the radioactive material is utilized in the body. "Permissible body burdens" are listed in Handbook 69 and in the Report of Subcommittee II of the International Commission on Radiological Protection. (See References.) Such a burden would be the amount of the nuclide constantly in the body, which would result in an annual radiation dose to the whole body of 5 rad. Determination of dose in such a situation cannot be by a calculation of total $D_{\beta+\gamma}$ as discussed above, but must be for *every* day, hour, or minute.

Five rad in a year would be $\dfrac{5000 \text{ m rad/yr}}{365 \text{ days/yr} \times 24 \text{ hr/day} \times 60 \text{ min/hr}} =$ 0.01 m rad/min. From 9—(7) and 9—(15) $d_{\beta+\gamma}/\text{min} = C(3.55 \times 10^{-2}\overline{E}_\beta + 1.7 \times 10^{-5} \Gamma \overline{g})$ rad. The permissible body burden for a particular nuclide would be found by putting the dose per minute as 0.01 mrad = 10^{-5} rad, and using the proper values for $\overline{E}_\beta$ and Γ. $C = \mu Ci/70{,}000$ gm (whole body weight), and $\overline{g} = 120$ (whole body). Thus the permissible body burden for ^{42}K would be found from

$$10^{-5} = \frac{\mu Ci}{70{,}000} \, (3.55 \times 10^{-2} \times 1.42 + 1.7 \times 10^{-5} \times 1.4 \times 120).$$

From this $\mu Ci = 10$. If the individual had no other radiation dose, he could have 10 μCi of ^{42}K continuously in his body without exceeding the permissible level.

If an individual is known to have a constant body burden of a particular nuclide, the continuing dose can be found. For example, someone working with ^{131}I was found on a routine check to have 0.2 μCi of the nuclide in his thyroid gland. On investigating his working habits it was found that he had not been observing adequate precautions (see Chapter 12) so that it is probable that he had had this burden for some time. His thyroid dose during the past 3 months could be determined by calculating the dose per day and multiplying by 90 days. Assuming a 30 gm gland

$$d_{\beta+\gamma}/day = \frac{0.2}{30} \, (51.2 \times 0.18 + 2.4 \times 10^{-2} \times 2.2 \times 15) = 0.07 \text{ rad.}$$

In 3 months the total would have been about 6 rad. Obviously such an occupational exposure is unacceptable and correct laboratory procedures must be set up at once.

4. *Substitution of One Radionuclide for Another.* For many years radon, in the form of "seeds" deposited permanently in tissues, has been used in treatment of malignant lesions. Detailed dosage tables and charts are available and widely used. Recently there has been a search for other nuclides which could be substituted for radon in such a way that these tables could still be used. Radioactive gold, ^{198}Au, has been promising. To find the number of μCi of ^{198}Au equivalent to 1 μCi of radon, it will be assumed that in the small volumes of tissue usually considered, the γ rays from the two are equally absorbed, the decision as to equivalent amounts must be made on a basis of T and Γ.

	T	Γ
Radon	3.8 days	8.25 r/mc-hr at 1 cm
^{198}Gold	2.7	2.3

$D\gamma = CT \times 0.0346 \, \Gamma \, \overline{g}$. To find equivalent microcuries,

$$\frac{\mu Ci \, (Rn)}{gm} \times T \, (Rn) \times 0.0346 \, \Gamma \, (Rn) \, \overline{g} = \frac{\mu Ci \, (Au)}{gm} \times T \, (Au)$$

$$\times 0.0346 \, \Gamma \, (Au) \, \overline{g}.$$

Cancelling the common factors

$$\mu Ci\ (Rn) \times T\ (Rn) \times \Gamma\ (Rn) = \mu Ci\ (Au) \times T\ (Au) \times \Gamma\ (Au),\ or$$

$$\frac{\mu Ci\ (Au)}{\mu Ci\ (Rn)} = \frac{T\ (Rn) \times \Gamma\ (Rn)}{T\ (Au) \times \Gamma\ (Au)} = \frac{3.8 \times 8.25}{2.7 \times 2.3} = 5.$$

Thus 5 μCi of ^{198}Au should give the same effect as 1 μCi of Rn, if uniformly distributed through the mass. Hence a lesion that would have required 15 μCi of radon will require 75 μCi of ^{198}Au.

5. *To Decide Whether an Observed Differential Uptake between a Lesion and the Rest of the Body is Adequate to Permit Radiation Therapy with This Nuclide.* For adequate radiation therapy it is necessary to decide on the dose to be delivered to the lesion, and then determine whether, on a basis of the observed differential, the dose to the whole body would be tolerated. Obviously the whole body dose may be considerably greater than the permissible occupational exposure. On the other hand, it must not be lethal or likely to be so. It is believed that about 450 rad to the whole body would be lethal in half the cases, and probably seriously disabling in the rest. However possibly about half this amount, say 200 rads, could be accepted. For a carcinomatous lesion, the tumor dose would probably be about 6000 rads. On a basis of β dose alone

$$D_\beta\ (body) = C\ (body)\ T_e \times 73.8\ \overline{E}_\beta.$$
$$D_\beta\ (tumor) = C\ (tumor)\ T_e \times 73.8\ \overline{E}_\beta.$$

Assuming that T_e is the same for both, it is evident that the beta doses are just in the ratio of the concentrations. For the above doses

$$\frac{6000}{200} = \frac{C\ (tumor)}{C\ (body)},\ or\ the\ concentration\ in\ the\ tumor\ must\ be\ 30$$

times that in the rest of the body. If the γ dose is included the situation becomes worse, since $\overline{g}$ for the body is greater than for the tumor. Thus it will require even fewer μCi per gram to build up the body dose, or C can be smaller for the whole body, and the differential correspondingly must be greater.

Differential uptakes of this magnitude are seldom found except with iodine isotopes and functioning thyroid tissue. If a satisfactory result could be expected with a tumor dose of 2000 rad, obviously a differential of 10 times would be sufficient. If cure is not the aim, but palliation, then even smaller differences might be effective. But it is obvious that little can be hoped for with a differential of 2 or 3 times, as far as curative radiotherapy is concerned.

Summary of Dosage Formulas Developed in Chapter 9

Page

$\Gamma = 1.5 \times 10^5 \, \overline{E}_\gamma \, (\text{MeV}) \, \mu_\alpha \, (\text{cm}^{-1} \, \text{air})$ 107

$\Gamma = 5.4 \, \overline{E}_\gamma \, (\text{MeV}) \, (0.06 \text{ to } 2.0 \text{ MeV})$ 108

$d_\beta/\text{sec} = 5.92 \times 10^{-4} \, C \, (\mu\text{Ci/gm}) \, \overline{E}_\beta \, (\text{MeV}) \, \text{rad}$ 111

$d_\beta/\text{min} = 3.55 \times 10^{-2} \, C \, \overline{E}_\beta \, \text{rad}$ 111

$d_\beta/\text{hr} \, (T > 20 \, \text{hr}) = 2.13 \, C \, \overline{E}_\beta \, \text{rad}$ 112

$d_\beta/\text{day} \, (T > 20 \, \text{days}) = 51.2 \, C \, \overline{E}_\beta \, \text{rads}$ 112

$D_\beta \, (\text{total}) = 73.8 \, C \, \overline{E}_\beta \, T \, (\text{days}) \, \text{rads}$ 112

$D_\beta \, \text{during t days} = D_\beta \, (1 - e^{-\lambda t}) = D_\beta \, (1 - e^{-0.693/T \times t}) \, \text{rads}$ . . 112

$\text{Exp}_\gamma/\text{min} = 1.7 \times 10^{-5} \, \Gamma \, C \, (\mu\text{Ci/gm}) \, \overline{g} \, \text{roentgens}$ 116

$\text{Exp}_\gamma/\text{hr} \, (T > 20 \, \text{hr}) = 10^{-3} \, \Gamma \, C \, \overline{g} \, \text{roentgen}$ 116

$\text{Exp}_\gamma/\text{day} \, (T > 20 \, \text{days}) = 2.4 \times 10^{-2} \, \Gamma \, C \, \overline{g} \, \text{roentgen}$ 118

$\text{Exp}_\gamma \, (\text{total}) = 0.0346 \, \Gamma \, C \, \overline{g} \, \text{roentgens}$ 118

$d\gamma/\text{hr} = 21 \, CE\gamma \, (\text{A.F.})$ 123

$D\gamma = 72.8 \, CTE\gamma \, (\text{A.F.})$ 123

$D_{\beta+\gamma} = CT \, (73.7 \, \overline{E}_\beta + 0.0346 \, \Gamma \, \overline{g}) \, \text{rads}$.   (Assuming an exposure of
1 roentgen results in a dose of 1 rad.) 128

$d_{\beta+\gamma}/\text{min}$ for constant body burden $= C \, (3.55 \times 10^{-2} \, \overline{E}_\beta + 1.7 \times 10^{-5} \, \Gamma \, \overline{g}) \, \text{rad}$.   For any length of time the dose is the dose/min
multiplied by the time in minutes. 136

$$T_e = \frac{T_p \times T_b}{T_p + T_b} \qquad T_b = \frac{T_p \times T_e}{T_p - T_e}$$ 137

REFERENCES

HINE, G. J. and BROWNELL, G. L.: *Radiation Dosimetry*, Chapters 16, 18, and Appendices. New York, Academic Press, Inc., 1956.

GLASSER, O., QUIMBY, E. H., TAYLOR, L. S., WEATHERWAX, J. L. and MORGAN, R. H.: *Physical Foundations of Radiology*, 3rd Ed., Chapter 13. New York, Paul B. Hoeber, Inc., 1961.

International Commission on Radiological Protection: Report of Subcommittee II: *Permissible Dose for Internal Radiation*. New York, Pergamon Press, 1959.

National Committee on Radiation Protection, Handbook 69: *Maximum Permissible Body Burdens and Maximum Permissible Concentrations of Radionuclides in Air and Water for Occupational Exposure*. Washington, U. S. Government Printing Office, 1959.

VENNART, J. and MINSKI, M.: Radiation doses from administered radio-nuclides. Brit. Jour. Radiology, *35*, 372, 1962.

WAGNER, HENRY N.: *Principles of Nuclear Medicine*. Chap. XVII. Philadelphia, W. B. Saunders Co., 1968.

SPECIFIC REFERENCES

1. WITTEN, V. H., WOOD, W. S. and LOEVINGER, R.: The erythema effects of a polonium plaque (an alpha emitter) on human skin. Jour. Investigative Dermatology, *28*, 199–210, 1957.
2. ROSSI, H. H. and ELLIS, R. H.: Calculations for distributed sources of beta radiations. Am. Jour. Roentgenology, Radium Therapy & Nuclear Med., *67*, 980–988 1952.
3. HINE, G. J. and BROWNELL, G. L.: *Radiation Dosimetry*, New York, Academic Press, Inc., 1956, pp. 850–859.
4. MARINELLI, L. D., QUIMBY, E. H. and HINE, G. J.: Dosage determination with radioactive isotopes. II. Practical considerations in therapy and protection. Am. Jour. Roentgenology & Radium Therapy, *59*, 260–280, 1948.
5. HOECKER, F. E. and ROOFE, P. G.: Studies of radium in human bone. Radiology, *56*, 89–99, 1951.
6. SPIERS, F. W.: Alpha-ray dose in bone containing radium. Brit. Jour. Radiology, *26*, 296–301, 1953.
7. BUSH, F.: The integral dose received from a uniformly distributed radioactive isotope. Brit. Jour. Radiology, *22*, 66, 1949.
8. FOCHT, E. F., QUIMBY, E. H. and GERSHOWITZ, M.: Revised average geometric factors for cylinders in isotope dosage. Part I. Radiology, *85*, 151–152, 1965.
9. SMITH, E. M, HARRIS, C. C. and ROHRER, R. H.: Calculation of local energy deposition due to electron capture and internal conversion. Jour. Nuclear Medicine, *7*, 23–32, 1966.
10. ELLETT, W. H., CALLAHAN, A. B. and BROWNELL, G. L.: Gamma-ray dosimetry of internal emitters, II: Monte Carlo calculations of absorbed dose from uniform sources. Brit. Jour. Radiology, *38*, 541–544, 1965.
10a. BROWNELL, G. L., ELLETT, W. H., and REDDY, A. R.: Absorbed fractions for photon dosimetry. Jour. Nuclear Med. Supplement No. 1, February, 1968.
11. WIDMAN, J. C. and POWSNER, E. R.: Energy absorption in cylinders containing a uniformly distributed source. Jour Nuclear Medicine, *8*, 179–187, 1967.
12. LAWRENCE, J. H.: *Polycythemia, Physiology, Diagnosis, and Treatment.* New York, Grune & Stratton, 1955.
13. SINCLAIR, W. K., ABBATT, J. D., FERRAN, H. E. A., HARRISS, E. B. and LAMERTON, L. F.: A quantitative autoradiographic study of radioiodine distribution and dosage in human thyroid glands. Brit. Jour. Radiology, *39*, 34–61, 1956.
14. MARINELLI, L. D. and HILL, R. F.: Radiation dosimetry in the treatment of functional thyroid carcinoma with I-131. Radiology, *55*, 494–502, 1950.
15. ROBERTSON, J. and GODWIN, J. T.: Calculation of radioactive iodine beta radiation dose to bone marrow. Brit. Jour. Radiology, *27*, 241–242, 1950.
16. SEIDLIN, S. M., YALOW, A. A. and SIEGEL, E.: Blood radiation dose during radioiodine therapy of metastatic thyroid carcinoma. Radiology, *63*, 797–813, 1954.
17. DYCHE, G. M. and MACKAY, N. R.: Techniques for the intracavitary treatment of bladder neoplasms with radioactive solutions contained in a rubber balloon. Brit. Jour Radiology, *32*, 752–756, 1959.

10

Biological Effects of Ionizing Radiations

THE first part of this chapter will be devoted to a discussion of observable effects of ionizing radiations. In the second part, some of the basic theoretical considerations will be reviewed.

PART I

GROSSLY OBSERVABLE EFFECTS

General Phenomena. When radiation falls upon living matter, it produces changes which may be more or less profound, depending on the radiosensitivity of the system and the quantity of radiation. Grossly, four broad stages may be noted:

(*a*) For a small dose of radiation there will be no visible effect. It is true that some changes of at least a temporary nature have been induced in some of the cells, but there is nothing detectable by present means.

(*b*) For somewhat larger doses of radiation there will be observable pheneomena, very slight, or fairly obvious, but from which there will apparently be complete recovery. In cells there will be increased permeability of the membranes, with swelling, increased acidity and granularity of the protoplasm, clumping of chromosomes, and halting of cell division. In the entire organism, especially of mammals, there may appear the syndrome called radiation sickness—nausea, vomiting, malaise, possibly ac companied by changes in the blood picture, decreased white count usually being the first thing observed. Such localized phenomena as erythema or epilation also may be produced. However, none of the changes is permanent, and after a time it is again impossible to observe anything to indicate that radiation has been administered.

(*c*) With still larger doses, all these effects are increased, and now complete recovery is impossible, although the worst symptoms may be alleviated. At the cellular level, reproduction or cell division is permanently altered. At the organism level, general debility may be accompanied by profound changes in the blood picture, with depression of all the elements— red and white cells, platelets and hemoglobin. Intractable anemia may develop, and if the gonads have been heavily irradiated, sterility may result. Heavy irradiation to the eyes may lead to cataract formation.

141

Epilation will be permanent instead of temporary, possible skin changes are many and varied. Occasionally there may be malignant degeneration of some cells, with cancer formation.

(d) At a still higher dose level, all the results mentioned are increased beyond the point where the organism can combat them. Death results.

These various effects will be discussed in some detail in the following sections.

It is interesting that, except for fantastically high doses, no *immediate* result of irradiation is observable. There is always a longer or shorter *latent period*, whose duration depends on the effect to be observed, the quality of the radiation, the magnitude of the dose, and its rate of administration. With moderately large doses delivered at a single exposure, radiation sickness may appear in a few hours, a skin erythema in one day, blood changes in a few days, or even sooner, epilation in a week or two. Even with really large doses, radiation death may not occur for a month or more. Such delayed effects as leukemia or cancer formation may not be evident for years. Yet the *immediate* effect of irradiation, the production of ion pairs, occurs only while the irradiation is going on. The ionization results in the production of abnormal atomic or molecular fragments; this condition is, however, very transient; positive and negative ions quickly recombine to form neutral atoms or molecules. Yet during the brief instant of ionization, physicochemical changes can be initiated in living matter which may ultimately lead to detectable radiation changes. Once initiated, this chain of biological events is apparently irreversible except under very special conditions. The search for antidotes, or means to reverse the effects of radiation doses after their delivery, is one of the fascinating fields of current radiobiological research.

Units of Radiation Dose. Radiation dose has been discussed in Chapter 9. The dose unit, the rad, represents an energy absorption of 100 ergs per gram of absorber, and results in the ionization of something like one tissue atom in 20 billion. This is a very small amount of energy; it would raise the temperature of soft tissue by only about two-millionths of a degree centigrade. A really large therapeutic dose would be less than ten thousand times this; that is, it would result in a temperature rise of less than two one-hundredths of a degree. Nevertheless, this would result in profound and irreversible changes in the living organism.

Classes of Biologic Effects. The most obvious effects are, of course, those arising in the irradiated individual. These are called *somatic*. However it is also true that certain changes can be transmitted to future generations, if they arise in the germ plasm. Such effects are called *genetic*.

Factors Influencing Somatic Radiation Effects. Some somatic radiation effects are observable after a relatively small dose of radiation, say 50 rads, while others require some hundreds of times as much. A number of other factors besides the actual dose enter into the degree of the final reaction produced.

1. *The rate at which the dose is administered:* Living tissues are not inert; as soon as any degree of damage has been produced, a corresponding repair process sets in. If a particular dose is spread out over a long time, it is possible that repair may keep up with damage, and no visible change ever be observed; whereas if it had been given all at once, a violent reaction might have been provoked. Even within relatively short periods the effect of a given dose is less, the longer the irradiation time. Or, conversely, to produce a specified effect, more radiation is required for a long irradiation period (days or weeks) than for a short one. Irradiation need not be continuous during this time. The fact that it is given in small daily increments is sufficient. However, there are some forms of biological damage, notably gene mutation, in which this time factor apparently is less effective.

2. *The extent of the body irradiated.* If the whole body receives a large or moderate dose of radiation, a severe and possibly fatal illness will ensue. Smaller doses to the whole body may not produce any prompt effects, nor some of the late ones due to larger doses. On the other hand, if only a small fraction of the body is irradiated, as in x-ray therapy, systemic effects are mild, even for very large doses. Local effects may be quite severe in these cases, and there may be some degree of permanent local change in the tissues.

3. *The part of the body irradiated.* General reactions are much more severe if the dose of radiation is delivered to the upper abdomen, or possibly to the spine, than if a field of similar size elsewhere is exposed to the same dose.

4. *The age of the individual.* In general, physically immature individuals are somewhat more sensitive to the effects of radiation than are adults.

5. *The biological variation among individuals.* While experience makes it possible to set an *average* dose for the production of a certain effect, individuals may vary greatly in their response. For instance, it requires 600 rads in a single dose to result in death within 30 days of half of a group of a certain strain of rats (MLD 30 days). However, some of the same rats will die after 400 rads and some will survive after 800.

Sources of Information Regarding Radiation Effects. Sources of information regarding radiation effects are varied. Of course, it is not possible deliberately to experiment with human beings. Animal experiments are fruitful; all radiation effects produced in man can be produced in animals. However, dose-effect relations are not necessarily the same, so the data thus obtained need such checks as are possible with human experience. This is of three types:

1. *Occupational.* Early radiological workers received small doses from x or gamma rays at fairly constant rates over long periods. In many instances it has been possible to evaluate these fairly accurately and correlate them with observed changes, if any. Painters of luminous dials ingested paint containing radioactive material, much of which was retained in the skeleton; many of these developed serious damage years later.

Some miners in uranium mines worked in an atmosphere containing high concentrations of radioactive gas and subsequently developed lung cancer. In atomic energy plants a very few accidents have occurred in which individuals were exposed to a flash of nuclear radiation.

2. *Medical.* X rays and radium rays have been used for over 60 years in diagnosis and in treatment of cancer and other diseases. For nearly 20 years, radionuclides have been administered internally for diagnosis and treatment of disease. Observations on these patients have provided data.

3. *Atomic Bomb.* Although fire and blast caused most of the damage in the Hiroshima and Nagasaki bombings, about 15 to 20 per cent was caused by gamma and neutron radiations emitted during the explosions. Since 1946 the United States has had an Atomic Bomb Casualty Commission, studying the immediate and long-term effects on the population of those cities. In 1954 during atom bomb tests in Bikini, a heavy fall-out of bomb debris was experienced by dwellers in neighboring islands. Here doses could be quite accurately evaluated; they were much less, of course, than those in Japan. All exposed individuals are being carefully followed and studied.

Radiation Doses to Produce Particular Effects. Radiation effects are usually classified as early or immediate, and late. As has been pointed out, even the early reactions have a certain latent period, but if this is only days or weeks, the response is called immediate. These are the effects usually observed in animal research and in treatment of human beings.

For human beings, a dose of 500 rads given in a short time to the whole body would be very drastic; many individuals would die from its effects. Within a few hours after such an exposure, the individual would probably be violently sick, with nausea and diarrhea. Exhaustion, fever and delirium might follow, and death ensue. On the other hand, there might be a fair degree of recovery for a week or two, followed by a second cycle of sickness, with loss of hair, hemorrhages from skin and mucous membranes, profound anemia and low white blood count, loss of ability to combat infection, and again, possibly death. Both these cycles of illness would be classed as immediate effects. Those who survived would have a long slow convalescence, and probably never be really well. Years later there might be the development of leukemia, or of tumors or cataract. These last would be the late effects.

Half of those exposed to 500 rads would be expected to die. With smaller doses, fewer people would develop severe symptoms and the illness would be less severe. For 100 rads probably not more than 15 per cent of the population would be really sick, and few would die. For 25 rads it is probable that no one would observe any serious symptoms.

If only a small part of the body is exposed, very much larger doses are tolerated, and it is rare that death ensues, even after several thousand rads in a small region, unless this involves very sensitive vital organs. Such doses are regularly given in the treatment of cancer, not in a single exposure, but within a few weeks.

Delayed effects may appear years after the exposure, and may follow a period in which no radiation effect was observable. These effects include local tissue breakdown, sometimes leading to cancer, development of leukemia and possibly anemia, cataract formation, and possibly shortening of life.

The knowledge that such delayed effects may be produced by radiation indicates a need for a statistical study. It must be found out, from mortality data, how often any one of these conditions appears in the absence of exposure to radiation in addition to that from unavoidable internal sources and background radiation. This figure is to be compared with the incidence of the same condition following radiation exposure. If an increase is demonstrated, the frequency with which the condition develops at different levels of radiation dose must be determined, and the relationship between dose and incidence of the disease must be evaluated. Only in this manner will it be possible to assess the hazards, if any, associated with different doses of radiation. Some of these effects will be reviewed briefly.

Effects on Skin. This information is mostly obtained by following patients treated with x rays. Doses up to 1000 rads or so, given within a few days, leave little or no permanent mark of any kind. For two or three times this, there may be permanent tanning and some superficial blood vessel damage. Hair loss may be permanent and sweat glands destroyed. Above 3000 or 4000 rads the skin may remain somewhat thin, covered with dilated blood vessels, sensitive, and subject to infection. Cancer may develop following this type of single large dose, but this is extremely rare. More often (though still not really frequently) it follows a long series of much smaller doses, repeated over months or years.

Effects on Blood. Anemia is a very rare late sequel of large doses to the bone marrow. This may be so damaged as not to be able to produce red cells in sufficient numbers. A much more common effect is the depression of white blood cell production, resulting in a leukopenia which may be transient or protracted. Platelet count may also be depressed. The final result of serious damage to the blood-forming organs may be the development of some form of leukemia. This is a disease in which uncontrolled over-production of the white blood cells occurs. It is apparently always fatal, although some forms may run chronic courses over many years, and long remissions may be produced by various types of therapy. The disease may follow a single large exposure or several smaller ones. In Nagasaki and Hiroshima up to 1955 there had been 93 proven and 15 suspected cases among those present at the time of the explosion and still living in one of those cities at the time of the diagnosis. Vital statistics would predict about 25 deaths from leukemia in a comparable unexposed population. This is too big a difference to be merely statistical. Furthermore, the distribution of the 93 cases within the radiation zone is instructive. For persons within 1000 meters of the center of the explosion, the incidence is at a rate of 128 per 10,000 population; at greater distances the numbers decrease fairly rapidly, until at more than 2000 meters the incidence is 2 per 10,000, which is not statistically different from the unirradiated group. Here the dose was probably of the order of 10 to 50 rads to the whole body. For those close to the center it is impossible to make even approximate estimates of dosage, for shielding of buildings, etc, is in all cases an unknown factor. Such shielding certainly existed; the unprotected individual close to the center of the blast did not survive. The first cases appeared within 2 years after the bomb exploded; from that time until 1951–53 the annual incidence increased; it then maintained a plateau for about 3 years, but now since 1957 appears to be definitely on the decline.

Repeated smaller whole body exposures have been given in the treatment of certain non-cancerous diseases. A careful study in England of a group of such patients showed a steadily increasing incidence of leukemia with dosage to spinal marrow from 2 per 10,000 with a dose less than 500 rads to 17.6 per 10,000 with a dose exceeding 2750 rads. The expected rate in an unirradiated population would be $\frac{1}{2}$ per 10,000. The average time between first x-ray treatment and diagnosis of leukemia was 6 years, but some patients had had several series of treatments.

Long-continued chronic exposure of the type received by some early radiologists might also be expected to lead to leukemia. There is some evidence that the death rate from leukemia among senior American radiologists is considerably higher than among the general population, but accurate statistics are not available. It would be expected that this difference would disappear with current knowledge and adequate planning for protection of the radiologist.

Induction of Cancer. Occasionally long after a single large dose of radiation or a long-continued series of small ones, there will be malignant degeneration of some cell system, with cancer formation. This may have been preceded by serious local effects, but in many cases the immediate local effects were very mild. The malignant transformation may arise in the blood-forming organs, with leukemia development, as just described, or it may be local in skin and other regions. Such changes leading to cancer formation occur only rarely in human beings, although in certain strains of inbred animals they can be produced regularly. Very little is known regarding the special trigger that sets off this type of transformation; it is regarded as being probably some form of cell mutation.

Lung cancer has been reported among Austrian uranium miners, a very high incidence arising among those who had continued to do this work for a long time. The average interval between beginning of work and cancer development was 17 years, and in this time the average dose to the lungs was about 1000 rads. However, the possibility of inhalation and lodgement of highly active particles, resulting in very high local doses, cannot be ignored. No other record of production of lung cancer in man is found. Occasionally lesions can be produced in laboratory animals under special conditions.

This is also true for the assimilation of bone-seeking radionuclides such as radium, strontium, or plutonium. Bone cancer can be produced at will in animals by these materials. In man, such cancers have arisen in individuals who had painted luminous dials with radioactive materials. It was their custom to point the brushes between their lips, thus ingesting some of the material. The latent period was of the order of 15 years, and the individuals developing cancer apparently all had retained at least 3.6 μgm of radium or its equivalent. A few similar effects have been observed in individuals long ago given radium compounds internally for treatment of disease, and in people who have consumed large amounts of radioactive water, containing small amounts of radium salts in solution. The radium concentrates in the bones, and there continues to give off its radiations all through the lifetime of the individual.

A number of cases of cancer of the thyroid gland have been reported in children who had some years previously received x-ray treatment for enlargement of the thymus gland, infected tonsils, and other disorders. These treatments frequently were given in early infancy. Some years ago this was very popular; it has now been practically discontinued except in real emergencies,—which are *very* rare. The dose of radiation was always much smaller than that mentioned earlier as causing skin cancer, sometimes only 300 or 400 rads. The possibility of an additional hormonal factor cannot be overlooked, but it has not been demonstrated.

Induction of Cataract. X rays can produce cataract, but the necessary dose is at least some hundreds of rads. Of 98 cases of cataract among survivors of the Hiroshima explosion, 85 occurred in persons within 1000 meters of the center. Here the neutrons accompanying the explosion probably were mainly responsible; it is well known that they are several times as effective as x rays in producing cataract. Of the cases mentioned, two later developed leukemia. A detailed study was made by Merriam and Focht of 100 cases of radiation cataract following radiotherapy to regions including the eyes, and 73 cases similarly treated who showed no radiation damage. (Am. Jour. Roentgenol. & Rad. Ther., 77, 759; May 1957.) Doses were carefully determined for the various clinical procedures. Of those who had single treatments, one cataract developed many years after a dose of 200 R from a radium applicator. However, the majority in this group received from 500 to 700 R. With divided treatments over 3 weeks to 3 months, the smallest dose resulting in cataract was 400 R; in the series whose treatments were spread over more than 3 months the smallest cataract-producing dose was 550 R. The average time for onset for the smaller doses was about $8\frac{1}{2}$ years; after considerably larger doses the average time of appearance was about $4\frac{1}{2}$ years.

Effects of Exposure During Pregnancy. After a large dose of radiation, probably more than 1000 rads to the pelvic region, a pregnant woman may have a miscarriage or a still-birth, although several cases are on record of women receiving more than this for treatment of cancer and producing normal children. Of 98 pregnant women in Nagasaki who were within

1000 meters of the center, about 23 per cent of those who had severe radiation sickness miscarried, compared to 4 per cent of those who were not sick, and 3 per cent of those 3000 or 4000 meters away.

Children irradiated *in utero* may be abnormal. The stage of pregnancy during which irradiation occurs is significant. There are few data on the effects of small doses of radiation on human pregnancy, but careful studies on mice by various workers are very suggestive. In these animals the fetus is much more radiosensitive during the period of development of organ primordia by differentiation from primitive cell types. This, in the human, is from the 18th to the 38th day. During this period it appears that a dose of the order of 50 R might produce serious abnormality. Later in pregnancy much larger doses would probably be necessary to produce the same defects. Relatively large doses, such as those employed in radiotherapy, would be expected to result in overt damage, if the fetus survived. It is true that from time to time cases are reported of the birth of apparently normal children after intensive radiotherapy. There are also, however, many reports of various abnormalities, especially microcephaly. There are not enough of such reports for statistical evaluation. The Japanese records show an abnormally high percentage of mentally retarded children, and of microcephaly among those exposed before birth at distances of the order of 1000 meters from the center. In the group exposed at 5000 meters, no variation from the unexposed population was found.

Sterility. Permanent sterility may be produced in either man or woman by doses of the order of 500 R to the reproductive organs. This dose is close to the lethal one for the whole body, and would produce serious radiation sickness. Sterility is sometimes deliberately induced for medical reasons; in this case the radiation is closely confined to the critical organs. Under modern conditions of occupational exposure, for instance among radiologists and atomic energy plant workers, there is no evidence of any impairment of fertility. It should be pointed out that impotence is not produced by even large doses of radiation.

Shortening of Life Span. A number of reports based on observations made on animals suggest that exposure to ionizing radiations may lead to a reduction in the expectancy of life. In animals this can be demonstrated with chronic exposure at low doses. In man, definite statistical evidence is lacking. A widely quoted statement that in radiologists the average age at death is less than for the general population has been shown to be based on unsatisfactory evidence. A careful analysis of all available data leads to the conclusion that, at even the earlier permissible dose rates for occupational exposure, there is no statistical evidence of life shortening. A figure often quoted is one day of life shortening per accumulated rad of whole body dose. In the individual case this could not be demonstrated, and it is doubtful if it could be sorted out statistically at the present time.

Genetic Effects of Radiation. Recently the subject of genetic damage—harm to future generations—has assumed an important place. Unlike the systemic or somatic damage just discussed, there seems to be no lower level to the amount of radiation which can produce at least some order of gene mutations. It is not possible in such a discussion as this to go into much detail in the matter of genetic damage. However, there are certain points to be brought out.

It is hardly necessary to review the fact that in man, and all higher animals, every individual arises from a single cell formed by the fusion of two germ cells from the two parents. Each cell contains a nucleus, which in turn contains a number of microscopic, thread-like structures called chromosomes. Each chromosome is an aggregate of sub-microscopic structures, the genes, which determine the hereditary nature of the individual. The germ cell receives half its genes from each parent, and these determine the family likenesses.

However, occasionally a sudden change occurs in a gene; this is called a mutation, and the characteristic which it governs may be passed on in a new form to subsequent generations. Some mutations are *dominant*; that is, they can change the characteristic in the next generation, if either parent develops the mutation. Others are *recessive;* in this case the characteristic must be passed on by both parents for it to appear. This is an over-simplification of course; there are various possible combinations of which these might be considered the two extremes.

The hereditary variation found among human beings is the result of mutations which have occurred in past generations. As far as is known, all genes are subject to mutation, and over the population as a whole, mutation is constantly occurring at a definite but very low rate. Natural selection tends to eliminate harmful genes from the population, but they are again replenished by new mutations, so that in general a state of equilibrium exists. Evolution has occurred slowly by successions of small variations from the average. The cause of these natural mutations is not completely known; some are doubtless produced by cosmic rays and other unavoidable radiations, but these are apparently not responsible for all.

In animals the production of gene mutations by radiation has been studied; the mutation rate is proportional to the radiation exposure; there seems to be no lower threshold and little or no recovery. There is no valid information about genetic effects of ionizing radiations in man, but it is reasonable to suppose that they follow the same general pattern.

The genetically effective dose to a population and to future generations depends on the ages of the exposed individuals as well as on the dose. If they are past the reproductive age, there is of course no effect. It is apparently the *frequency* of gene mutations that is increased by radiation; there is no evidence and little likelihood that radiation produces any new kinds of change. Damage to genetic material is cumulative and essentially irreparable, and is carried on from generation to generation. Long continued exposure to radiation of low intensity apparently induces approximately as much gene mutation as a single exposure to an equal dose of

11

higher intensity. This is unlike the recovery previously described for damage to the individual or to his organs,—the so-called *somatic* damage.

Genetic mutation is spoken of as damage; it is considered to be generally undesirable. True, the human race has arrived at its present state as a result of mutations, but in the generations during which these developments have taken place natural selection has also acted to get rid of many other, probably less desirable, mutations.

The increase in damage to be expected from radiation is usually discussed in terms of a "doubling dose." This is the dose that would eventually cause a complete doubling of gene mutations. The total effect in the population would, of course, depend on the kinds of mutations, and the interdependence of the various characteristics. It is impossible to assess this with any degree of accuracy, but certain general lines can be followed.

In any analysis of genetic changes in human beings it must be remembered that accurate data are completely lacking. There is a good deal of information on fruit flies and mice, both as to natural and radiation-induced mutations, but extrapolation to man must be done with caution. Such differences as total number of genes, total length of reproductive period during which mutations can be collected, and so on, complicate the picture. Accordingly, at the present time numerical data must be taken as probably of correct order of magnitude and broadly illustrative, not as rigidly factual.

The Doubling Dose. There are two effects to be considered if all individuals in the reproductive age receive a "doubling dose" of radiation; first, the effect on their immediate offspring; and second, that on their later descendants and on the population as a whole.

The effect on various types of inheritance of doubling the mutation rate can be analyzed in some detail. Here, however, only the extremes of dominant and recessive mutations will be considered briefly. For a dominant trait, doubling the number of mutations in one generation would almost double the number of cases in the next. In successive generations the excess would be eliminated, and return to equilibrium established. However, if the doubling rate persisted generation after generation, equilibrium would eventually be established at double the original rate. In case of a recessive trait, a single doubling dose would produce an extremely small increase in the first generation; at a permanently doubled rate it would take more than 50 generations to increase the incidence by 50 per cent. Of course there are various intermediate sorts of inheritance, such as those requiring specific combinations of genes; the whole problem is very complex.

From one point of view the simplest way to discuss genetic effects due to radiation is to consider the total number of tangible serious genetic damages in presently living individuals,—damages such as epilepsy, idiocy, congenital malformation, defects in vision or in endocrine organs, etc.,—and then see how the population would be expected to be affected by radiation. Roughly 2 per cent of all live births in the United States have genetic defects of this sort not due to radiation. If every member of the population were subjected once to a doubling dose of radiation, this level would rise in the first generation, but would return to equilibrium. If the doubling dose were continued generation after generation, the figure would, after many generations, rise to the double level. Numerically, in the United States at present there are about 100 million children born in a generation; of these about 2 million will have genetic defects as a result of "spontaneous" unavoidable genetic changes which have occurred during the generations of their ancestry. If a doubling dose of radiation were applied to the total population for many generations, this would eventually rise to 4 million defectives. This would take a very long time; perhaps 10 per cent of the increase, 200,000 new defectives would be found in the first generation. If the added doses were $\frac{1}{5}$ of the doubling dose for each generation, the first generation casualties would be 40,000 in the total 100 million, and the ultimate additional load 400,000 in the 100 million.

Dominant damaging mutations are much rarer than recessives,—perhaps only 1 per cent as common. The risk of one of these occurring spontaneously in any individual parent is almost negligible,—possibly 1 in 2000,— and even after a doubling dose of radiation it is still very small. For the more frequent recessive traits, *if* a parent carries the mutated gene the chance is 1 in 2 that a child receives it, 1 in 4 for a grandchild, and so on. Furthermore, every human being carries his natural load of harmful recessive genes received from his own ancestors; the addition of a few more by a doubled rate during his lifetime will be only a "drop-in-the-bucket" of the whole story. Therefore, any particular individual need not fear that just because he has received such a dose of radiation, he will run an appreciable risk of starting a bad line of descendants.

If a relatively small group of prospective parents receives the doubling dose of radiation, no noticeable effects will be produced in the sum total of the first generation or of any subsequent one. *For levels of radiation up to the doubling dose and even definitely beyond it, the genetic effects of radiation are only appreciable when reckoned over the population as a whole.*

For determining the doubling dose for human beings there are really no data which have any quantitative significance. Man is not a pure species, like a pure strain of fruit flies or white mice. The Japanese bomb cases are being studied carefully, to be sure, but little accurate information is available about the dosage, the regular incidence of mutations in the unirradiated population, and so forth. Furthermore, so far, in a single generation of a few individuals, only a very few types of mutations can be observed.

Various lines of argument lead to estimates of from 25 to 150 rads for the doubling dose, with the probability that it lies between 30 and 80 rads. This dose can be delivered all at once or in many small portions during the reproductive period.

PART II

EFFECTS AT THE MOLECULAR LEVEL

When ionizing radiation traverses matter, the first interaction is the production of ion pairs. Subsequent to this there may be various radiochemical phenomena, followed by direct or indirect effects on cells or cell components. All the immediate reactions are completed in less than a second; however, there is a *latent period* ranging from minutes to weeks before any change can be observed.

Energy Absorption from Ionizing Particles. When a charged particle passes through matter, it leaves a "track" of ionized and excited atoms and molecules. These tracks are comparable to those seen in the cloud tracks of Figure 7–3 except that, when the medium is denser than air, the tracks are shorter. For fast beta particles the ions are separated relatively widely, for slower ones the path is more dense. It is generally assumed that radiobiological effects are due to ionizations occurring in specific regions of cells. It is conceivable that a single ion pair produced in such a critical region as a chromosome might bring about a definite effect (a break). On the other hand, some effects require the accumulation of considerably more energy in a small region.

Linear Energy Transfer. The rate of energy release along a track is described by the energy lost by the particle per unit length of path, usually specified in keV per micron of track. This is called *linear energy transfer* (LET). The number of ion pairs per micron is obtained by dividing LET by 34 eV, the average energy lost by the ionizing particle per ion pair produced.

Direct and Indirect Effects. The effects of radiation may be either *direct*, as a result of ionization produced in the material, or *indirect* as a result of transfer of energy to the material from ionization produced in the surrounding medium. Certain chemicals and biological organisms, when irradiated in the dry state, require a great deal more radiation to produce a given degree of inactivation than when they are dissolved or suspended in water. For instance, when purified dry catalase is irradiated, it requires about 1000 times as much radiation to produce a given inactivation as when the material is irradiated in dilute solution.

Activated Water. This is usually explained on a basis of "activated water," the water molecule being first ionized and then dissociated more or less in the following sequence:

$$H_2O + energy \rightarrow H_2O^+ + e^-$$
$$H_2O^+ \rightarrow H^+ + OH^{\cdot}$$

and at a distance the e^- interacts with another water molecule

$$H_2O + e^- \rightarrow OH^- + H^{\cdot}$$

The H$^+$ and OH$^-$ combine to form water again. The H$^.$ and OH$^.$ radicals are highly reactive fragments of molecules. They may also combine to form water, but it is likely that they will enter into other combinations. They may interact directly with molecules they encounter, or they may combine to give rise to molecular hydrogen and hydrogen peroxide.

$$H^. + H^. \rightarrow H_2$$
$$OH^. + OH^. \rightarrow H_2 O_2$$

These are strongly reducing and oxidizing agents and can diffuse to an appreciable distance through the water, and so exert their effects over a wider area than that available to the original ionization.

Mean Lethal Dose. Suppose a biological sample contains N_o individual biological entities, and the whole sample receives a small dose of radiation dD. This will inactivate a number of entities which should be proportional to the dose, and also proportional to the number of entities present. This may be expressed (as in radionuclide decay)

$$- dN = \frac{1}{k} N \, dD \qquad\qquad 10-(1)$$

Integrating

$$N = N_o \, e^{-D/k} \qquad\qquad 10-(2)$$

N now represents the number of unaffected entities remaining. This equation is analogous to the radionuclide decay equation, where D corresponds to t and 1/k to λ. With constantly increasing dose there is constantly increasing inactivation. If every interaction resulted in an inactivation, then N_o interactions would result in complete inactivation. However, in such a preparation not every interaction will be effective. If an entity has already been inactivated, a second attempted interaction within it will do no more; the energy of this interaction will then be "lost" in terms of final effect. Thus as more and more entities are inactivated, the chance of further interaction becomes less, and in fact, if exponential survival is accepted, it will never be possible to inactivate every one. A dose of interest is that which would have inactivated every one if each had undergone an interaction and none had been "lost." In this case dN must equal N (all entities changed) whence dD must equal k (total dose to produce complete inactivation if no interference). In the case of actual exponential decrease, if $D/k = 1$ be introduced into equation 10−(2), then

$$N = N_o \, e^{-1}, \text{ or}$$
$$N = 0.37 \, N_o \qquad\qquad 10-(3)$$

That is, in a population which has undergone enough interactions to kill all, if all had been equally exposed, actually only 67 per cent have been killed and 37 per cent survive. These may be said to have been "protected" by the cells which received more than one "event." The dose thus derived is called the *mean lethal dose*. This is, then, the dose that is required on the average to place one inactivating event in each entity, but after which actually 37 per cent remain unaffected.

Further discussion of this topic is beyond the scope of this book. The interested reader is referred to texts on radiobiology.

REFERENCES

ALEXANDER, PETER: *Atomic Radiation and Life*, London, Penguin Books, 1957.

BACQ, Z. M. and ALEXANDER, P.: *Fundamentals of Radiobiology*, 2nd Ed., London, Butterworth, 1961.

British Medical Research Council: *The Hazards to Man of Nuclear and Allied Radiations*, London, Her Majesty's Stationery Office. First Report, 1956; Second Report, 1960.

DU SAULT, L. A.: The influence of the time factor on the dose-response curve, Am. Jour. Roentgenol., Radium Ther., & Nuc. Med., *87*, 567, 1962.

ERRERA, M. and FORSSBERG, A. (eds.): *Mechanisms in Radiobiology*, Vol. 11, New York, Academic Press, Inc., 1960.

GRAY, L. H.: *Cellular Radiobiology*, Radiation Research, Supp. 1, p. 73, 1959.

HOLLAENDER, A. (ed.): *Radiation Biology*, New York, McGraw-Hill Book Co., Inc., 1954.

LEA, D. E.: *Actions of Radiation on Living Cells*, 2nd Ed., New York, Cambridge University Press, 1956.

National Bureau of Standards: *Handbook 59, Permissible Dose from External Sources of Ionizing Radiation*. Washington, D.C., U.S. Superintendent of Documents, 1954.

PIZZARELLO, D. J. and WITCOFSKI, R. L.: *Basic Radiation Biology*, Philadelphia, Lea & Febiger, 1967.

STERN, CURT: *Principles of Human Genetics*, 2nd Ed., San Francisco, W. H. Freeman, 1960.

United States National Academy of Science: *The Biological Effects of Atomic Radiations, Summary Reports*. Washington, D.C., National Research Council, First Report, 1956; Second Report, 1960.

United States National Academy of Science: *The Biological Effects of Atomic Radiations; A Report to the Public*. Washington, D.C., National Research Council, First Report, 1956; Second Report, 1960.

11

Radiation Hazards and Their Avoidance

Historical Introduction. Within a short time after the discovery of x rays and of radioactive substances, it was recognized that the radiations were potential health hazards. Skin areas repeatedly exposed to them became dry, scaly, ulcerated, and as years went by cancer developed in some of these ulcers. Experiments with animals showed that other types of lesions could be produced, that life could be shortened, and even that the progeny of the irradiated creatures could show defects. A relationship was demonstrated between quantity of radiation received and degree of damage, and there were radiation levels below which no effects could be detected. These effects have been discussed in some detail in the preceding chapter.

The idea of setting up levels of "safe" exposure for radiation workers began to be developed in the 1920's, but it was not until after 1930 that radiation measurements were adequate to put "radiation-safety" standards on a workable basis. The first approach to a numerical value was based on surveys of existing installations, where individuals had been working for considerable periods under conditions such that their exposures could be evaluated, at least approximately. Based on the observation that no detectable radiation effects had been produced in a group of individuals who had been receiving radiation at rates definitely higher than 1 roentgen per week, this limit was adopted in 1934 by the International Commission on Radiological Protection. In the United States in 1936 this was lowered to 0.1 roentgen per day, partly as a result of the belief that there was not an adequate factor of safety in the 1934 recommendation.

In 1946 the National Committee on Radiation Protection, of the United States, undertook a review of the whole problem of permissible exposures. Up to that time, the level set earlier had been described as a "tolerance dose," namely a dose which could be tolerated by anyone without expectation of harm. As more information became available about radiation effects, it became a question whether there was such a thing as a tolerance dose; it appeared more likely that *any* amount of radiation might produce some damage, and that it would be necessary to balance this possible damage against the known benefits. Therefore the term *tolerance dose* was rejected, and in its stead came the expression *maximum permissible dose* (MPD). The Committee then undertook to set up such permissible limits, with the understanding that these might be subject to revision as more information became available.

155

During the decade between the 1936 recommendations and the time of the study, new and more powerful sources of x rays had been developed, artificially radioactive nuclides had become available, the conditions under which persons might be exposed to radiation became more numerous and varied, and more was known about biological effects of radiations. At this time the permissible whole-body exposure to gamma rays and x rays in the usual energy range was set at 0.3 roentgen per week. This reduction was made in spite of the fact that, so far as was known, there was not a single case on record where an individual whose exposure did not exceed the previously established maximum had developed any detectable injury that could reasonably be attributed to that radiation exposure. National Bureau of Standards Handbook 59, *Permissible Dose from External Sources of Ionizing Radiation,* contains a detailed treatment of these recommendations.

Present Recommendations. Nevertheless a further reduction in maximum permissible dose was agreed upon by national and international organizations in 1956. This is still not based on any positive evidence of damage at the earlier levels, but is rather in accordance with trends of scientific opinion. It is recognized that there are many uncertainties in the available data, and it is believed that there will be a large future increase in radiation uses.

Until the current recommendations, no overt attention was paid to the genetic problem. It was recognized that genetic damage could be produced, but it was felt that the great mass of the population received so little radiation that the contribution to the genetic *average* by the dose received by radiation workers would be negligible. However, with the greatly increasing use of medical x rays and the widespread applications of atomic energy, this may no longer be the case. Accordingly the entire populace has been divided into two groups, a small one consisting of those who work with radiation or radioactive substances under the supervision of a radiation safety officer, and a very large one consisting of everyone else. The recommendations for radiation workers (occupational exposure) apply to all medical users of radioactive nuclides and to their patients except when these are receiving treatments or tests designed to benefit them; they apply to personnel in departments where radiation use is adequately controlled, but not to the general hospital or office staff nor to casual visitors. They are given in detail in subsequent paragraphs.

Present Sources of Radiation to Which Human Beings are Exposed. Sources of radiation may be divided into *natural,* over which little or no control can be exerted, and *man-made,* which could be subject to modification.

Natural sources are cosmic rays, radiations from earth and building materials, and radioactive substances regularly found as constituents of the body. Cosmic rays increase in intensity with altitude, the dose rate being about twice as great in places a mile or so high as at sea level. Environmental radiation depends on the type of soil or rock upon which the individual lives, and on the material (stone, brick, or wood) of which his buildings are constructed. Inside a stone house on a granite base there may be more than twice as much radiation as in a wooden house on deep soil. The radioactive content of the average human adult is about $\frac{1}{7}$ μCi of potassium-40, $\frac{1}{17}$ μCi of carbon-14, and a trace of radium. The total radiation to the average individual from all these natural sources, external and internal, is in general from 100 to 200 millirads per year, and this dose is received by everyone.

Of man-made sources, for those who are not actually radiation workers, by far the most important is medical and dental x rays, and here, of course, the variation among individuals is tremendous. In addition there are small contributions from various luminous devices and other equipment containing radioactive material, from nuclear power plants and related activities, and from fall-out from nuclear weapons. This last is often greatly exaggerated. For individuals in the United States, now and in the foreseeable future (unless there is nuclear war), it amounts to something like $\frac{1}{5}$ of the dose received from cosmic rays.

In the preceding chapter it was pointed out that genetic changes were the only ones of real concern for the general population, and that these depended on the *average* exposure to all prospective parents throughout their reproductive lifetimes. If the medical, dental, and occupational exposures of part of the population are averaged for everybody, and the fallout contribution included, the result is approximately equal to the exposure from natural sources.

If any individual is engaged in an occupation involving use of x rays, radioactive substances, or nuclear reactors, the somatic rather than the genetic hazard is to be considered; it is now a question of individual welfare rather than that of the race. Since radiation workers are only a fraction of 1 per cent of the total population, they may be considered as a very special class. Users of radioactive nuclides, of course, fall into this class, and the control of their exposures will be considered at some length.

Maximum Permissible Dose Recommendations for Occupational Conditions (MPD's in Controlled Areas). The basis of the present recommendations is the *total* accumulated dose in an individual's lifetime, rather than a daily or weekly allotment. The unit is the *rem;* this is the quantity of any ionizing radiation which has the same biological effectiveness as 1 rad of x rays in the usual energy range. Various radiations have various *relative biological effectiveness* (*RBE*), which differ according to the specific ionization; the dose in rems is equal to the dose in rads multiplied by the RBE for the radiation in question. Since for all beta and gamma radiations from radioactive nuclides considered in this book, the RBE is unity, it is satisfactory to use rads in thinking of the recommendations, although they will be quoted below in rems.

The maximum permissible accumulated dose at any age, to the whole body, the gonads, or the lens of the eye, in rems, is equal to five times the number of years beyond 18, provided no annual increment exceeds 12 rems. Thus the accumulated MPD = 5(N-18) rems, where N is the age and greater than 18. (Occupational exposure should not start before age 18.) This implies an *average* weekly dose of 0.1 rem if the exposure is a regular part of the occupation. However, there are provisions for fluctuations as long as the annual total is kept at about 5 rems. A permissible weekly whole body dose of 0.3 rems may be maintained for an appreciable period, provided that in another period the dose is enough less to keep the total for the year within the set limit. Even the 0.3 rems in a week may be exceeded for short periods but in this case the total accumulation in 13 consecutive weeks must not exceed 3 rems. Again, such a period of high exposure must be compensated for by an adequate period of low.

In radiation work the hands and forearms are often exposed to more radiation than any other part of the body. Since hands and forearms do not constitute a critical region involving either gonads or vital organs, it is permissible for them to receive considerably more radiation. Their annual maximum permissible dose has been set at 75 rem; fluctuations may be treated in the same manner as for whole body doses. For individuals starting radiation work at ages greater than 18, who might be presumed to have a "back-log" of permissible radiation, a level of 12 rem per year is established. This is to prevent undue exploitation of the older worker. Even in this situation, the limit of 3 rem in any 13 consecutive weeks must be maintained.

Maximum Permissible Dose Recommendations for the Whole Population. (MPD's for the General Public.) For the general population the significant dose is that to the gonads during the entire period from conception to the end of reproduction. This must include all radiation from both natural and man-made sources. The present statement is that the genetically significant dose during the first 30 years of life should not exceed, on the average, 5 rems plus the lowest practicable contributions from medical exposure and background, all of which amounts to a maximum of about 10 rems. This is now generally accepted as the permissible average population dose for the first 30 years of life; thereafter, until the end of child-bearing it is usually taken as 5 rems per decade. It must be kept in mind that in the genetic picture it is the *average* to all prospective parents that counts; there may be very wide variations among individuals.

Dosage Due to Internal Emitters. Radiation levels for radionuclides deposited within the body must conform to the same general principles as for external irradiation. For occupational exposure the dose to the gonads or to the total body shall not exceed 3 rems in any period of 13 consecutive weeks, or 5 rems in 1 year. The dose to any single organ except gonads, bone, skin, and thyroid shall not exceed 15 rems in 1 year. Skin and thyroid may receive twice this amount. One-half of the annual dose limit may be accumulated in any period of a quarter of a year; in this case the dose for the rest of the year may not exceed the other half. For non-occupational exposure, the permissible doses are usually taken as 1/10th of the occupational. Internal radionuclide exposure outside controlled areas can only occur from drinking contaminated water or inhaling contaminated air, and therefore is related to disposal of radioactive waste. This subject will be considered in the next chapter.

Methods for determining dose from radioactive material within the body have been discussed in Chapter 9, and their application to protection problems will be discussed later in this chapter.

All medical uses are considered as coming more or less under controlled area regulations. However, when it is a question of radionuclide therapy, or of diagnostic procedures from which the patient is expected to receive some advantage, it is evident that these limits cannot be imposed, any more than they can in diagnostic and therapeutic applications of x rays. Here the matter of the benefit to be obtained from the radiation must be weighed against the possible harm, and the patient's doctor must make the final decision. On the other hand, in research, where normal (or even diseased) individuals are to be used in studies with radioactive material every effort must be made to keep the dose at the lowest practicable level.

Radiation Protection Supervisor (RPS). In any institution where radioactive nuclides are used for medical or research purposes, there must be a Radiation Protection Supervisor (RPS) who is responsible for safe use of all radioactive material. His duties include responsibility for determining radiation exposure to anyone concerned with radioactive nuclides, the supervision of disposal of radioactive waste, and the removal of any radioactive contamination if it should occur. He should check safety of all laboratory procedures, and of all activities connected with care of patients who are receiving radionuclides. All procedures discussed in the remainder of this chapter should be subject to his review and approval.

Radiation Monitoring for Personnel and Area Safety. This subject is treated in some detail in Chapter 21. It should be noted here that continuing records of radiation exposure are required for all persons subject to occupational exposure. They are usually obtained by film badges worn for specified times and suitably processed. For relatively brief periods, small ionization-chamber instruments are available. For establishing adequacy of shielding, or for checking on local contamination, various types of dose- or dose-rate meters may be used.

Consistent carrying out of both types of monitoring, and careful inspection of the records of these measurements, make it possible to insure that the chance of over-exposure is very low. If a film badge does show too high a reading, it should be possible to find out quickly whether this was the result of a genuine over-exposure, or of such a mistake as wearing the badge on a laboratory coat while dental x rays were taken, or possibly of an error in the processing laboratory. In any case, the trouble must be promptly identified and its repetition avoided.

The Radionuclide Laboratory. The laboratory must be designed to provide all necessary safety. Some specific suggestions will be presented in Chapter 11; various books and AEC publications supply more details. A few points sometimes given insufficient emphasis may be mentioned.

All surfaces should be smooth, non-porous, and waterproof. Floor covering should be asphalt, rubber or vinyl tile, or linoleum; concrete and wood are highly undesirable. Walls, especially around sinks and other critical areas, should be covered with high-gloss enamel paint. Bench tops should be stainless steel, especially where radioactive solutions are to be handled. In any case, operations should be carried out on easily cleanable plastic or metal trays.

In most such laboratories a fume hood is installed, although this is seldom necessary for handling solutions at room temperature. The hood must be of such design that eddy currents cannot return contaminated air to laboratory space. It is necessary for the hood to be mounted on a base sturdy enough to support considerable shielding, if appreciable quantities of gamma emitters are to be handled. The hood must not discharge into a general institutional duct system, but must have its own exhaust high enough above the roof of the building to ensure that contaminated gases cannot re-enter through windows.

Sinks should be of stainless steel or alberene stone, with separate drainboards for clean and dirty glassware. Water valves should be controlled by foot or knee levers.

For manipulating moderate amounts of beta emitters, a "gloved box" is convenient. This is rarely necessary in the medical radionuclide laboratory, but is frequently useful in radiochemical and radiobiological procedures. It is simply a closed container with a suitable ventilation and exhaust system, into which shoulder-length gloves have been built. The operator, outside the box, inserts his hands and arms into the gloves, and can then carry out procedures inside the box without danger of contamination.

Safety Procedures with External Beta-Particle Emitters. Beta rays *per se* never constitute a whole-body external radiation hazard; their range in tissue seldom exceeds a few millimeters. Ranges in water and in glass, in relation to maximum beta energy are given in Figure 11–1. Thus it is seen that ^{32}P betas ($E_{max} = 1.7$ MeV) cannot traverse more than 9 mm of water or tissue; a glass bottle with 3 mm walls will stop most of them.

However, it must be remembered that in traversing matter these beta rays give rise to bremsstrahlung. It was stated in Chapter 7 that the fraction of the beta energy appearing as external bremsstrahlung is approximately equal to $\dfrac{ZE}{3000}$, where E is the maximum beta energy and Z the atomic number of the absorber. Thus the 3 mm glass which stops the beta particles serves as a source for penetrating x rays whose maximum energy is over a million volts. Only about 1 per cent of the total energy will emerge in this way, but for a large quantity of the nuclide this would not be negligible. Therefore appreciable quantities of radioactive nuclides emitting penetrating beta particles should be stored in shielded containers.

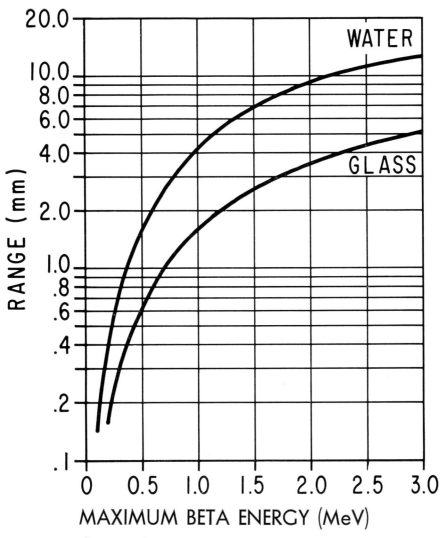

FIG. 11–1.   Ranges of beta particles in water and in glass.

A gamma emitter may have low energy gammas but higher energy betas, so that the bremsstrahlung is more penetrating than the gamma rays. In this case the heavy shield against the gamma rays (see below) should have a lining of low atomic number material to reduce the quantity of bremsstrahlung. For instance ^{42}K has 3.58 MeV betas and 1.5 MeV gammas. An aluminum lining in the lead shield stops the betas and greatly reduces the bremsstrahlung.

One of the greatest hazards with beta-emitters is the handling of uncovered vessels containing the material. In Chapter 9 a method is given for calculating dose due to beta-emitting flat sources. In an open solution of ^{32}P with a concentration of 1 mCi per cu cm the dose rate at the surface is about 13 rads per minute and this will not be appreciably reduced by attenuation in a few centimeters of air. Obviously a hand or face over such an open container may receive a considerable dose of radiation in a short time.

Safety Procedures with External Gamma Ray Emitters. Gamma rays are in general much more penetrating than beta rays, and accordingly require more precautions in handling. Two methods are available for reducing radiation intensity, increasing the distance between the radiation source and the recipient, and interposing a barrier to absorb the radiation.

The decrease in intensity due to increased distance results from the geometrical phenomenon known as the *inverse square law*. Consider a point source of radiation at the center of a sphere of radius r. The surface of this sphere is $4\pi r^2$ sq cm, hence 1 sq cm will receive $\dfrac{1}{4\pi r^2}$ times the total energy emitted. On the surface of a larger sphere, of radius R, 1 sq cm will receive $\dfrac{1}{4\pi R^2}$ times the total.

Hence

$$\frac{\text{radiation per unit area at distance r}}{\text{radiation per unit area at distance R}} = \frac{\dfrac{1}{4\pi r^2}}{\dfrac{1}{4\pi R^2}} = \frac{R^2}{r^2},$$

or, the intensity of the radiation is inversely proportional to the square of the distance from a point source. For sources which are not points, the actual falling off of intensity with distance is slower.

In general it is not feasible to carry out all operations at considerable distances from radiation sources, and so shields or barriers are interposed. In the case of radioactive nuclides these barriers usually take the form of containers of lead or other heavy material in which the radioactive substances are placed. The thickness of lead necessary depends on the quantity of the nuclide, the energy of the gamma radiation, the distance to the person, the duration of the expected exposure, and the specific gamma ray constant Γ.

For any number of millicuries, N, the dose rate at 1 cm from a point source is $N\Gamma$ roentgens per hour, and at any other distance d cm it is $\dfrac{N\Gamma}{d^2}$ R per hr. For example at 50 cm from 20 mCi of ^{131}I the dose rate would be $\dfrac{20 \times 2.20}{(50)^2} = 0.017$ R per hr or 17 milliroentgens per hour.

Working conditions should be based on the MPD of 0.1 rem per week for constant exposure. For a 40-hour week this corresponds to 2.5 mR per hour. To reduce 17 mR per hr to 2.5 mR per hr would require a barrier cutting down the intensity by a factor of 7 times. In calculating barrier thicknesses it must be remembered that one half value layer of the barrier material reduces the radiation to one-half, two half value layers to one-fourth, three to one-eighth, and so on.

Table 11–1. Lead Half Value Layers and Specific Gamma Ray Constants for Various Radioactive Nuclides

Element	Atomic Number	Mass Number	HVL Cm Lead	R /mCi-hr at 1 Cm
Bromine	35	82	1.2	14.6
Calcium	20	47	1.1	5.95
Cesium	55	137	0.5	3.1
Chromium	24	51	0.2	0.15
Cobalt	27	60	1.2	13.0
Copper	29	64	0.4	1.1
Gold	79	198	0.3	2.3
Iodine	53	130	1.0	12.1
Iodine	53	131	0.6	2.20
Iodine	53	132	1.4	9.4
Iridium	77	192	0.6	5.1
Iron	26	59	1.1	6.4
Manganese	25	52	1.2	18.5
Mercury	80	203	0.3	1.2
Molybdenum	42	99	0.5	1.29
Potassium	19	42	1.2	1.4
Radium (in equil.)	88	226	1.3	8.25
Selenium	34	75	0.3	1.76
Silver	47	110m	1.3	14.3
Sodium	11	22	1.1	13.0
Sodium	11	24	1.6	18.7
Tantalum	73	182	1.2	6.8
Tellurium	52	121	0.5	4.2
Tin	50	113	0.3	3.4
Zinc	30	65	1.0	2.9

Lead is usually employed in the construction of barriers and shielded containers, since for a given reduction in radiation its bulk will be less than that of any other practicable material. In Table 11–1 are listed half value layers in lead for radioactive materials likely to be employed in hospitals. together with the gamma dose rate constants.

For any particular situation, with a specified amount of any radionuclide, the R per hr at the position is calculated as just indicated:

$$\text{R per hr} = \frac{N\Gamma}{d^2}. \qquad 11-(1)$$

The attenuation which must be supplied by the barrier (attenuation factor) is then found by dividing this value of R per hour by the permissible R per hour for the situation in question.

$$\text{Att. Fact} = \frac{\dfrac{N\Gamma}{d^2}}{\text{Permissible dose rate per hour}}. \qquad 11-(2)$$

From this factor the necessary number of half value layers is immediately obtained. Table 11–2 is useful for this purpose.

Table 11–2. Relation between Attenuation Factor and Number of Half Value Layers

Att Fact	1	2	3	5	7	10	15	20	30	50	75	100
No HVL	0	1	1.6	2.3	2.8	3.3	3.9	4.3	4.9	5.6	6.2	6.6

In deciding barriers for any particular set of conditions, a *work factor* may be employed. For instance, the technician will not spend an entire 40-hour week 50 cm from strong radiation sources. If the entire radionuclide laboratory is to be maintained at 2.5 mR per hour or less, this factor must be used for all barrier calculations. In this case the dose level at the worst location will be 2.5 mR per hr and will be much less throughout most of the area. If, on the other hand, she spends a maximum of 10 hours a week close to sources, and the rest of the time in rooms with radiation levels less than 1 mR per hr, the activity at the working position may be about 10 mR per hr.

The barrier to be employed will usually be selected according to the total radionuclide load. Because some nuclides emit much more penetrating radiations than others, it may not be the greatest number of millicuries that sets the limit. As an example, consider a laboratory where on different days the working space will have to accommodate in one week

$$200 \text{ mCi of } ^{131}\text{I},$$
$$150 \text{ mCi of } ^{198}\text{Au},$$
$$20 \text{ mCi of } ^{24}\text{Na},$$
$$15 \text{ mCi of } ^{32}\text{P}.$$

The average distance for the period of actual manipulation is about 50 cm; less than half an hour will be spent in this position with each nuclide. However, 2 hours may be spent at an average distance of 1.5 meters with the sodium and the iodine. In addition it is expected that 10 hours will be spent in a region of possibly 2.5 mR per hr. Out of a 40-hour week, then, about half is at set levels of activity and the 100 mR may be divided among them. The phosphorus may, of course, be neglected in planning gamma ray barriers.

If the 50-cm dose rate is maintained at 15 mR per hour, three half-hour exposures add to 22.5 mR. The 1.5 meter distance dose rate automatically drops to $\frac{1}{9}$ that at 50 cm, or 1.7 mR per hour. Four hours at this level total 6.8 mR. Ten hours in a general 2.5 mR per hour field total 25 mR. Thus all the exposures mentioned add to just about half the weekly permissible exposure, leaving a good margin of safety. The necessary barrier is set by the manipulation at the work table with 50 cm distance for one-half hour.

For 200 mCi ^{131}I, $\quad \dfrac{200 \times 2.20}{2500} = 0.176$ R per hr.

150 mCi ^{198}Au, $\quad \dfrac{150 \times 2.3}{2500} = 0.138$ R per hr.

20 mCi ^{24}Na, $\quad \dfrac{20 \times 18.7}{2500} = 0.150$ R per hr.

To bring these exposure rates to 15 mR per hr, the attenuation factors are

For the ^{131}I, $\quad \dfrac{176}{15} = 11.7$, requiring 3.5 hvl or 2 cm Pb.

^{198}Au, $\quad \dfrac{138}{15} = 9.1$, $\qquad$ 3.2 hvl or 1 cm Pb.

^{24}Na, $\quad \dfrac{150}{15} = 10$, $\qquad$ 3.3 hvl or 5 cm Pb.

Obviously the sodium barrier is the important one, and if 5 cm of lead are used, the radiations from all the other radionuclides will be reduced much below the necessary level. It might then be inquired what the result would be of using only 3 cm of lead as a barrier. This is only two half value layers for the sodium, so that during the half hour of exposure to this nuclide the dose would be 18.5 mR. However, the dose rates for the iodine and the gold would still be reduced to very low levels, so that this reduction would be justified if there were a reason for reducing barrier weight or thickness.

It is obviously unreasonable to insist on providing such a barrier that the radiation everywhere is reduced to 2.5 mR per hr or less. If an analysis of the expected work load is carried out as indicated, with a reasonable factor of safety for occasional exposure, there will be adequate protection.

It should be pointed out that mere interposition of a barrier between the source and the operator may not be sufficient. If the source is close to a

12

wall, and there is no barrier between source and wall, a considerable amount of radiation may be scattered back into the room. Similarly, if the source is on a table, the bottom of the container should be shielded to prevent scatter from the floor. Of course protection must always be provided for occupants of rooms beyond walls or under floors.

Although the body of the operator is protected by shields, his hands and face may not be, as manipulations are carried out. Care must be taken to keep containers closed and adequately covered with lead except during actual pipetting or diluting. Pipetting by mouth should *never* be done, and pipettes or other instruments should be tilted so that the hand does not come over the open container. Forceps and other tools should have adequately long handles, but not so long as to cause awkwardness. There are many special tools available on the market; this is not the place to describe them.

The Accidental Radioactive "Spill." It is inevitable that, in a busy laboratory or hospital, radioactive material will some time be spilled on floor, furniture, or personnel. If a container has been upset, it should immediately be righted, care being taken not to touch wet parts with bare hands. Paper towels should immediately be dropped on spilled liquid to keep it from spreading, but further operations usually need not be done in a hurry. The first thing is to make sure that no person has become contaminated. If he has, he must immediately get rid of contaminated clothing and scrub contaminated skin. (Detailed instructions for these and other procedures will be found in National Bureau of Standards Handbook 48, Control and Removal of Radioactive Contamination in Laboratories, which should be in the hands of every user of appreciable quantities of radioactive nuclides. See also page 180.)

An important part of cleaning up the spill is to prevent its spread. As much as possible of the spilled material should be taken up with damp papers, which must be handled with forceps and deposited immediately into a container for contaminated waste. After as much as possible has been removed in this way, the surface should be washed with damp—not wet— rags, always working toward the center rather than out from it. Monitoring should be carried out throughout the procedure. Reduction of counting rate over 1 or 2 square feet to 5 times background, or over a few square inches to 10 times background is usually satisfactory, especially for short-lived nuclides.

Transportation of Radioactive Material within the Institution, and Administration of Doses to Patients. When radioactive material is to be transported from one part of the hospital to another, the thickness of the portable lead container will depend on the amount and kind of nuclide and the time in transit. Very heavy containers for large doses of radioactive gold or iodine should be mounted on wheeled carts or tables.

In administering radioactive material to patients by mouth, different procedures may be used depending on the quantity of radionuclide. Tracer and small therapy doses are available from commercial suppliers in capsule form; in this case the patient handles the capsule and swallows it with an adequate amount of water. When the tracer dose is in solution, it is usually poured into a paper cup, the bottle rinsed two or three times, the rinsings added to the liquid in the cup, and the whole given to the patient to drink, followed by more water poured into the same cup. For a therapy dose the bottle is not taken out of its shield. The patient drinks the active solution through a beverage straw; water is then poured into the bottle and drunk through the same straw, and the process repeated to be sure that no radioactive residue remains. All used cups, straws, and wipes of any kind are taken back to the radionuclide laboratory for proper disposal.

For intracavitary colloidal gold, the infusion apparatus is usually transported on the same cart with the gold, and after the procedure all of the the contaminated equipment is returned to the laboratory.

The Radioactive Patient. The patient who receives radioactive material now becomes a potential source of radiation and must be treated accordingly. No tracer or test dose will make a patient active enough to demand any precautions, and this is also true for therapy doses up to a few millicuries, *as long as the material remains in the patient.* Radioactive vomitus or excreta can cause contamination; in a hospital personnel should be instructed as to precautions to be taken in disposing of the material. Some details will be given in the next chapter. At home, a single small therapeutic dose would never lead to a hazardous situation.

For larger doses more definite precautions are necessary, both in the hospital and at home. The criterion in all cases is to keep the exposure to all other persons below the maximum permissible levels.

In any institution where radioactive nuclides are employed, there must be a Radiation Protection Supervisor (RPS) responsible for establishing procedures for the safe use of these materials, as mentioned above. He should be informed prior to the administration of any therapeutic dose, and should decide whether special precautions are needed. It has been agreed (NCRP Report No. 36) that the following doses of short-lived nuclides do not ordinarily need special precautions: ^{131}I, 8 mCi; ^{198}Au, 23 mCi; Radon, 5 mCi. For doses larger than these, or for any dose of longer-lived gamma-emitting nuclides, the radiation exposure rate at 1 meter from the patient, due to his radioactive dose, should be determined immediately after administration. This can be done by calculation on the basis of the Γ factor, or by measurement with a suitable survey instrument; the resulting data should be entered on the radioactivity tag attached to the patient's chart and to his bed or his person.

Permissible Times for Attendance on Radioactive Patients. On the basis of this information, precautions can be established. In institutions having relatively few patients treated with radioactive nuclides (including radium) it should be possible to maintain all personnel within the non-occupational exposure levels of 0.5 R per year. This will be the situation in many hospitals. On the other hand, there is an appreciable number which have relatively large radionuclide services, where it may be necessary to consider nurses and orderlies as radiation workers. In this case they must be instructed and monitored in the same manner as other radio-nuclide personnel.

Nursing attendance rules for either level of exposure will be based on exposure rates as determined at the time of dose administration. Some helpful data are given in Table 11–3. Here are listed the exposure rates in milliroentgens per hour at 1 meter from 100 mCi of various nuclides, based on the data of Table 11–1. The radiation from a patient containing this much nuclide will always be somewhat less than the calculated value, due to absorption of some of the radiation in the body of the individual, so their use furnishes a small factor of safety.

Table 11–3. Milliroentgens per Hour at 1 Meter from 100 mCi of Several Radionuclides

Radionuclide	MR/Hr at 1 Meter (=3.27 Feet)
Iodine-131	22
Gold-198	23
Iridium-192	51
Cobalt-60	130
Cesium-137	31
Radium or Radon	83

The permissible personnel exposure will depend on whether occupational or non-occupational levels are sought. The occupational level of or 20 mR per day (for a 5 day week), or the non-occupational level $\frac{1}{10}$ of this, could be maintained continuously. Exposure times leading to the occupational level are given in Table 11–4, for a number of nuclides and of distances from the patient, calculated from the data of Table 11–3. Thus from 100 mCi of ^{131}I or [198]Au, 20 mR would be received in 20 minutes at 2 feet, 45 minutes at 3 feet, 80 minutes at 4 feet, or 3 hours at 6 feet. For other quantities the relative times would be inversely proportional to the amounts. That is, for 50 mCi all times would be twice as long, and so on. For non-occupational exposure rates, all times would be $\frac{1}{10}$ of those listed.

When this table is used for calculating permissible nursing times, the rapid decay of some nuclides must be taken into consideration. That is, the quantity of [198]Au that was 100 mCi on the first day, will be reduced to half of that by the third day and to half again after the sixth. Obviously the time for 20 mR increases as the quantity of the radionuclide decreases. On the other hand, for the long lived material, the daily exposure rate will remain constant. If exposure to such a radioactive patient occurs only at intervals, daily permissible doses may be two or three times as high as those listed, as long as the permissible quarterly dose is not exceeded. In special cases where higher exposures may be unavoidable, nursing duty should be divided.

Table 11–4. Approximate Times for Exposure of 20 mR from 100 mCi of Various Radionuclides at Four Distances

Time for Exposure of 20 mR

Radionuclide 100 mCi	2 Ft. (min.)	3 Ft. (min.)	4 Ft. (min.)	6 Ft. (min.)	(hr.)
Iodine-131 . . .	20	46	82	184	3
Gold-198	20	44	78	176	3
Iridium-192 . .	9	20	35	80	1.33
Cobalt-60 . . .	3.3	7.5	13	30	0.5
Cesium-137 . .	15	34	60	136	2.67
Radium or Radon .	5	12	21	48	0.8

In the institution having few radiation cases, the annual permissible dose to the general population may be the basis for nursing planning. If a nurse were not to be expected to care for more than 3 such patients a year, and to have no other radiation exposure, she might be allowed to accumulate $\frac{1}{3}$ of her annual permissible dose of 0.5 R, or 170 mR, per patient. Consider a patient with 60 mg of radium, on the ward for 5 days. The permissible daily exposure would be $\frac{1}{5}$ of 170 mR = 34 mR. This would be acquired at 2 feet in 14.5 minutes ($\frac{34}{20} \times \frac{100}{60} \times 5$) and at 4 feet in 58 minutes. Obviously there is plenty of time for the necessary care,— but this should not be repeated for a few months.

General Precautions. As stated above, the Radiation Protection Supervisor is responsible for directing all necessary precautionary procedures. However, some general instructions may be listed. Radioactive materials should not be allowed to come into contact with the skin. Rubber or plastic gloves should be worn whenever such contact is possible, as for instance in handling bedpans for these patients. Articles or utensils suspected of being contaminated should be turned over to the safety officer for monitoring; disposable materials such as paper handkerchiefs should be put into non-porous paper garbage bags until they can be thus disposed of. No precautions are usually necessary for dishes, instruments, or utensils, unless contamination (as by vomiting) is known to have occurred. Standard items of nursing care, such as basins and bedpans, should be thoroughly washed with soap and running water; the nurse or orderly should wear heavy rubber gloves while doing this. The same items should be used for an individual patient until his treatment is considered terminated. If they were used for a patient who had received a large dose of ^{131}I, they should be monitored before being returned to stock. If the patient vomits, is incontinent, or leaks material from a drainage wound (especially in the case of radioactive gold), the RPS should be summoned at once. In the meantime all unnecessary people should be removed from the contaminated neighborhood, and every effort made to confine the contamination until it can be dealt with as discussed in "spills" above.

Protection of Other Patients from Radiation. Whenever a patient has received such a dose that radiation precautions are required for nursing care, attention must also be paid to the possibility of his irradiating other patients. Bed or patient separation must be such that no other patient can receive more than 0.5 R in 1 year. It is desirable to reduce this to 0.2 or 0.3 R from a single patient, because of the possibility of a second exposure.

In the usual case, exposure of one patient by another will be for a determinable time. A patient with 60 mg of radium, at 6 feet from his neighbor, will irradiate him at the rate of 15 mR per hour. If both are confined to bed, with this separation, the dose will amount to 360 mR in 24 hours. This is an unacceptably high rate of exposure. However, in general, it is not likely that during the whole period exactly the 6-foot separation will be maintained. It is accordingly evident that any good approximation of such patient doses must depend on knowledge of their relative movements, as well as on bed separation. When there is any question about such a case, the RPS should make a careful study of it and establish appropriate procedures.

Visitors for Radioactive Patients. There is seldom need of restricting visits by adults, but they may be cautioned to sit a few feet away from the patient. Children or pregnant women should not be permitted to visit, unless it seems extremely desirable.

Discharge of Radioactive Patients from the Hospital. It is recommended by the AEC that any patient carrying a dose of more than 30 mCi of any nuclide should be hospitalized. However, in the light of the preceding discussions, it appears that this can often be liberalized, while at the same time it should be tightened in certain areas. Hospitalization need not be required for patients receiving less than 8 mCi of ^{131}I (see page 167). Patients receiving larger doses should be hospitalized for at least 24 hours; during this period most of the nuclide not utilized will have been excreted. In the case of intracavitary colloidal instillation it is recommended that the patient be hospitalized for at least 48 hours to make sure that the puncture wound is healing.

Following these delays, or in other instances where no delay may be necessary, patients who have received therapeutic doses of radioactive nuclides having lives less than 100 days shall be governed by the following provisions:

A. If all persons with whom the patient expects to have appreciable contact are over 45 years of age, the patient may be discharged if the maximum integrated exposure at a distance of 1 meter from the patient, for continous exposure, does not exceed 5 R in 1 year.

B. If individuals under the age of 45 years must be considered, for these individuals the integrated exposure must not exceed 0.5 R in one year

The initial exposure rates at 1 meter, or initial millicuries which will result in an integrated exposure of 5 R are listed for several nuclides in Table 11–5; for an integrated exposure of 0.5 R of course the amounts are all $\frac{1}{10}$ of those in the table.

Table 11–5. Initial Exposure Rate, or Initial Millicuries which Result in an Integrated Exposure of 5 R at 1 Meter, Computed for Complete Decay

Radioactive Nuclide	Milliroentgens per Hour per mCi at 1 Meter	Initial Exposure Rate Leading to 5 R Total (mR/Hr at 1 Meter, Approx.)	Corresponding Radioactivity (Millicuries Approx.)
Iodine-131 . . .	0.22	20	80
Gold-198	0.23	50	230
Radon . . .	0.825	40	50

It is highly unlikely that any person will be permanently as close as 1 meter from the patient, so that even larger doses would be permissible in the usual case. Assume that one person might spend 2 hours at 50 cm in certain nursing procedures, and the rest of the time at an average distance of about 6 feet (about 2 meters). Two hours at 50 cm equal in exposure 8 hours at 1 meter. Sixteen hours at 2 meters equal 4 hours at 1 meter. Similar considerations lead to the fact that essentially any likely dose of the first three nuclides offers no hazard to the older individual. For longer-lived nuclides special rules must be set up.

For the integrated exposure of 0.5 R permitted to individuals less than 45 years old the amounts at 1 meter would all be $\frac{1}{10}$ of those in the table. For these persons a table of more specific data has been compiled (Table 11-6). Here two types of "contact" are listed:—no contact and 1 hour per day. No contact means that the distance between the patient and the individual under 45 years of age should be greater than 2 meters. The

Table 11–6. Approximate Times for Permissible Exposure at Indicated Distances from Patients with Indicated Initial Exposure Rates at 1 Meter, or Indicated Radionuclide Content (for Persons under 45 Years of Age)

I Radioactive Nuclide	II Exposure Rate at 1 Meter at Time of Discharge from Hospital mR/Hr	III Approx. Activity at Time of Discharge mCi	IV No Contact (2 Meters) Weeks	V 1 Hr/Day (1 Meter) Weeks
Iodine-131 . . .	11.0	50	1st	2–4th inc.
Gold-198 . . .	11.5	50	1st	2nd
Radon	16	20	1st	2nd

second period is self-explanatory. Holding of children or infants should not be allowed until the period listed in Column V is past, and then only for a brief period each day.

For somewhat smaller initial exposure rates or doses, observation of the same times will result in a larger margin of safety, and this is probably simpler than trying to make adjustments in the table. If the initial rates are as little as half those tabulated, obviously times in each category can be doubled, or distances reduced to $\frac{3}{4}$.

For initial exposure rates appreciably exceeding those tabulated, corresponding reductions must be made in the permissible times.

Handling of Bodies Containing Radioactive Nuclides. It will occasionally happen that a patient requires emergency surgery shortly after receiving a therapeutic dose of radioactive isotope. Or the patient may die, in which case an autopsy may be desired, or the body will be embalmed. The handling of such bodies may pose problems of radiation exposure for the surgeon, the pathologist, or the embalmer. This subject is treated in detail in NCRP Report No. 36. Precautions in the Management of Patients Who Have Received Therapeutic Amounts of Radionuclides.

Here it may be briefly stated that a patient whose radionuclide content is not more than 5 mCi of any radioactive material does not constitute a hazard for any of these procedures. If surgery or autopsy is to be done on an individual at a time when the radioactive content is greater than this, the RPS should advise as to procedures, in accordance with information in the handbook. If the body is to be embalmed, when there is an appreciable radioactivity content, it is advisable to have the procedure carried out in the hospital morgue, with the advice of the R.P.S.

Safety Considerations for Radionuclides Administered Internally. When radioactive nuclides are administered internally for therapeutic purposes, of course there is no thought of keeping the dose to the patient within the permissible levels. However, when they are used for diagnostic studies, and particularly for research in normal human beings, every effort should be made to maintain low levels. Permissible levels for internal irradiation in occupational and nonoccupational situations have been specified above (page 158). Such exposure may arise from a single dose of a radionuclide or from continuous intake of contaminated water or air. In the latter case the individual is said to have a certain "body burden" of the material. The "permissible body burden" is the amount continuously present in the body which would never result in a dose greater than the permissible one.

Calculation of Dose from Body Burden. In calculating doses from body burdens the previously developed formula for $D_{\beta+\gamma}$ does not apply. This is for the case of a single dose administered and eventually totally decayed or eliminated. For material constantly taken in and eliminated, the procedure must be to calculate the dose per minute from a given burden, and then multiply by the number of minutes in a year. To determine the permissible burden, it is necessary to find the concentration which gives the permissible dose per minute. For the whole body, for occupational exposure, this is

$$\text{Dose (permissible)/min} = \frac{5 \text{ rad/yr}}{365 \text{ days/yr} \times 24 \text{ hr/day} \times 60 \text{ min/hr}}$$

$$= 9.5 \times 10^{-6} \text{ rad/min.} \qquad 11-(3)$$

From page 139 the dose per minute is

$$\text{d/min} = 3.55 \times 10^{-2} \text{ C } \overline{E}_\beta + 1.7 \times 10^{-5} \text{ C } \Gamma \, \overline{g} \text{ rads.}$$

For example, to find the permissible body burden for ^{137}Cs,

$$9.5 \times 10^{-6} = \frac{\mu\text{Ci}}{70{,}000} (3.55 \times 10^{-2} \times 0.242 + 1.7 \times 10^{-6} \times 120 \times 3.1).$$

$$\mu\text{Ci} = 44.$$

A great deal of information regarding dosage from internal emitters is given in the Report of Committee II on Permissible Dose for Internal Radiation (see References). Here are listed maximum permissible body burdens for whole body and for certain critical organs, and concentrations of radionuclides in air and water which may be continuously inhaled or ingested and maintain the same levels. Data are given regarding the part of the dose remaining in the whole body, or deposited in the critical organ, the metabolism and effective half life. Often, however, only the element is listed and it is not stated whether all compounds behave in the same manner or to which the data apply. Therefore effective half lives thus listed should not be used without some indication as to their applicability.

Permissible Tracer Doses. None of the tables in this Report gives information about permissible single doses such as tracers; this, however, is a problem with which the physician is likely to be concerned.

The recipients of deliberately administered radionuclides are usually considered at the occupational level,—they are aware that they are receiving radioactive material and their exposures are under the cognizance of a radiation protection supervisor. The permissible dose then would be the quantity to deliver not more than 3 rads in a quarter or 5 in a year. However, for a tracer it would not usually be desirable to use up the whole annual permissible dose in a single test, unless it was extremely important. A reasonable starting point would be to permit 1 rad to the entire body, or 3 to a definite organ, if necessary. In this case the formula for $D_{\beta+\gamma}$ is applicable, and the number of microcuries to give the specified dose is readily calculated.

It must be borne in mind that if the nuclide has a very long effective half life, so that the dose is not all delivered within a few months, the residual radioactivity may complicate other testing for a long period. For instance, with ^{60}Co in the liver, it is estimated that T_e is about 2 years. Then only about $\frac{1}{4}$ of the total dose is delivered within the first year and appreciable activity will persist for several years. Obviously in this case it would be very advantageous to switch to a shorter-lived isotope of cobalt.

It is apparent from the foregoing considerations that for any radionuclide the permissible dose depends on the chemical form in which the material is administered, the critical organ, the route of administration, the rate of elimination, and other factors. Any attempt at tabulating permissible doses for many nuclides under practical conditions of administration would involve a much broader survey of physiologic procedures than can be undertaken in such a text as the present one. However, the data in Appendix E, giving the total dose in the critical organ for 100 μCi of various radionuclides administered, can be used to advantage. For instance, if 100 μCi of ^{197}Hg give 1.65 rads in the kidneys in a year, and 3 rads are to be permitted, the permissible tracer is $\frac{3}{1.65} \times 100 = 180\,\mu$Ci. On the other hand, for ^{203}Hg, the permissible dose at the same level is $\frac{3}{11} \times 100 = 27\,\mu$Ci.

General Safety Routines. It is a relatively simple matter to calculate barriers and working distances to control radiation levels. Shielded equipment and long-handled tools can be bought. But in the last analysis the safety of the worker depends on his understanding of the problem and his adherence to the rules. The following suggestions may be used as a basis for day-by-day procedure:

1. Maintain "good house-keeping" at all times. Keep the laboratory neat; wash glassware regularly; do not let waste or contaminated material accumulate.

2. Wear rubber gloves and laboratory coat for all operations in the "hot" laboratory.

3. Make all possible set-ups on easily cleanable trays.

4. Cover all trays and all other work surfaces with disposable absorbent paper. (Good material of this sort is commercially available.)

5. Make sure that all containers of radioactive material are properly labeled at all times, both with a statement of the kind and quantity of radionuclide, and with a suitable radioactivity label. (Such labels are commercially available.)

6. Keep all active solutions covered.

7. *Never* pipette solutions by mouth.

8. Have available a paper sack pedal-operated garbage can for immediate disposal of all contaminated waste, including paper wipes.

9. Try out all new procedures with dummy runs not involving radioactive material.

10. Never allow eating, drinking or smoking in the "hot" laboratory.

11. Monitor all work areas regularly.

12. Employ standard personnel monitoring with either film badges or monitor ionization chambers, and keep careful records of all exposures.

13. Give immediate attention to cleaning up any contamination. (See next chapter.)

The Atomic Energy Commission and the "Agreement States" require that in any institution where a radionuclide program exists there should be a radiation protection supervisor, whose duties are to make sure that all procedures with radioactive materials are safely carried out. He may be a staff member or a consultant; he may be a physicist, a radiologist, or other professional individual, but he must be thoroughly conversant with basic safety procedures. His name and qualifications are filed as part of any application for a radionuclide license. He is to be depended upon for checking all routine procedures and for advising on any new developments. He must know where to look for radiation hazards and how to avoid or overcome them. His duties cover the laboratory and clinical uses of radioactive material, the disposal of radioactive waste, and the removal of radioactive contamination if it should occur. These last topics will be discussed in the next chapter.

The Federal Register, in Part 20, lays down regulations governing permissible levels, precautionary procedures, waste disposal, records and reports. Every user of radionuclides should be familiar with these; the suitable excerpt from the Register is available from the Isotopes Division of the Atomic Energy Commission. Every one holding a license to possess radionuclides is subject to inspection by the Commission's agents, and is expected to comply with these regulations.

The Atomic Energy Commission has turned over control of radionuclides to a number of states whose authorities agree to abide by essentially the same regulations. In these so-called "agreement states" licensure and inspection are by state rather than by AEC officials, but all procedures are in accordance with those established by the AEC. It is the hope that eventually all such control will lie with the states.

Radioactive Fall-out from Atomic Bombs. Consideration of the hazards to the human race resulting from the peace-time testing of nuclear weapons has been confused by the tremendous emotional impact of the possibility of war. A dispassionate effort should be made to separate the two, and to look at such facts as are available regarding the irradiation from this source as a part of the general picture of irradiation of the population. Fall-out contributes a certain amount of external irradiation from radioactive material in the air and on the ground; it was earlier mentioned that this was equal to only a small part of the natural background. It is not expected to reach as much as 10 per cent of background unless the testing programs of all nations possessing nuclear weapons are markedly increased. It is evident therefore that as far as the external irradiation hazard is concerned, fall-out is negligible.

More serious fears arise from the fact that two of the principal components of fall-out, radioactive strontium and radioactive cesium, have long lives. After falling to the ground they are taken into growing plants, which serve as foodstuffs for man or cattle. In the latter case they enter the human foodchain via the milk. Strontium in particular, since it is metabolized in much the same way as calcium, is built into the bones and gives off its radiation there, becoming a long-time menace. The question is, how great a menace? Not genetic, for these materials do not deposit in the gonads, and do not deliver, from other sites of deposit, enough radiation to the gonads to be significant. The dangers usually spoken of are the production of leukemia and bone cancer, and possible life shortening. Calculations of dose from internally deposited fall-out products at levels prevailing in the United States in the last few years, lead to values of the order of 30 millirads per year to the bones or bone marrow, or a total of about 1 rad in 30 years. In the preceding chapter it was pointed out that no cases of leukemia or bone cancer had been demonstrated to follow less than a few hundred rads administered in a relatively short time. There is no evidence of life shortening resulting from chronic irradiation at or well above fall-out levels.

Those who maintain that these small doses can result in leukemia or bone cancer base their assertions on the (completely unproven) statement that there is no threshold dose which must be reached before the condition can develop, but that the incidence of these somatic changes, like genetic ones, is proportional to dose, down to the lowest possible levels. If this postulate is accepted, the number of additional cases of these two diseases to be expected annually can be calculated from presently available statistics regarding radiation-produced leukemia and bone cancer. These numbers turn out to be such small percentages of the present incidences that it would be statistically impossible to find them; year-by-year fluctuations in mortality statistics are greater. The difficulty of ever obtaining significant human data for such low doses is almost insuperable. The only permissible conclusion at present is that it cannot be demonstrated that these conditions *cannot* be produced by fall-out,—neither can it be demonstrated that they *can*.

REFERENCES

Advisory Committee on Biology and Medicine, G. Failla, Chairman. Statement on Radioactive Fallout. American Scientist, Vol. 46, pp. 138–150, June, 1958.
Braestrup, C. B. and Wyckoff, H. O.: *Radiation Protection*, Springfield, Charles C Thomas, 1958.
British Medical Research Council. *The Hazards to Man of Nuclear and Allied Radiations. Second Report.* London, Her Majesty's Stationery Office, 1960.
Federal Register, National Archives of the United States, Washington, D. C. (Part 20, 1956).
Glasser, O., Quimby, E. H., Taylor, L. S., Weatherwax, L. J. and Morgan, R. H.: *Physical Foundations of Radiology*, 3rd Ed., Chapter 20, New York, Paul B. Hoeber, Inc., 1961.

International Commission on Radiological Protection, Report of Subcommittee II on Permissible Dose for Internal Radiation. New York, Pergamon Press, 1959.

MORGAN, R. H. and CORRIGAN, K. E.: *Handbook of Radiology*, Section 6, Chicago, Yearbook Publishers, Inc., 1955.

QUIMBY, E. H.: *Safe Handling of Radioactive Isotopes in Medical Practice*. New York, The Macmillan Co., 1960.

SCOTT, W. G. (Editor): *Planning Guide for Radiologic Installations*, Chicago, Year Book Publishers, Inc., 1953.

VENNART, J. and MINSKI, M.: Radiation Doses from Administered Radio-nuclides. Brit. Jour. Radiology, *35*, 372, 1962.

National Bureau of Standards Handbooks:

42. *Safe Handling of Radioactive Isotopes.*
52. *Maximum Permissible Amounts of Radioisotopes in the Human Body, amd Maximun Permissible Concentrations in Air and Water.*
59. *Permissible Dose from External Sources of Ionizing Radiation.*
69. *Maximum Permissible Body Burdens and Maximum Permissible Concentrations of Radionuclides in Air and Water for Occupational Expense.*
73. *Protection against Radiations from Sealed Gamma Ray Sources.*
80. *A Manual of Radioactivity Procedures.*
92. *Safe Handling of Radioactive Materials.*

National Council on Radiation Protection and Measurements: Report No. 36. *Precautions in the Management of Patients Who Have Received Therapeutic Amounts of Radionuclides.*

12

Disposal of Radioactive Waste and Removal of Contamination

General Considerations. For most medical users of radioactive nuclides, waste disposal problems will not be serious. Material to be disposed of will in general be short-lived; for longer-lived substances, quantities will be very small. Methods of disposal are by putting the radioactive waste into sewage or garbage, by incinerating it, by burying it underground or dumping it at sea, or by returning it to the Atomic Energy Commission. Factors influencing the choice of method will be the half life of the radionuclide, the chemical form and solubility of the material, and its bulk. (Bulky waste is generally limited to contaminated equipment and animal carcasses.)

There are two general methods of handling the material, which may be described as *dispersion* and *concentration*. The principle of disposal is so to manage that nobody can, under the worst circumstances, receive as much as a permissible dose of the radionuclide. *Dispersion* is accomplished by mixing the radioactive material with so much diluting substance— water, air, or other—that constant intake of the diluted mixture will not result in accumulation of a permissible dose. This is the basis in the first three methods mentioned above. *Concentration* is accomplished by reducing the volume as much as possible, and is the necessary first step for burial or sea disposal.

Atomic Energy Commission Rules. At the present time the Atomic Energy Commission has control over waste disposal of all radionuclides obtained from its facilities. They accept only two procedures without special permission, release into sanitary sewage systems, or burial in the soil.

Sewage disposal is applicable to soluble or readily dispersible material, so long as certain specified concentrations are not exceeded. These are tabulated in Title 10, Part 20 of the Federal Register, and are in general the concentration for constant intake for a 40-hour week (Hb 69). The disposer must therefore know the average water flow from his institution, and the proposed disposal of all radionuclides. In the United States the average hospital water flow is about 1000 liters per day per bed. It is apparent that except for very small institutions or very large disposals, hospital and laboratory waste, if it is soluble, presents no problem. The matter is further simplified by the fact that excreta from individuals undergoing medical diagnosis or therapy with radioactive materials are exempt from even these limitations.

Burial in soil is permissible under conditions which would be difficult to apply in practically any urban institution. It would be useful for large laboratories located in the country, with extensive grounds over which complete control could be exercised.

Incineration would appear to be the logical method for disposal of combustible materials, and similar considerations could be applied to the exhaust stack gases as to the water outflow from the institution. Permissible concentrations of gaseous radionuclides in air are also listed in the Federal Register. However, the possible radioactive residual in the ashes must be considered, as well as deposits in chimney soot. Therefore in any particular institution the problems must be analyzed as to quantity and type of radionuclide, final disposal of ashes, nature of prevailing winds, vicinity of other buildings, and so on, and application made to the AEC for permission to incinerate under these conditions. While this can usually be obtained, sometimes after various adjustments in the procedures, it is sometimes simpler, for small quantities of short-lived nuclides, to store the waste until its activity is only slightly above background, and then burn it. For paper wipes used in procedures with ^{131}I, for example, storage for a few weeks is seldom a problem. On the other hand, for animal carcasses with appreciable quantities of ^{32}P, several months in a freezer might be necessary, and this puts a strain on facilities.

Because of these problems, certain commercial waste disposal groups have been authorized by the AEC to collect waste materials from institutions and dispose of them according to procedures set up under their licenses. This type of service is very useful in the institution where a good deal of research is carried out with long-lived nuclides, or resulting in insoluble waste—animal carcasses, insoluble chemicals, and so on.

Stable Isotope Dilution. A disposal method sometimes practicable for relatively small quantities of radioactive isotopes of common elements is stable isotope dilution. The AEC does not recommend it, but under certain circumstances might accept it. To any preparation of a radioactive isotope enough "carrier," stable isotope of the same element in the same chemical form, can be added, so that if this mixture furnished the whole source of the element for an individual, his body burden would never reach the permissible level. In this case, no disposal precautions are necessary. With small quantities of long-lived materials this is a desirable procedure. Dilution by sewage water may be adequate at the date of disposal, but if successive quantitites are thrown away, there may be a reconcentration in the sludge of a sewage treatment plant, such as would not develop with a short-lived radionuclide.

Data in Handbook 52 facilitate the calculation of the necessary amount of carrier. This may be illustrated with ^{45}Ca. The handbook gives the daily intake of calcium as 0.8 gm, of which all is in the 7000 gm of skeleton, in a concentration of 0.15 gm Ca per gm of bone. There are therefore $0.15 \times 7000 = 1050$ gm of calcium in the body. The permissible body burden of ^{45}Ca is 65 μCi or 1 μc for every 16 gm of stable calcium. Admixture of carrier at this level would do away with need for *any* disposal precautions. At a somewhat lower level it might be a worthwhile precaution against too severe reconcentration.

Deceased Patients Containing Appreciable Quantities of Radioactive Material. As stated in the last chapter, this matter is discussed in detail in Report No. 36 of the National Council on Radiation Protection. In brief, the permissible exposure will never be reached for anyone handling the body of an individual who has received only a tracer or small therapeutic dose of a radionuclide. If a patient dies soon after receiving a large therapeutic dose, and the body is to be interred or cremated without embalming, there will be no radiation hazard from the necessary external handling. However, when the body is embalmed, radioactive fluids may be removed during the procedure, and care must be taken that these are properly disposed of (usually into the sanitary sewer) without contaminating persons or surroundings. For this reason it is advisable to have the embalming carried out in the hospital morgue, with the advice of the RPS. He can also monitor the proceedings, if he deems it advisable, to make sure that no one is exposed to an undesirable amount of radiation. If the body is to be cremated, no additional precautions are necessary unless the radionuclide in question is very long-lived. Implants of ^{192}Ir, or ^{182}Ta should be removed in the hospital, prior to release of the body.

Radioactive Contamination and Decontamination. Where procedures with radioactive materials are carried out in accordance with the rules suggested in the last chapter, there is little likelihood of serious personnel contamination. Apparatus and floors may be contaminated by an occasional accidental spill, patients who vomit or are incontinent may present problems in the hospital. The entire subject is dealt with in National Bureau of Standards Handbook 48, *Control and Removal of Radioactive Contamination in Laboratories;* familiarity with this should be mandatory for all isotope users.

Certain general rules may be indicated. In the laboratory, if bottles and equipment are maintained on trays as suggested, contamination, if it occurs beyond the tray, is likely to be at a low level. If it is on person, clothing, or floor:

1. Drop towels or absorbent material on spill.

2. Get out of contaminated clothing; put it on a large paper for future check. Put on a clean laboratory coat.

3. Scrub hands well with soap or detergent, not highly alkaline and not abrasive. Do not scratch the skin surface.

4. Put on fresh rubber gloves.

5. If the spill is on floor or table, take up as much as possible with

blotters or absorbent paper, using forceps to hold the material. Place it immediately into a receptacle for radioactive waste. Clean further with a damp cloth and detergent; avoid spreading the contamination by sloshing water. Levels to which cleaning must be carried are given in the Handbook.

6. Monitor contaminated material to determine whether clothing may go to the laundry and mopping material to the incinerator, or whether they must be stored for decay. The Handbook gives suitable levels.

If a larger contamination occurs in the hospital as a result of vomiting or excretion after a large dose of ^{131}I or a leak or spurt back from an injection of radioactive colloid, so that patient and bedding are involved, the following procedures are indicated:

7. Call the Radiation Protection Supervisor *at once.*

8. While awaiting his arrival, immediate steps should be taken to prevent spread of the contamination. An area containing the entire region of possible contamination should be marked off, and no person permitted to walk through this. No person should leave it without being monitored. The number of persons involved in the clean-up should be kept to a minimum.

9. If the RPS or his deputy is not immediately available, further steps should be taken to control the contamination. Procedures outlined in Steps 1 through 4 are applicable here. If there is contamination of the patient or other persons, clothing and bedding should be removed and stored within the circumscribed area. Contaminated skin should be scrubbed using a washroom in this area or wash basins brought there for this purpose. Contaminated material should not be removed from this area until the arrival of the RPS.

10. As an aid in preventing spread of contamination, and to reduce possible radiation exposure, after the liquid material has been taken up, it is a good idea to cover the region of the spill with a plastic bed sheet and about $\frac{1}{2}$ inch of absorbent material, such as two thick blankets. This will protect personnel from beta radiation exposure. If, in addition, personnel remain at least 6 feet from the covered spill, this will be adequate to protect against gamma radiation until the arrival of RPS.

11. If the contamination is due to breakage of a radium needle, the possibility exists of airborne radioactive particles. In this case all ventilators and windows should closed (if possible) and the room evacuated at once. The region immediately outside the room should be designated as a radiation hazard area until the RPS arrives to take charge; all persons evacuated from the room should remain here until monitored by the RPS.

12. The RPS on arrival will issue detailed instructions, depending on the nature and magnitude of the spill. He will treat contaminated floors and furniture as specified in item 5.

13. All contaminated material should be taken to the "hot laboratory" for checking. It may be spread on a large piece of paper, and individual pieces separated by picking out with forceps, and tested. The decision

13

has to be made whether to store this material for decay, or to try to decontaminate it. If the latter, pieces may be dropped, a few at a time, into a utility sink filled with water and detergent, lifted, stirred, and manipulated with sticks, rinsed and rewashed until the remaining activity is low enough to permit sending them to the laundry. (See Handbook 48.) If such levels cannot be attained, material can be dried on disposable lines, with pans and papers to catch the drippings, and stored for decay, or they can be turned over to a suitable waste disposal agent. Individuals carrying out such decontamination procedures should be constantly monitored; if levels are high the work should be done by a team.

14. Everyone who has been concerned with clean-up procedures should be carefully monitored for residual radioactivity; if any is found, the RPS must institute suitable procedures.

Special Case of Internal Personnel Contamination. If good housekeeping practices are adhered to in the "hot" laboratory, no one will ever ingest radioactive material. If pipetting by mouth is done, sooner or later radioactive material will be swallowed. If smoking is permitted during radionuclide handling, it is inevitable that contamination will go from fingers to cigarette to mouth. Measurable levels of ^{131}I have repeatedly been found in the thyroid glands of some individuals who persisted in this practice, insisting that they could do it "cleanly." It is desirable to monitor at intervals the thyroid glands of all those who work regularly with radioactive iodine.

REFERENCES

National Bureau of Standards Handbooks:

42. *Safe Handling of Radioactive Isotopes.*
48. *Control and Removal of Radioactive Contamination in Laboratories.*
49. *Recommendations for Waste Disposal of Phosphorus-32 and Iodine-131 for Medical Users.*
52. *Maximum Permissible Amounts of Radioisotopes in the Human Body and Maximum Permissible Concentrations in Air and Water.*
53. *Recommendations for the Disposal of Carbon-14 Wastes.*
58. *Radioactive Waste Disposal in the Ocean.*
65. *Safe Handling of Bodies Containing Radioactive Isotopes.*
69. *Maximum Permissible Body Burdens and Maximum Permissible Concentrations of Radionuclides in Air and Water for Occupational Exposure.*

National Council on Radiation and Measurements. Report No. 36. *Precautions in the Management of Patients Who Have Received Therapeutic Amounts of Radionuclides.*

Federal Register (Part 20) National Archives of the United States. Washington, D. C. 1956.

Part II

INSTRUMENTATION AND LABORATORY METHODS

By Sergei Feiltelberg and William Gross

13

Radiation Detectors: Principles of Operation

EACH disintegration of a radioactive nuclide is accompanied by a burst of radiant energy. This radiant energy may be electromagnetic radiation of very short wavelength (gamma rays), it may consist of elementary particles like electrons—negative or positive (beta rays or positrons), nuclei of helium (alpha rays), or any combination of some of them in extremely rapid succession. The interaction of these types of radiations with matter makes them detectable although the energy of each burst is almost inconceivably small when compared to the energy of events with which we deal in every-day experience. The disarrangement of orbital electrons when radiation interacts with gases is basically liberation of electrons from the confines of the gas atoms, which is called ionization, and which permits gases to conduct electricity although they are ordinarily non-conductors. The conductivity of gases due to ionization by radiation is one of the basic processes used in the detection of radiation bursts accompanying the disintegration of radioactive nuclides and hence in the observation of the occurrence of such disintegrations. The processes involved in the interaction of ionizing radiation with solid matter are more complex, but the sequelae of a variety of these processes can be also observable. A number of crystals, for instance, emit visible light when ionizing radiation is absorbed, and this light can either be observed directly or be measured by devices sensitive to visible light. Halogen salts of photographic emulsions form latent development centers which can be transformed by reducing agents to visible agglomerations of metallic silver (photographic image). In a variety of substances the disarrangement of orbital electrons results in a change of color or the emission of visible light when heated or exposed to ultraviolet radiations. In semiconductors electrical conduction occurs in a manner similar to that which occurs in a gas.

Radiation detectors have been made using any of the mechanisms listed above. The selection of the type of detector will depend on a great variety of factors as, for instance: whether the *number of disintegrations* in a given sample or the *overall intensity* of the radiation has to be determined; whether the radiation consists of penetrating gamma rays or of easily absorbed beta particles.

185

An understanding of the mechanism of radiation detectors is therefore essential not only for their intelligent and efficient use, but also for the selection of the best instrument for a given problem.

Ionization Chambers. We shall examine first the detection of radiation in a gas. When a beta particle with a range of several feet traverses air, it will ionize a large number of air molecules. This number will be different if one foot or two feet of its path are observed. To eliminate this first and elementary ambiguity, the volume of air under observation must be defined; the simplest way of doing it is by using some container of definite volume. This container or its inner walls must be an electric conductor, since the ionization produced will have to be observed by induced conductivity of the enclosed air. In order to observe this conductivity, a second piece of conducting material has to be introduced into the box and insulated from it. Conductivity of air will be measured by connecting the wall of the box and the second component (electrode) to a source of electric potential, for instance to a battery, and to a measuring instrument which will indicate the flow of electric current (*see* Fig. 13–1).

If there is no ionization inside the box, no current will flow and the meter will show no deflection. When a beta particle traverses the air, a large number of air molecules will be ionized: there will be floating along the paths of the beta rays free electrons and the remainders of gas molecules. The gas molecules were originally electrically neutral; since they have lost negative electrons, they have now positive charges. Ion pairs have been formed, consisting of a (negative) free electron and the positively charged residue of the molecule.

Two different things can happen to the ion pair. The two parts, coming originally from the same or from different molecules, may meet; they are attracted to each other as are any opposite electric charges and they may recombine to form again a complete and electrically neutral gas molecule.

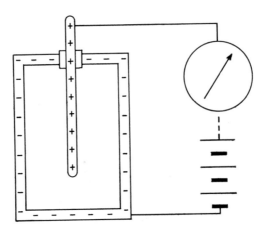

FIG. 13–1.   Schematic illustration of an *ionization chamber* and of the associated electric circuit.

An event of this sort will not affect the electric circuit and will not be observable on the meter. It is possible, however, that free electrons which are repelled by the negative electrode, the box wall for instance, and attracted by the positive electrode, which may be a rod inside the box, will reach the rod and be drawn into the electric circuit. The positive remainder of the molecule will drift to the negative wall and become neutral by getting an electron from the conducting wall, since this, being negative, has a supply of free electrons. In this second case there will be a charge pulse in the electric circuit and this could be detected in the meter if it were sensitive enough.

Which of the two possible processes will occur—inside recombination or external collection—will depend on the electrostatic attraction by the electrodes in the box. If this attraction is increased by increasing the battery voltage, for instance, the free electrons will be collected more quickly by the central rod, and they will have less time and therefore less chance to recombine with the positive remainders of the molecules. A larger proportion of the ion pairs formed during the passage of a beta ray will contribute to the charge flowing through the electric circuit and indicated on the meter. Thus with increasing voltage, the ratio of collected to recombined ion pairs increases, until almost all ion pairs produced are collected, and the deflection on the meter becomes a good measure of the total ionization produced. At this point a further increase of voltage will have no appreciable effect on the collection efficiency. The device has been saturated as seen from the external circuit, and the voltage range for this condition is called *saturation voltage*. The changes in the charge collected for each beta ray traversing the box for varying voltage are represented in Figure 13–2. The figure also indicates the relative magnitude of charge flow which occurs when different rays pass through the air. Specific ionization (number of ion pairs per unit length) along the path of a beta ray is very much less than for an alpha particle. Thus, when an alpha particle reaches the inside of the box, more ion pairs are produced and the charges flowing through the circuit are more numerous than for the beta ray.

The device discussed here has therefore one very remarkable and useful property: when it is operated with saturation voltage, the current (charge flow rate) going through the meter is a direct measure of the total number of ion pairs produced per unit time in the enclosed air space, and is therefore a measure of the ionization due to radiation. It is called an *ionization chamber* and it is one of the best instruments for the measurement of ionization. One of the problems which we are trying to solve here, however, is to observe each radiation burst separately; and for this purpose the charge pulses occurring in the external circuit, even when an alpha particle is the radiation to be observed, are too small for any available electric meter. The limitation of electric meters is not so much their sensitivity, but the speed of their response to a fast electric pulse; as a general rule the

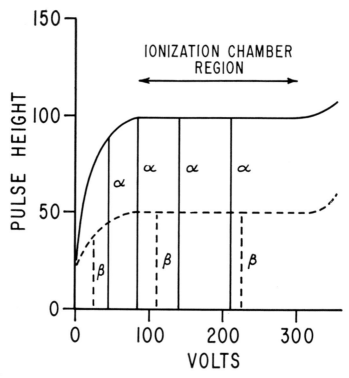

Fig. 13–2.   Height of electric pulses due to passage of beta and alpha particles through an *ionization chamber* (pulse height scale in arbitrary units, as in Fig. 13–3 and Fig. 13–4).

sensitivity can be increased only at the expense of speed.   Ionization due to a radiation burst from a disintegrating nuclide occurs over an extremely short interval of time; the collection of ion pairs takes more time, but it is also accomplished very quickly.   When a large number of ionizing events occurs in the ionization chamber, electric measuring instruments of several kinds can be used to measure either the amount of electric charge equivalent to the total number of ion pairs produced during the time of observation (total ionization, which is a measure of radiation dose), or the current, which is equivalent to the number of ion pairs produced per unit time (a measure of the dose rate).

To summarize: an ionization chamber is an instrument which is well suited to measure dose and dose rate of ionizing radiations, but the current pulses due to radiation bursts, produced when individual disintegrations of radioactive atoms take place, are generally too small to be observed.

Proportional Counters.   This pulse size difficulty can be overcome by taking advantage of a phenomenon occurring in the gas during the ionization process, when the applied voltage is increased beyond the saturation range.

Ion pairs are produced due to radiation; the free electron and the positive remainder of the molecule are attracted towards the anode and cathode. In moving through the gas they collide repeatedly with other gas molecules. The positive remainder of the molecule, which is heavy (nucleus of the atoms plus whatever orbital electrons are left), drifts relatively slowly towards the cathode. The electron, however, being very light, will acquire a considerable velocity which will depend on the electric field acting on it: this velocity will be therefore increased when the voltage is raised. Ultimately the velocity attained by the electrons between collisions reaches a value at which their kinetic energy is high enough to ionize the gas molecules with which they collide. Then these electrons produced during the primary ionization process will in their turn form secondary ion pairs, that is, liberate secondary electrons by impact. These secondary electrons will be accelerated also and produce tertiary ion pairs resulting in more free electrons; this process will continue in the form of an avalanche until a whole cone of ionized gas is formed, starting at the site where each primary electron was formed and ending at the anode. The ionizing effect of electrons accelerated by the increased collecting voltage may seem puzzling at first, but it is the same effect which is observed when beta particles pass through a gas, since beta particles are also electrons of high energy, moving at a high speed.

The crucial result of the avalanche formation insofar as it affects the charge flowing through the external circuit of Figure 13–1 is that for each primary liberated electron, a large number of additional electrons is liberated, and the pulse through the electric circuit, and hence through the meter, is greatly amplified. Since this amplification occurs in the gas of the detector itself, it is called the gas amplification factor.

This gas amplification factor depends on the energy which was imparted to the liberated electrons by the electric field and therefore on the applied voltage. The electric pulse through the circuit will therefore increase with higher voltage, as illustrated in Figure 13–3.

The pulse will also depend on the total number of avalanches occurring simultaneously; and since each primary ion pair gives rise to an avalanche, the pulse will depend on the number of primary ionizations produced by the passage of the radiation burst through the gas. Since this ionization is higher for an alpha ray than for a beta ray, the amplified pulse will also be greater for an alpha ray than for a beta ray; the pulses will be proportional to the primary ionization. This device is therefore called a *proportional counter*.

The great advantage of a proportional counter is that the pulse produced by the ionizing event due to the passage of a single radiation burst is much greater than in an ionization chamber; it is large enough to be detected by available electronic devices. Since the pulse height is proportional to the ionization, the pulses can be sorted out in the electronic measuring device, and alpha particles, for instance, can be observed separately and inde-

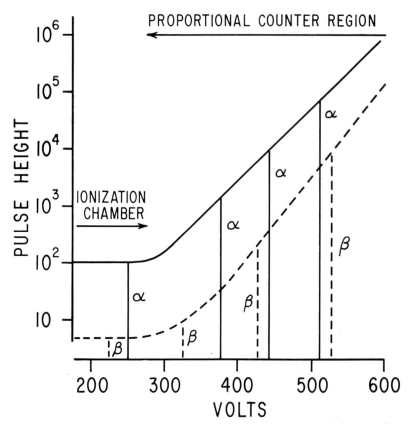

Fig. 13–3.   Height of electric pulses due to passage of beta and alpha particles through a *proportional counter* (see legend to Fig. 13–2).

pendently of beta particles. There are, however, two disadvantages. First, the electric pulses, though amplified, are still quite small and their observation requires rather elaborate and somewhat delicate electronic devices. Second, the magnitude of the electric pulses, as seen in Figure 13–3, varies with the applied voltage, and unless this voltage is maintained sufficiently constant, the pulse height will vary with it and affect the observations.

Geiger-Mueller Counters.   If the voltage applied to the counter is increased still further, a third process begins to play a significant role which at the lower voltage occurs so infrequently that it can be neglected.

This process has to do with other interactions of electrons with atoms than those leading to ionization. When the energy of secondary electrons is high enough, radiative collisions with gas atoms will occur and bremsstrahlung of low energy photons (visible and ultraviolet light) will be produced.

With higher applied voltage the number of secondary electrons in each avalanche increases, as can be seen in the increased size of the electric pulse. The number of radiative collisions will also increase. These photons of visible and ultraviolet light will traverse the counting volume, and when they reach the enclosing walls they will be absorbed and may release electrons by the photoelectric effect. These electrons will be accelerated by the potential inside the counter and form avalanches in their turn.

When this process begins to occur with significant frequency, the number of avalanches becomes greater than the number of the ion pairs formed during the primary ionization process due to the radiation bursts, which we are interested in detecting. The proportionality between the primary ionization and the electric pulses is lost. The counter does not behave any longer strictly as a proportional counter and this region is called that of limited proportionality. Further increase in voltage will lead to an even more frequent occurrence of radiative collision within the avalanches; there will be more and more avalanches due to photoelectrons released by light photons from these collisions, and finally these processes will increase to a point when ionization will spread through the whole enclosed gas volume. Beginning at this voltage, the device is called a Geiger-Mueller counter. It shows quite a remarkable behavior: once any ionizing event occurs in the gas, ionization is no longer localized. The electric pulse through the circuit will have a higher value than in the proportional region; a very high gas amplification factor is reached, of the order of a million to a billion. This pulse will be independent of the size of the original ionizing event (all proportionality is lost); it still will be dependent on applied voltage, but much less than in a proportional counter. The advantages are therefore the large size of the electric pulse, which is easy to observe, and the decreased dependence on the variations in the voltage supply. The disadvantage is that there is no proportionality between pulse height and the intensity of the ionization produced by the radiation bursts under observation: the pulses are the same whether they are released by alpha or beta radiation. The voltage at which the proportionality between the size of the primary ionizing event and the size of the electric pulse is lost, and where the Geiger-Mueller region begins, is called the *threshold voltage* (*See* Figs. 13–4 and 16–2).

The voltage cannot be increased indefinitely beyond the threshold value without destroying the ability of the counter to detect radiation, since eventually the electric field will reach a value at which it has enough force to tear away by itself an orbital electron from an atom. Depending on the pressure, either an electric spark or a gas discharge will occur, and current will flow through the circuit without ionization due to radiation. The voltage at which this occurs is called the self-discharge voltage.

The positive ions have been neglected so far, but they play also a relevant role in the behavior of a Geiger-Mueller counter. Since they are much heavier than the electrons, they acquire a correspondingly lower velocity and move relatively more slowly towards the cathode than the electrons toward the anode, and therefore arrive later at their destination. The

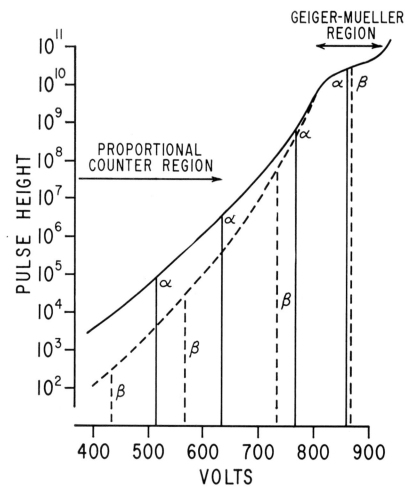

Fig. 13–4. Height of electric pulses due to passage of beta and alpha particles through a *Geiger-Mueller counter* (see legend to Fig. 13–2).

presence of such an accumulation of positive ions in the counter volume creates a cloud of positive charge which counteracts the potential gradient created by the applied voltage. This can effectively stop the discharge; when this happens, the positive ions will reach the cathode and become neutralized. Until this occurs, the counter has effectively no potential gradient inside the gas and it cannot respond to another ionizing event; it is "dead" and the time which this neutralization takes is called its "dead time."

The neutralization of positive ions at the cathode can occur in two ways. One is by disassociation, if the gas contains polyatomic molecules. Such disassociation occurs without the emission of any radiations, and the counting discharge is quenched as described in the preceding paragraph. Such counters are called *self-quenching*. But in some other gases, a radiative neutralization may also occur which acts in the same way as radiative collisions in the avalanches: ultraviolet and visible light quanta (photons) are emitted, and they release photoelectrons which form additional avalanches. The discharge process perpetuates itself and continues until it is quenched externally by disconnecting or reducing the voltage applied to the counter; this is called a non-self-quenching counter. Most counters in use today are of the self-quenching type.

In order to recapitulate what happens in an enclosed gas volume when an ionizing ray passes through it, the processes are listed in the following paragraphs. The voltage applied to the electrodes in the gas volume is increased for each subsequent paragraph:

1. Some of the ion pairs formed are collected; some recombine.

2. Ionization chamber at saturation voltage. All ion pairs formed are collected. Pulses due to single radiation bursts are generally too small to be detected singly but are measurable when many are combined.

3. Proportional Counter. Acceleration of primary electron is great enough to produce secondary ionizations and localized avalanche discharges. Primary ionization pulse is amplified by this gas amplification factor and is large enough to be detected; it is proportional to the amount of primary ionization. Pulses due to rays of different ability to ionize gases can be differentiated and observed independently.

4. Geiger-Mueller Counter. Radiative collisions in the avalanche become sufficiently frequent to release enough photoelectrons from the cathode so that ionization spreads through the whole counter volume. Maximal gas amplification and highest electric pulses are independent of the intensity of the primary ionizing event. Positive ion cloud terminates the discharge in self-quenching counters. In non-self-quenching counters, discharge is self perpetuating due to radiative recombination and must be quenched externally.

Scintillation Counters. So far, ionization processes in radiation detectors have been discussed as they take place in gases. They are comparatively simple, since ion pairs formed can move freely in a gas. But the density of a gas is low, the chances of interaction with a beam of γ or x radiation therefore small and the inherent sensitivity of such gas detectors is not high. Far greater radiation absorption takes place in solid matter of similar volume, so that solid radiation detectors are potentially much more sensitive. This is particularly important in the detection of highly penetrating gamma radiation. The phenomena involved are, however, more complex than in a gas.

A variety of organic and inorganic crystals undergo a process which is analogous to what was called radiative collision in gases; they emit photons, quanta of visible light, as a result of absorbing ionizing radiation. This luminescence is one of the oldest known effects of radiation on matter; its observation led Roentgen to the discovery of x rays; it was the phenomenon by means of which Rutherford originally investigated the nature of radium disintegrations, and it is in everyday medical use in fluoroscopy.

When a crystal, which has this property of emitting light when absorbing radiation, is hit by a single burst of radiant energy, and some or all of this energy is absorbed by it, a light pulse of short duration is produced. If the crystal is transparent, the light pulses occurring not only on its surface, but also inside of the crystal will become visible. Such light pulses are called *scintillations;* they are often of sufficient intensity to be seen. This intensity is proportional to the energy absorbed by the crystal from the impinging radiation. The number of pulses is a measure of the frequency with which radiation bursts impinge on the scintillating crystal, and therefore a measure of the disintegration rate of a radioactive nuclide, if this is the source of the radiation.

Visual observation and counting of these scintillations are obviously too laborious and too slow for practical purposes. For this reason, scintillating crystals were not generally used as radiation counters until a way was found to observe and register the occurrence of scintillations automatically.

The obvious way to achieve this was to use a photoelectric cell for the conversion of light pulses into electric ones. The difficulty was, however, that photoelectric cells were not sensitive enough to translate scintillations into electric pulses of useful intensity, even with the use of electronic amplifiers. It was only after the invention of the photomultiplier tube that the potentially extremely useful property of scintillation detectors could be employed in practice.

A photomultiplier tube utilizes secondary emission of electrons. Figure 13–5 illustrates schematically a single stage photomultiplier tube. Let us examine first the cathode and the first electrode (called a dynode); they form a conventional photocell. The cathode is formed by a thin, transparent coating of a conducting material on glass and a potential of about 100 volts

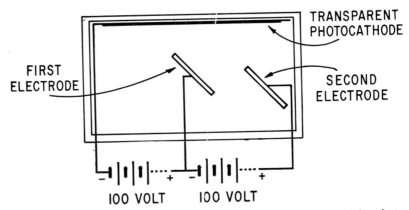

FIG. 13–5. Schematic illustration of a *photomultiplier tube.* Only one multiplier electrode is shown; in actual design there are usually ten or more such electrodes.

is applied between this coating and the first electrode. The whole glass envelope is evacuated to a high vacuum. The electric field attracts the electrons from the cathode, but is not strong enough to pull them out. When light strikes the photocathode, some of its energy is transferred to the electrons, and this added energy liberates them from the coating. These electrons will fly towards the first electrode, attaining speed and hence energy when they impinge on it, depending upon the potential between this electrode and the coating. This will allow some current to flow in the circuit formed by the photocathode, the battery and the first electrode.

The next step involves events between the first and second electrode which characterize the photomultiplier. Let us examine what happens when a single electron, emitted from the photocathode and accelerated by the first battery, impinges on the first electrode. It will be absorbed, that is, its energy will be transferred to the atoms and electrons in the first electrode. These electrons, however, are attracted by the second electrode which is at a positive potential with respect to the first electrode due to the second battery. Again, the field by itself cannot pull electrons out of the first electrode; when they acquire additional energy from the electrons arriving from the photocathode, they are able to leave and fly to the second electrode. A single photoelectron can set free several of them. Then the current which will flow through the circuit formed by the second battery and the first and second electrodes will be several times greater than the current flowing between photocathode and first electrode. This secondary emission has *amplified* the original photocurrent. The amount of this amplification is determined by the applied voltage; it cannot be increased indefinitely, however; if the voltage is too high it will be able to pull out electrons from the electrodes without help from electron bombardment, current will flow when no light strikes the photocathode and will be, therefore, no measure of light intensity. In practice, four secondary electrons for one primary electron is approximately the limit. But further amplification is possible by arranging an additional electrode after the second one, with an additional battery as another voltage supply. This will give again an amplification of four, or a total amplification of sixteen. This can be repeated and practical photomultiplier tubes contain ten or more such electrodes and have a total amplification of over a million. When the light flash of a scintillating crystal reaches such a phototube, the electric pulse has a value approaching the output of a Geiger-Mueller counter in size.

The emission of light by a scintillator after the absorption of ionizing radiation occurs by processes which are fundamentally different in inorganic and organic materials. In the former, light emission is a property of the crystal, while in the latter it is a property of the organic molecule. Thus organic scintillators can retain their ability to emit light even when dissolved in liquid or plastic solvents.

Selection of a scintillator involves several factors. Among these are the interaction of the ionizing radiation and the scintillator, the light output per unit of energy absorbed, the size and the cost. Inorganic scintillators such as thallium activated sodium iodide contain high atomic number constituents. Thus, they are far better absorbers of gamma radiation than the organic materials (see Chapter 3). In addition the inorganic scintillators have a higher density so that for the same size there are more grams of scintillator available for interaction when inorganic material is used. However, because the light emission is a property of the crystal an inorganic scintillator must be a single crystal which requires special techniques to fabricate. Also, scintillators such as NaI(Tl) are destroyed by contact with the water in the air and must therefore be packaged in air tight con-

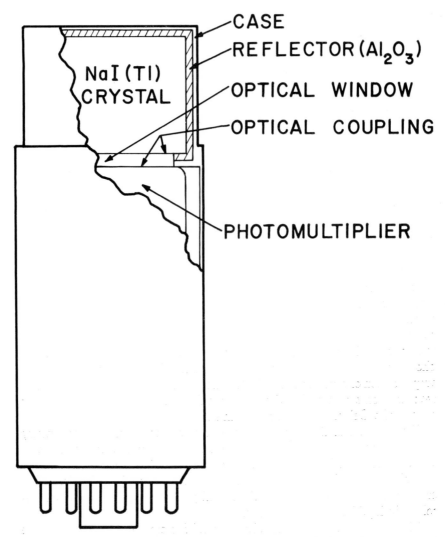

Fig. 13–6.   Cutaway view of a thallium activated sodium iodide scintillation counter.

tainers. Both these requirements raise the cost of such scintillators. Thus, for very large counters (whole body) the organic scintillator may be chosen by price. For charged particles, such as alpha or beta rays, an organic scintillator is slightly more absorbent than is an inorganic scintillator of equal weight. Thus, for these radiations the organic materials may be preferred. Where the radioactive material is mixed with the scintillator (liquid scintillation counters) only the organic scintillators can be used.

A complete NaI(Tl) scintillation counter is shown in Figure 13–6. The crystal, packed in an air-tight housing, is surrounded by a layer of aluminum oxide powder except on the face contacting the photomultiplier. The powder serves as a shock absorbent material as well as a diffuse light reflector. The crystal is optically coupled to the photomultiplier tube envelope. The photocathode is deposited directly on the inside surface of the envelope so that the light is very efficiently transported to the photocathode. Electrical connections to all the tube electrodes are made via the tube base at the far end of the counter.

Solid State Detectors. The main advantage of scintillation counters over gas detectors is that the crystal is a solid and absorbs, therefore, much more energy from an impinging radiation than a gas of equal volume. Its disadvantage is the complexity of the mechanism which consists in the three steps: 1. Absorption of ionizing energy, 2. Conversion of this energy into light pulses, and 3. Conversion of the light pulses into electric pulses by a photocell. It would be desirable to have a solid state detector which combines the advantages of high absorption for ionizing radiation with the simplicity of a gas detector which converts the absorbed energy directly into an electric pulse.

Such a detector is available. A device closely related to the transistor is used, in which a highly purified semiconductor such as silicon or germanium is modified by the addition of controlled impurities. The conductivity of this semiconductor is altered by the absorption of ionizing radiation. When properly connected to an external source of voltage such a solid state detector behaves very much like an ionization chamber; the electric pulse is proportional to the energy absorbed. Unlike the ionization chamber whose volume is determined by its walls, the region from which ions are collected in the solid state detector is determined in part by the applied voltage. This region is called the depletion region and its size increases with increasing applied voltage. The ions in the semiconductor consist of negative electrons, as in a gas, and of positive "holes." Unlike the positive gas ions these holes move through the semiconductor under the influence of the applied voltage with velocities comparable to those of the electrons.

In a fashion similar to gas detectors semiconductor detectors can be used as pulse devices or as ionization chambers. In this latter use the detector, a battery and a sensitive current meter form the entire instrument. Such

14

devices are extremely simple and are useful whenever the radiation intensity is sufficient such as in the case of the calibration of bulk nuclide
shipments.

Semiconductor detectors used as pulse devices for charged particles have
depletion regions which extend essentially to the surface of the detector
and of depth greater than the particle range. Thus, the entire energy of
the charged particle is expended in the depletion region and the electrical
pulse height is therefore proportional to the particle energy. These
charged particle detectors are called planar surface barrier detectors and
are generally prepared from a silicon base.

The requirements for a gamma ray detector are somewhat different.
Here, the absorption is a two step process, *i.e.* the creation of a charged
particle (electron or positron) followed by ionization in the detector. The
first process must occur frequently if the detector is to be efficient. (It is
for just this reason that the scintillation counter is an efficient photon
detector while the proportional and Geiger-Mueller counters are not, particularly at higher photon energies.) To obtain high efficiencies solid state
gamma-ray detectors are prepared from germanium rather than silicon.
The higher atomic number (32 rather than 14) and the greater density
(5.3 rather than 2.3) both increase photon absorption in germanium. In
addition, to be efficient a large depletion volume in the crystal is required.
This can be achieved either in planar or coaxial regions. However, in order
to use these gamma-ray detectors they must be operated at low temperatures. This condition is met by cooling with liquid nitrogen which requires
somewhat complex equipment. It is this complexity along with a detection
efficiency small compared to that obtained with scintillation counters which
has limited the application of solid state photon detectors in medicine and
biology. Silicon charged-particle detectors require no cooling.

The major advantage of these solid state detectors over scintillation
counters lies in their energy resolution, *i.e.* how well the device can separate
particles which deposit almost the same energy. A scintillation counter can
distinguish between two photon emitters whose energy is about 600 keV
only if these energies differ by at least 40 keV. The solid state detector is
ten times better than this. However, this advantage is obtained only with
very special amplifiers and the more complex cooling equipment. High
energy resolution is not generally required in medical applications and thus
the solid state gamma ray detector does not play too large a role at this
time.

A few special applications of the solid state pulse detectors in the medical
area have involved detectors small enough to be inserted into the patient's
body. These have included brain probes and gastrointestinal detectors,
each of which is very small and used to detect a beta ray emitter. These
devices are more satisfactory than the scintillation or Geiger-Mueller
counter devices which they replace.

Photographic Emulsions. The blackening of a photographic plate by x rays and by other ionizing radiations is at least as familiar to the reader as luminescence, although the processes involved are far from simple. The essential difference between the two mechanisms is that in a scintillation counter the changes due to absorption of radiation are fully reversible. After the emission of a light pulse the original state of the crystal is restored, while the phenomena which occur in the photographic emulsion are longer lasting chemical changes. For this reason, a photographic emulsion is of no use when the rate of radioactive disintegrations has to be detected, but it is a simple and convenient device to measure the accumulated amount of radiation, that is, the dose. It is of course also of unique value in the determination of the spatial distribution of radiation sources.

The first step in the absorption of radiation by a photographic emulsion is probably the emission of an electron from the electronegative halogen ion. This electron is then captured by an electropositive silver ion. Capture of an electron is chemically a reduction. The reduction of electropositive silver ions in the silver-halogen molecule forms development centers of the latent image. The latent image is made visible by further reduction during the development, when metallic silver particles are produced in visible conglomerations. The amount of metallic silver can be measured quantitatively by a densitometer. The observed density is a measure of the total radiation absorbed by the emulsion.

Other Solid State Devices. Other processes occur in solids which are irradiated by ionizing radiation. These can be detected and used as a measure of the quantity of radiation. After exposure certain glasses will emit visible light while irradiated with ultraviolet. The quantity of light emitted is proportional to, among other things, the quantity of ionizing radiation to which the glass was exposed. This process is called photoluminescence. Some materials when heated emit light proportional to the amount of ionizing radiation which they have absorbed. This is called thermoluminescence. Chemicals can be oxidized by ionizing radiation, *e.g.* ferrous sulfate to ferric sulfate, and these reactions are quantitative. All these devices, however, are useful primarily as radiation dosimeters at dose levels above those normally encountered in the procedures of nuclear medicine. They will, therefore, not be considered further in this work.

Summary. Some general properties of the different types of radiation detectors can now be summarized.

Ionization chambers can be used to measure both dose rate and total dose. They do not allow the observation of single radiation bursts during the disintegration of a radioactive isotope.

Proportional counters give electric pulses when they are traversed by radiation bursts. The height of the electric pulse is proportional to ionization occurring during such bursts.

Geiger-Mueller counters give electric pulses when ionizing events occur in the sensitive volume in a similar manner to a proportional counter, but the pulse height is independent of the ionization intensity of the initiating radiation burst.

Scintillation counters which are made of solids or liquids absorb more radiation energy than the devices containing gas; they have the highest sensitivity for penetrating radiation such as gamma or x rays. The light intensity of each scintillation depends on the absorbed energy of the radiation.

Solid state detectors have many of the advantages of scintillation counters but require more sophisticated auxiliary equipment.

Photographic emulsions can be used only to measure directly the total dose, in addition to their particular properties of localizing radiation sources by image formation. Other changes in solids can also be used for dose measurement.

14

Auxiliary Instruments

THE description and explanation of auxiliary apparatus for nuclear measurement present a dilemma. At first it seems reasonable and perhaps necessary to offer a complete presentation of function, design and construction to satisfy an interested and critical reader. But on second thought the background of the reader has to be considered. The training of the physician or biologist may cover some physics but usually no electronic engineering. Knowledge of electronics cannot be presupposed. The first part of this chapter ought to contain, therefore, an elementary treatise on this branch of engineering. It is not possible to do this satisfactorily within the framework of the present book. Prior attempts have met with little success. Cursory explanations of the operation of a transistor or vacuum tube quickly followed by diagrams of flip-flops and similar circuits do not clarify matters for the neophyte and are too elementary for the engineer. The technical complexities of the instruments are too great for a casual, semi-popular short treatment.

The approach selected for this chapter is perhaps best explained by an analogy. To drive a modern automobile well it is not necessary to understand the construction of cam shafts, the design of the automatic transmission, the intricacies of the electric ignition system, the response and damping of the suspension springs and shock absorbers. What is necessary is a full understanding of the functions and controls of the car: conversion of combustion energy of fuels into mechanical power; what happens when accelerator, brake and steering are operated. Knowledge beyond these functional operations is not necessary for driving, but is essential of course for repairs when the car breaks down. However, cars are today quite reliable pieces of machinery: they do not break down often when they get adequate servicing, and when they do break down, there are enough service stations to get them going again. Neither was true forty years ago. At that time a driver had to know a great deal about the mechanism, or he would too frequently get stranded and helpless on the road.

The situation with nuclear equipment has had a very similar development. About twenty years ago this equipment was rather experimental. It would have been foolhardy to use it without knowing how to take it apart and how to repair it. Its use was limited to technically trained people or those who were willing to get this technical training. Today this equipment is reasonably reliable and service facilities are generally available, so that knowledge of the engineering construction is no longer essential.

It is still essential, however, to understand the functions of the various controls and components. This is so because otherwise the instruments cannot be used intelligently and reliably, malfunctions will not be detected and observations may become misleading.

During the past few years a minor revolution has occurred in nuclear instrumentation. Vacuum tubes have almost entirely been replaced by transistors. While similar in function to the vacuum tube, the transistor does not depend upon the emission of electrons from a heated electrode. Conduction occurs in a solid semiconductor rather than in a vacuum and the potentials used are tens instead of hundreds of volts. The net result is that far less power is dissipated, less heat produced, and the instrument operates at lower temperature. Lower power and temperature insure longer and more stable life to all the circuit components. Also smaller components can be employed and grouped for unit replacement for service. Further, transistors tend to fail catastrophically while vacuum tubes often deteriorate gradually. It is generally easy to notice when some function of an instrument fails completely; when deterioration is gradual it is possible to work for some time with an apparatus without realizing that it is not functioning properly and is giving erroneous readings.

Further developments in the instrument field promise even more desirable equipment in the future. Modular instruments are now commonplace, i.e. each portion of a complex piece of equipment is separate and fits into an overall container or bin. Even more desirable is the bin standardization among manufacturers so that instrument components of different makes may be used in the same bin. This standardization has been pioneered by the Atomic Energy Commission and is a boon to the instrument consumer as it avoids expensive duplication of power supplies. It also permits an instrument to be tailored to a specific use without special engineering or purchase of unnecessary functions.

The integrated circuit is another recent development which deserves mention here. This device incorporates in a single small package the function of several transistors, resistors and capacitors, i.e. complete circuits. These are gradually replacing the separate component transistor circuits. While smallness of packaging does not necessarily improve function, in this case the elimination of external connections does greatly enhance reliability.

These remarks may appear to indicate that almost all instrumental difficulties have been, or shortly will be, eliminated. Unfortunately this is not true. Technological developments have improved circuit reliability but concurrent with these improvements has been a vast increase in instrument sophistication. This has resulted from a desire to perform more complex tasks and of course does create more possibility for instrument failure.

However, the overall picture is bright. Properly designed instruments work very well over long periods of time.

This chapter will be devoted, therefore, mainly to the functional description of the auxiliary instruments and to the purpose of their different components. The reader who would like to gain insight into the actual mechanisms and technical details is referred to specialized textbooks on electronics and instrumentation.

Ionization Chambers. Ionization chambers are not suitable for the observations of single radiation bursts occurring during the disintegration of a radioactive nuclide, but they are inherently stable and simple devices to measure dose or dose rate, a problem which is of great practical importance in radioactive nuclide work, particularly for purposes of health protection and standardization. We shall discuss first methods of measuring dose rate and then methods of measuring total dose.

Dose Rate Meters. The three integral parts of such an instrument are (a) ionization chamber, (b) source of electric potential, and (c) sensitive current measuring device.

The ionization chamber itself is an enclosure, defining the gas volume in which ionization occurs. The larger the gas volume, the more ion pairs it will contain when it is exposed to a given intensity of radiation, and the larger therefore will be the current observed. The sensitivity of the whole instrument can be increased by increasing the volume. This is limited by inconvenience of handling a bulky chamber, and the size of practical ionization chambers is usually not larger than a sphere of several inches in diameter or a cylinder about 6 to 8 inches long and a few inches in diameter. The ionization chamber must contain two conducting electrodes; as a rule the inside walls of the chamber are made conducting and serve as one electrode, and a metal or graphite rod in the center of the chamber serves as the second. The walls of the chamber have to fulfill a variety of physical conditions in order that they do not affect unduly the measurements. One such condition is that the walls have proper thickness. Absorption of primary γ radiation, production and absorption of secondary electrons by walls of different thicknesses and material may give a wide variation of ionization in the chamber when it is exposed to the same radiation intensity of different γ-ray energies. By suitable choice of wall thickness and material the ionization can be made directly proportional to the dose in tissue over a gamma-ray energy range between about 0.1 MeV and a few MeV. Beta rays present a different problem owing to their low penetration and limited range.

A few hundred volts are required to obtain saturation in an ionization chamber. In portable instruments this can be supplied either directly by high voltage dry cells or from an electronic supply powered by low voltage dry cells.

For radiation intensities of interest to us, the current through an ionization chamber cannot be measured directly by ordinary pointer type meters,

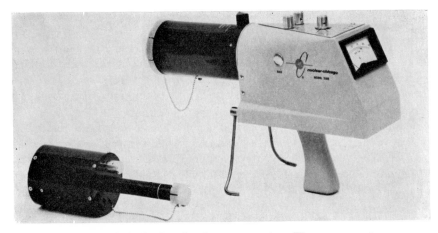

FIG. 14–1. Portable ionization chamber *survey* meter. The exposure rate ranges are 25, 250 and 2,500 milliroentgens per hour full scale. The large ionization chamber of 500 cc volume can be removed and a small chamber 5 cc (also illustrated) plugged in; this increases the range to 2.5, 25 and 250 roentgens per hour. In addition it can be used as an exposure meter covering a full scale range of 0.25 mR to 25 R using both chambers (courtesy of Nuclear-Chicago Corporation).

since they are not sensitive enough, and amplifiers have to be used. Such amplifiers can have a wide range of sensitivity and complexity. They can be made to give readings with a current flow of only a few electrons per second (vibrating reed electrometers, stationary electrometers), but then they are quite expensive. Less sensitive portable amplifiers can be made using special miniature vacuum tubes or field effect transistors, which are sensitive enough for health protection measurements. Such an instrument is illustrated in Figure 14–1. It weighs only a few pounds and radiation exposure rates down to about 10 mR per hour can be measured.

Dose Meters. The total dose, as observed in an ionization chamber, is proportional to the total number of ion pairs produced in a given volume and it is independent of the time during which such an ionization occurred. The technical problem in measuring the total dose is therefore the measurement not of current (amperes, electrons per second) but of the number of electrons, which is expressed as "charge" and may be measured in several units. The unit corresponding to the ampere is a coulomb, which represents a charge equal to 6.25×10^{18} electrons. The unit of radiation exposure, the roentgen (R), is defined as that quantity of x or gamma radiation which will produce 2.58×10^{-4} coulombs per kilogram of air. If we use as an example an ionization chamber of 10 ml volume, it will contain about 13 milligrams of air and thus 1 roentgen will produce 2.58×10^{-4} coulombs per kilogram times 1.3×10^{-5} kilogram $= 3.3 \times 10^{-9}$ coulombs. This charge, small as it is, can be measured by a comparatively simple and robust device, a combination of a small electric capacitor and an electrostatic voltmeter (Fig. 14–2). To within a few percent the exposure mea-

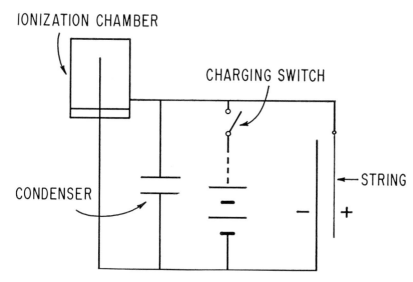

IONIZATION CHAMBER

CHARGING SWITCH

CONDENSER

←—STRING

FIG. 14–2. Schematic illustration of a capacitor type ionization chamber with string electrometer for total dose measurement.

sured in roentgens is equal to the absorbed dose in soft tissue measured in rads. For purposes of protection the two may be equated when dealing with x or gamma rays.

Capacitors can easily be made of such a small capacity that a voltage of the order of 20 volts will store in them not more than about 10^8 electrons. This also means that if 10^8 electrons are accumulated in such a capacitor, the voltage across it will change by 20 volts. One hundredth of a roentgen will produce in a 10-cc ionization chamber about 2×10^8 electrons. This number of electrons would change the voltage on the selected capacitors by 40 volts. Such a voltage change can be measured by observing through a low power microscope the electrostatic attraction of a thin quartz string to an oppositely charged support. Rather small doses can be measured, therefore, with such an arrangement. The inconvenience of the device shown in Figure 14–2 consists in the need for a steady supply of high voltage (a battery, for instance). This inconvenience can be reduced by changing the arrangement slightly as illustrated in Figure 14–3. Here the source of voltage is separate from the ionization chamber and the electrometer, and is connected only for charging. The string will indicate when the desired charge is reached. As soon as this charge is accomplished, the charging device is disconnected and can be removed entirely. Another way to handle the problem of a bulky charging device is that for the measurement process of this sort, only a small amount of "electricity," that is, of electrons, is needed, and this can be supplied by electrostatic friction generators of a simple kind. The charge on the ionization chamber, and hence the string deflection, will remain unchanged as long as no ionization occurs,

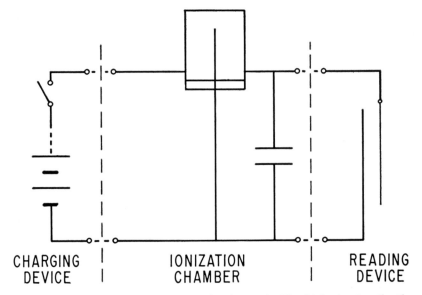

CHARGING   IONIZATION   READING
DEVICE   CHAMBER   DEVICE

Fig. 14–3. Capacitor type ionization chamber as in Fig. 14–2, showing the three basic components as they can be separated in actual construction. Such instruments have been designed in every possible combination of the components.

provided insulation in the instrument is perfect and no leakage takes place. As soon as ion pairs are produced in the ionization chamber, they will be collected by the electrodes, neutralize the charge on the capacitor and reduce the potential. The degree of this discharge will be a measure of ionization produced and it can be observed on the electrometer string. The microscope scale can be calibrated in milliroentgens directly. The notable feature of this scale is that zero radiation dose corresponds to full charge, that is to a full deflection of the string: this position is marked "O," corresponding to "no radiation received." As radiation dose increases, the string moves towards the discharge position and the scale markings show *increasing* dose reading, while the charge decreases.

A dose rate instrument is usually self-contained: ionization chamber, voltage source, amplifier and meter are one integral unit. A dose measuring instrument, which consists of an ionization chamber, capacitor, charging device and electrometer, can be made in separate parts. The capacitor and ionization chamber are usually combined in one unit* but otherwise the following combinations will be found:

a. Ionization chamber separate, charger and reading device combined.

b. Ionization chamber and reading device combined, charging device separate.

c. All three elements combined.

* Such units are often referred to as "condenser" chambers. The word condenser is an improper replacement for the term capacitor.

The first arrangement allows for optimal precision and reliability and is generally used for dosage purposes in radiotherapy. The second and third arrangements are preferable for health protection measurements, where precision better than 10 to 20 per cent is not essential, but portability and convenience are important. The ionization chamber and reading device are made in the size of a fountain pen for personnel monitoring. Because the reading device is carried with the chamber, the dose received by the wearer can be ascertained in the field.

Counting Circuits. Radiation detectors with sufficient sensitivity to record single bursts of radiation of a disintegrating element have the purpose of determining the disintegration rate of the radioactive sample. Not every disintegration will reach the detector and produce a "count," but as a rule there will be a straightforward, proportional relationship between the disintegration rate, or activity in millicuries, and the counting rate as observed by the detector and associated counting circuit. This relationship will be discussed in detail in later chapters. In this chapter we will discuss how the counting rate can be observed and determined.

A radiation detector, whether it is a proportional counter, a Geiger-Mueller counter or a scintillation counter, needs a supply of constant voltage of about one to two thousand volts. The pulses which occur when the counter "sees" radiation are rather small and must be amplified. An amplifier will increase not only the pulses produced in the counter, but all other electric "noises" which may originate in the circuit. A device must be incorporated to discriminate against this noise and to pass the amplified counter pulses. Finally the pulses must be counted and the time for which they are counted determined. The counting rate is finally obtained by dividing the observed counts by the time of observation and expressing it as counts per second or counts per minute. The electronic counting apparatus is generally called a "scaler," or scaling circuit. However, it has become accepted usage to describe the complete "black box" containing all auxiliary devices just mentioned as "scaler." We shall discuss these separate components of the scaler in a little more detail.

High Voltage Supply. The simplest source of high voltage is a dry cell battery. This is occasionally used in portable counters, but not in standard stationary laboratory scalers because it is quite expensive in use and requires continuous replacement. The conventional way to get the high potential is to step up the alternating line voltage of 115 volts by a transformer to about 2000 volts and then to rectify it and smooth and stabilize it against line voltage fluctuations by suitable electronic methods. The voltage attained in this way fluctuates very little. The stability attained by modern equipment is routinely better than 0.1 per cent and this is sufficient for all but the most critical applications. The voltage necessary to operate a given counter varies for different types of radiation detectors and for individual tubes. A Geiger-Mueller tube may require a supply of from 900 to 1500 volts, whereas a scintillation counter or a proportional counter may require up to 1000 volts more. A scaler must be able to supply, therefore, a variable potential. A coarse and fine control of this voltage is provided on the panel, and a voltmeter is built in so as to read the voltage used and to make it possible to adjust this whenever necessary. For very precise applications the voltage is determined by the settings of several dials. In this way the uncertainty of reading the voltmeter is avoided.

Amplifiers. Amplifiers required to increase the size of the electrical pulse from a radiation detector vary markedly depending upon the application. For Geiger-Mueller counting the total amplification required is less than 10 when using transistor circuits, the maximum frequency to be passed by the amplifier is of the order of 10,000 Hertz (cycles per second), and the amplification does not have to remain very constant. On the other hand, to take full advantage of a solid state detector, amplification of more than 10,000 may be required, frequencies greater than 10 Megahertz may have to be amplified and stability must be of the order of 0.1%. The proportional and scintillation counters demand amplifiers between these extremes. Some of these requirements may seem quite severe but linear amplifiers (*i.e.* amplifiers whose output pulse height is directly proportional to the input pulse height) are available to satisfy all these requirements.

Preamplifiers. Proportional counters and solid state detectors have very small output pulses when compared to those of a Geiger-Mueller counter. When using these low output detectors an additional amplifier is required which is placed ahead of the main amplifier and is therefore called a preamplifier. Such preamplifiers are placed close to, or integral with, the detector and are specially designed to have a very low inherent noise level. They are also designed to operate effectively with long cables to the main amplifier. For this reason a preamplifier is also quite often used with a scintillation counter even though the output pulse here is generally large. More recently "charge sensitive" preamplifiers have become available. In these devices the output pulse height is proportional to the charge delivered from the detector rather than to the voltage of the pulse from the detector. Their use permits longer cables between the detector and the preamplifier and they also feature a lower noise output than do the older amplifiers.

Discriminator. The function and the purpose of a discriminator are identical to the threshold phenomenon in sensory perception, it passes on to the counting circuit proper only pulses which exceed a certain ("threshold") value. Thus spurious pulses originating within the measuring device itself and not coming from the outside are not counted. The equivalent purpose served by the visual and acoustic threshold is to prevent the cortex from being swamped by endoptic and endaural phenomena. It is always desirable to set the discriminator threshold as high as possible in order to have maximum rejection of unwanted electric noise; but it is of course not possible to set this threshold too close to the value of the counter pulse itself, since one has to be sure that all proper counts are transmitted. With Geiger-Mueller counters it is easy to find a compromise; most scalers have, therefore, no external control for the discriminator, but have a rarely adjusted internal control. Other detectors yield pulses whose size depends upon the energy absorbed and here when a discriminator is used, an external adjustment is desirable. The proper use of a discriminator control is discussed more fully below.

Counting Mechanisms. After the electric pulses are amplified and "cleaned" from electric noise by the discriminator, they are counted in the scaling circuit in the narrow sense of the word.

Basically the scaling or counting circuit has the same function as a hand tally counter, used for the counting of blood cells. This is a device with a set of numerals which advance by one unit whenever a lever is depressed by the finger. The only difference is that in the counting circuit this advance is achieved electrically. In its simplest form an electromagnet performs this function. Although such an electromechanically operated counter is very simple, it has one serious limitation: it is slow, and it cannot follow counts which occur more frequently than 10 to 20 times per second (some specially constructed ones have achieved maximum speeds of 130 counts per second). Disintegration rates in samples to be observed are frequently much higher; counting rates in radiation detectors therefore exceed usually the limitations of electromechanical counters. Electronic devices using transistors, vacuum tubes or other similar components are capable of much higher speeds and can be built to approach a counting rate capacity of several million per second.

From the point of view of the user, the electronic counters can be divided into two classes: decade and binary.

A decade counter displays the result in our conventional decimal notation in several ways. It may have a row of lights, labeled from 0 through 9 for each decade. There are also several special counting and indicating tubes where either a light dot moves from side to side or around the periphery of the tube, and each position is labeled by the numbers 0 to 9 (glow transfer tubes). Indicator tubes are available which actually display the arabic numerals. The advantage of these decade counters is that they indicate the counts in the conventional, decimal notation. The disadvantage is the complexity of the electric circuits.

Electrically the simplest counting circuit is the binary counter; its disadvantage is that the binary system of notation is not familiar, and rather puzzling at first, although it is basically simpler than our decimal system. It is in general use in electronic computing machines. While binary indicating scalers are only infrequently encountered in present-day equipment, binary counters are often used. Binary coded decimal equipment is widely available. Thus, an understanding of the binary number system is desirable.

It can be best explained by an examination of the decimal notation. What do we mean by writing down say:

$$8052?$$

We know the answer of course:

$$8 \times 1000 + 0 \times 100 + 5 \times 10 + 2 \times 1$$

Or, remembering that any number raised to the power zero equals one, so that $10^0 = 1$:

$$8 \times 10^3 + 0 \times 10^2 + 5 \times 10^1 + 2 \times 10^0$$

We see that the *position* of a digit designates the power of ten by which it has to be multiplied:

$$\begin{array}{cccc} 8 & 0 & 5 & 2 \\ 10^3 & 10^2 & 10^1 & 10^0 \end{array}$$

If there are five digits, the first on the left, which will be the fifth from the right or unit digit, will indicate ten thousands or 10^4 and so on. To summarize: in the decimal system the position of each digit indicates by what power of ten it has to be multiplied. This is of course what we are doing when we use this system.

In the binary system powers of two are used instead of powers of ten. If we write

$$1011$$

the positions will denote

$$\begin{array}{cccc} 1 & 0 & 1 & 1 \\ 2^3 & 2^2 & 2^1 & 2^0 \end{array}$$

or, if the powers of two are spelled out:

$$\begin{array}{cccc} 1 & 0 & 1 & 1 \\ 8 & 4 & 2 & 1 \end{array}$$

which means, in complete analogy to decimal notation

$$1 \times 8 + 0 \times 4 + 1 \times 2 + 1 \times 1 = 8 + 0 + 2 + 1.$$

We can, if we wish, add this up in decimal notation ("translate") to 11. There are naturally no limitations to the number of digits; the decimal number 1430 can be written down in binary notation as 10110010110:

$$\begin{array}{ccccccccccc} 1 & 0 & 1 & 1 & 0 & 0 & 1 & 0 & 1 & 1 & 0 \\ 2^{10} & 2^9 & 2^8 & 2^7 & 2^6 & 2^5 & 2^4 & 2^3 & 2^2 & 2^1 & 2^0 \end{array}$$

$$1024 + 0 + 256 + 128 + 0 + 0 + 16 + 0 + 4 + 2 + 0 = 1430$$

There are two features about binary notation which must be noted: First that we need more "places" to write out a given number: in the example four places are needed in the decimal notation and eleven places in the binary. This complication is one of the reasons why the binary system did not achieve widespread use prior to the introduction of electronic computers. Second we must note that only two "numbers" are needed, 0 and 1, instead of ten, 0 to 9. This alone permits a tremendous simplification in a counting circuit: we need no device to write out or to indicate the ten numbers of the arabic decimal notation and we can indicate every digit by a single lamp, by using for instance the code: lamp *off* indicates "0," lamp *on* indicates "1." The number 1430 would then appear on the scaler panel as

on	off	on	on	off	off	on	off	on	on	off
2^{10}	2^9	2^8	2^7	2^6	2^5	2^4	2^3	2^2	2^1	2^0

$$1024 + 0 + 256 + 128 + 0 + 0 + 16 + 0 + 4 + 2 + 0$$

The greatest advantage of the binary system goes much deeper, however, than the simplicity of an indicating system: the electric circuitry is inherently simpler; for the same capacity it requires fewer components (transistors, tubes, etc.) than a decimal scaler and is therefore cheaper and more trouble free. The complication of translating the binary numbers into decimal ones is unquestionably a nuisance, since necessary calculations are done in the decimal system (slide rule scales are of course so divided).

A combination of the binary and decimal number systems is most often used in the decade counter. Each decimal digit is separately stored electronically in its binary form within a decade counter. For example, the decimal number 279 will be stored in the form

Third Decade	Second Decade	First Decade
0010	0111	1001
2	7	9

Four binary counters are used in each decade. (Note that four binary counters are capable of storing the decimal numbers 0 to 15, but when used in this system are only used to store numbers from 0 to 9. This system is wasteful but has the advantage of easy decimal readout which most users prefer.) A set of indicator lights is operated from these four counters so that a number (0 to 9) is illuminated when the binary counter contains that number. A counter using this system is said to be a binary coded decimal (bcd) counter. Storage in binary coded decimal form is always used with scalers where a printout (typewriter, adding machine, etc.) is required.

Electronic counting circuits have no limitations in capacity, any number of counts can be counted by increasing the number of "digits," that is binary or decimal scaling stages. But it must be recalled that the purpose of using electronic counting stages was their high speed. The ultimate speed in measuring disintegration rates is limited, due to the limited ability of the radiation detectors themselves to record excessively high counting rates (see section on resolving time, p. 242). Most counters have a maximum counting rate limitation of between a few hundred and several thousand counts per second. A number of electronic counting stages which have a capacity of about 200 to 500 counts will reduce the counting rate of a detector of e.g. 2,000 counts per second to less than 10 pulses per second, so that subsequent counting stages need not have a high speed response and electronic counting stages can be replaced by much simpler and cheaper electromechanical tally type counters. Most modern scaling circuits have, therefore, a combination of electronic and electromechanical counting elements: the pulses arriving from the radiation detector are first counted by electronic counting stages; when these stages have divided the counts sufficiently so that the pulses passed by them are slow enough to be handled by electromechanical counters, these counters take over and carry out the further extension of the counts.

A common arrangement consists of three electronic decade counters followed by an electromechanical register. The register indicates one count for each thousand detector pulses and the decade counter lights show the number of counts over the last thousand indicated by the register.

Timing Mechanisms. The final purpose of nuclear measurements is the determination of the number of radiation bursts per unit time, and the purpose of the scaling circuit is to determine the counting rate. To achieve this, it is necessary to find in addition to the counts observed, c, also the time, t, in which the counts, c, accrued. Every reader is familiar with the measurement of time intervals with a stopwatch, and this is also used in scaling circuits; an electric stopwatch is either built into the instrument or it can be plugged in externally. The stopwatch is started and stopped simultaneously with the counting mechanism. The counting rate, R, is then calculated by dividing the observed counts by the elapsed time:

$$R = c/t.$$

It might be noted that time may be measured in seconds, minutes or hours, and the counting rate calculated in counts per second, counts per minute, or counts per hour. There is no theoretical reason to prefer any one of the units and the only guide for selection is convenience. For high counting rates, counts per second are more convenient since the numbers will have fewer zeros; for low counting rates, counts per minute are preferable since there will be fewer decimal places. Frequently the best guide to the selection of the units is the way the stopwatch happens to be calibrated. If it is calibrated in minutes and decimal fractions of a minute, counts per minute should be used, otherwise every result will have to be multiplied by 60, in order to convert it into counts per second.

For convenience and for reducing errors in starting and stopping, the counting mechanism and the stopwatch are electrically coupled in such a way that a single switch actuates both. Provision is further made to reset the counter and the timer to zero before a new observation is started. The resetting can be made in some instruments by operating a single switch or button, in others the timer and the counter are reset separately; the electromechanical counter has to be reset in some instruments mechanically. Separate resetting is a minor inconvenience.

Preset Time and Preset Count Features. A considerable inconvenience in working with scaling circuits is the necessity to watch the counts or the time and to stop the measurements when one of the two has reached the required reading. This is eliminated in most scalers by incorporating an automatic stopping of the measurement after the required time has elapsed or after the required number of counts have accumulated. The first is achieved by one of the familiar interval timers, which is suitably connected into the circuit to stop the counts when the preset time has elapsed; this is called the *preset time method*. The advantage of this method is that the timer can be preset for a convenient integral interval, say one or ten minutes. The calculation of the counting rate is then simply the division of the observed counts by one or ten. The second method is to stop the stopwatch after the desired number of counts has been accumulated. This is electrically as simple as the use of an interval timer. It is called *preset count method* and it has a basic advantage: by presetting a number of counts the precision of the observations is also preset, as will be discussed in the section on counting statistics. When making a series of measurements, a comparable precision of each measurement is usually desirable; preset count method can insure this automatically.

Time and Count Printers. With the scaling circuits discussed so far, after every measurement the elapsed time and the accumulated counts have to be read off the instrument panel and written down. Even with preset time or preset count circuits, the time or the counts have to be read and noted. When a large series of counting measurements have to be performed with an automatic sample changer, it is necessary also to record the readings automatically. For this purpose some scalers have provision for the connection of automatic printers, which print out on adding machine paper tape either elapsed time for a preset number of counts or the accumulated counts for a preset time interval. The advantage of such auxiliary printing devices is obvious with automatic sample changers: once such a sample changer is loaded, the instrument makes the observations automatically, it can operate during the night, and the results are recorded numerically. When using a preset time mode, *i.e.* when the number of counts accumulated is printed, all electronic scaling stages are generally used. The number of counts registered in an electronic decade can be "read" by a printer while those in an electromechanical register cannot. Thus, preset time counting may require as many as six decades of electronic scaling, but as these circuits are relatively inexpensive, this presents no great drawback to the method. There is a further use of such printers not

15

only where they are a convenience and a time and labor saving device, but where the required result cannot be obtained by simple manual counting. This situation presents itself if a phenomenon has to be observed where the radiation intensity changes so rapidly that it cannot be followed by manual counting. Several such examples will be encountered in clinical diagnostic studies, for instance in using radioactive sodium in peripheral vascular disease. A radiation detector is placed over some location of the human body and the appearance, increase and eventual decrease and disappearance of radioactivity is to be observed; these changes with time are the relevant information which is sought. If the time during which these changes occur is short, say a few minutes, it is difficult to count manually and to keep track of the time elapsed from the beginning of the experiment. An automatic printer, however, will register this information continuously and will give a record from which as many points for plotting a graph can be calculated as are desirable and as can be obtained with the average counting rate in the given experiment.

Rate Meters and Recorders. Sometimes the variations of radiation intensity are so rapid that it is inconvenient or perhaps impossible to observe them even with a printing device. In such situations rate meters can be used. A rate meter is an instrument which is basically different in design and construction from a scaler. It has in common with it a high voltage supply for the operation of the radiation detector, an amplifier and a discriminator; but instead of a counting circuit (the "scaling circuit" in the narrow sense of the word) it has a circuit which is made sensitive to the average frequency of the electric pulses, that is to the counting rate. Such electric and electronic circuits are well known and commonly used as frequency meters. Their output, usually a current of a few milliamperes, is proportional to the counting rate. If this output is connected to a meter, the counting rate at any given instant can be read on its dial. The output can be also connected to a strip chart recorder, which is similar to the recording part of an electrocardiograph, so that the time plot of counting rate is obtained directly. There is one feature of the rate meter circuit which should be clearly understood for its proper use and that is that it performs basically the same function as a scaling circuit; it observes counts and elapsed time and computes the ratio (counts per unit time) by electronic means. It does this in a manner essentially similar to the preset time method. The parameter in a rate meter which is analogous to time for which a scaler is "preset" is usually called "time constant." The longer the time constant, the more counts will the rate meter accumulate with a given counting rate to reach its final deflection, and the slower will its pointer or recording pen deflect in response to a change in radiation intensity. The time constant is also one of the factors which determine the precision; this will be discussed in connection with counting statistics. It may be useful to anticipate here the conclusion: the larger the time constant, the greater the statistical precision of the readings for a given counting rate; the higher the counting rate, the greater the precision with a given time constant. This determines the limitations of a rate meter in recording rapidly changing phenomena; a small time constant is required to observe rapid changes and this can be achieved only at the expense of precision, unless the observed counting rates are high.

One common use of counting rate meters is in radiation survey instruments. In this application low radiation intensities are of interest, and low counting rates have to be measured. The requirements for precision on the other hand are quite modest. A workable compromise between time constant and precision can therefore be easily achieved.

Coincidence and Anticoincidence Circuits. In certain counting applications it is required that not every pulse arriving from a radiation detector or some part of the auxiliary circuit is counted but only those pulses which occur simultaneously with some other pulse: coincidence counting, as for instance in positron scanning (see page 335). There are also applications where an opposite function is required, that is when only such pulses must be counted as occur alone and which should not be counted when they occur simultaneously with another pulse: anticoincidence counting, as for example in some background reduction circuits (see page 287) and in pulse height analyzers (see page 217).

Coincidence Circuit. Figure 14–4 illustrates the principle of operation in a coincidence circuit by an electromechanical model.

Two radiation detectors A and B are connected to two circuits A and B. The detectors A and B produce electric pulses and it is required that the pulse from detector A is counted only when detector B also produces a pulse simultaneously with the pulse of detector A, and that when a pulse occurs in detector A only, no count is registered in the counting circuit. The sources of pulses A and B need not necessarily come from two different

COINCIDENCE CIRCUIT

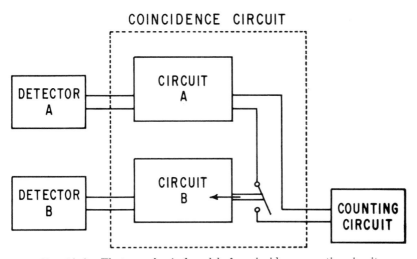

FIG. 14–4. Electromechanical model of a coincidence counting circuit.

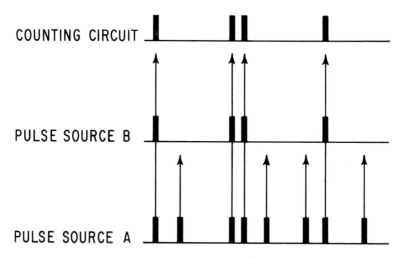

COUNTING CIRCUIT

PULSE SOURCE B

PULSE SOURCE A

FIG. 14–5.   Diagram of electric pulses in a coincidence circuit.

detectors; they may be generated in an auxiliary circuit source which produces two different pulses depending on the operating conditions of a single detector.

The pulses A and B are handled in circuits A and B, which contain, as required, power supplies, discriminators and amplifiers.

Circuit A passes the pulse from detector A after amplification and discrimination to the counting circuit, but there is a switch (relay contact) in series with this connection.   This contact is normally open so that the pulses from circuit A cannot reach the counting circuit and be counted, unless this contact is closed.

Circuit B operates the relay and closes the contact when and only when a pulse occurs in detector B, which after amplification passes through the discriminator of circuit B.

The result is that pulses originating in circuit A reach the counter only when the relay contact is closed by circuit B, due to a pulse in that circuit. Counts are registered therefore only when detector A with circuit A operate simultaneously (in "coincidence") with detector B and circuit B.

While it is quite feasible to build a coincidence circuit with a relay, as described, the usefulness of such an arrangement is limited due to the relatively slow action of an electromechanical relay.   In actual practice the same result is achieved by electronic means, which operate at the required high speed.

Figure 14–5 illustrates the performance of a coincidence circuit.

Anticoincidence Circuit.   Figure 14–6 illustrates a model similar to that shown for the coincidence circuit, arranged for anticoincidence operation.

Pulses passed by circuit A are here normally free to reach the counting circuit since the relay contact of circuit B is closed, unless circuit B pro-

ANTI-COINCIDENCE CIRCUIT

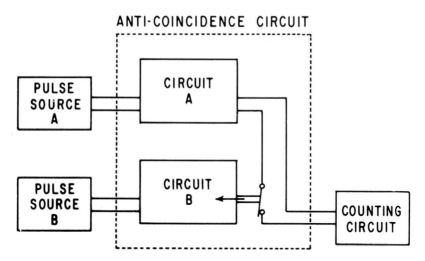

FIG. 14–6.   Electromechanical model of an anticoincidence circuit.

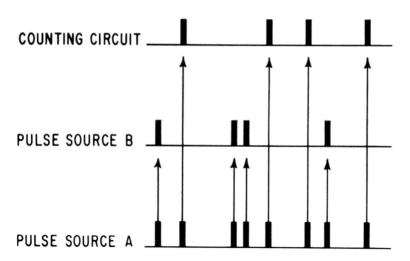

FIG. 14–7.   Diagram of electric pulses in an anticoincidence circuit.

duces a pulse originating in source B.   When this occurs, the relay contact opens and the pulse from source A-circuit A is blocked from the counting circuit and no counts can be registered.   The performance of the anti-coincidence circuit is illustrated in Figure 14–7.   As in a coincidence circuit the actual instruments use high speed electronic devices to block the pulses from circuit A when a pulse occurs in circuit B.

Pulse-Height Analyzers.   As discussed in the previous chapter the pro-portional counter, scintillation counter and the solid state detector all pro-duce output pulses which are proportional in height to the amount of

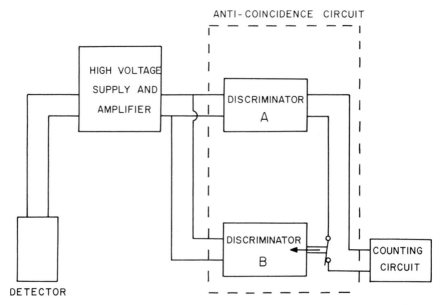

Fig. 14–8. A single channel analyzer using two discriminators in anticoincidence circuit. The threshold of discriminator A is set to V volt, that of discriminator B to V + △V volt. The counting circuit registers only pulses which have a voltage between V and V + △V.

energy absorbed in the detector. This property of these detectors can be used to advantage. However, this utilization requires additional electronic circuits which can sort the pulses according to their height. Such devices were originally called "kicksorters" (kick for pulse) and are presently called pulse-height analyzers.

The most elementary of these devices, the single channel analyzer (sca), is a combination of two discriminators and an anticoincidence circuit (See page 216) connected as shown in Figure 14–8. The amplifier output is connected to the two discriminators, labeled A and B, which are adjustable in a way to be described and whose outputs are connected to an anticoincidence circuit as indicated in the figure.

Let the two discriminators be adjusted in such a way that discriminator A passes pulses of V volts or larger and discriminator B operates only on pulses which are at least △V volts larger than those which just operate circuit A, i.e. on pulses of height V + △V or larger. Three types of events can occur:

1. Pulse is less than V. Neither of the circuits operates, no count is registered.

2. Pulse is larger than V but smaller than V + △V. Circuit A passes a pulse, circuit B remains inoperative; a count is registered.

3. Pulse is larger than V + △V. Circuit A operates, circuit B also operates and blocks the pulse of circuit A; no count is registered.

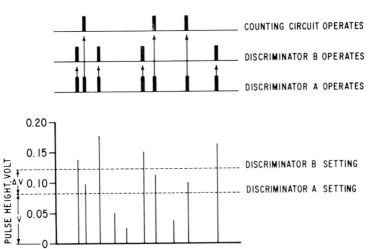

Fig. 14–9. The lower diagram illustrates the pulse heights as they come from the scintillation counter. The upper diagram indicates how the discriminators A and B operate in the anticoincidence circuit for different pulse heights. Note that when discriminator B operates, it blocks the pulses passed by discriminator A from reaching the counting circuit.

In short, only pulses which are between V and V + △V are counted. We thereby obtain the number of pulses within this range (changing the settings of the discriminators A and B makes it possible to determine the distribution of pulses according to their height. Hence the name of this circuit arrangement: pulse-height analyzer). Figure 14–9 illustrates the function of this analyzer diagrammatically.

For convenience of operation, the discriminator controls of A and B are coupled so that one control varies V in both circuits and another changes △V. These controls are usually labeled baseline or threshold and window respectively.

The terminology is apt. The single channel analyzer operates like a window. Only those pulses whose height put them over the "window sill" but yet within the window opening will produce an output. Thus, the baseline or threshold control varies the "window sill" height while the window control varies the "openness" of the window.

Some specially augmented versions of the single channel analyzer are worthy of note. One is an analyzer in which the baseline control is motor driven to permit a continuous, automatic increase in the value of V. When this device is used and the analyzer output pulses are fed to a rate meter connected to a recorder, a plot is obtained of count rate vs baseline setting. This provides a "spectrum" of the pulse heights useful for radionuclide identification.

Another specialized instrument employs several single channel analyzers each connected to its own scaler. All counts falling between V_1 and $V_1 + \triangle V_1$, V_2 and $V_2 + \triangle V_2$, etc. can separately and simultaneously be determined. Such a device is particularly useful when multiple radioactive nuclides are used and must be separately assayed.

The multiple single channel analyzer represents the transition between the single channel and the multichannel analyzers. Multichannel devices, while complex and expensive, are finding ever-widening use in the medical and biological area. A multichannel analyzer, as the name implies, is a device which is capable of measuring the number of pulses in many voltage or channel ranges simultaneously. The electronic circuits are such that these channels are adjacent and non-overlapping. Historically, these were indeed multiple single channel analyzers, but they now operate on an entirely different principle. The details of this principle are beyond the scope of this work and unnecessary to the understanding of the function of a multichannel analyzer. The principal advantage of the multichannel over the single channel analyzer is a time saving and this is a very significant factor in actual practice.

Modern multichannel analyzers can also serve another useful function. When employed in what is termed the "multiscale mode" each channel can be used as an independent high speed count register. Shifting from one channel to the next is accomplished either from an internal clock or an external signal. The analyzer in this mode can be used as a recorder to remember the number of counts received in each of a large number of time intervals for studies of the distribution of radioactive tracers with time (see p. 239 and Chapter 18).

15

Statistical Considerations of Radiation Counting

Basic Considerations. Radioactive disintegrations occur in a completely random manner. There is no way of predicting when a given individual atom will disintegrate; the only information we have about such an atom is that it has a 50-50 chance to disintegrate during the next half-life. The reliability of predictions about half-lives and disintegration rates of radioactive samples is based on the fact that even a minute fraction of a millicurie contains an extraordinarily large number of atoms, and that statistical predictions approach certainty when large numbers of events are involved.

Principles. When measurements of radioactive samples are made, the actual numbers of disintegrations which are observed by counting are not necessarily very large. Let us consider the measurement of a radioactive sample with some counting arrangement in which about five counts per second are observed. If we were to carry out our measurements until one million counts were accumulated, the uncertainty* due to the random nature of radioactive decay, that is the statistical fluctuations, would become negligible for any practical purpose. But such an observation would take 200,000 seconds, or over 55 hours. This is obviously impractically long, and therefore a certain amount of statistical uncertainty will have to be accepted in order to reduce this time.

The magnitude of the uncertainty which is acceptable is determined by the particular experiment. In measuring blood pressure for instance the acceptable uncertainty is a few mm of mercury, since physiological variations are of this order of magnitude and only larger deviations from the normal values have clinical significance. It is easy to build a manometer, which has an uncertainty of less than $\frac{1}{2}$ mm mercury, but the increased cost compared to a conventional sphygmomanometer will be wasted since the increased precision would be of no diagnostic value. On the other hand an uncertainty exceeding 10 mm mercury would not be acceptable, since such a difference approaches clinical significance. Similar consideration must lead us to decide what the tolerable uncertainties are in any particular use

---

* The word error is often substituted for uncertainty used in this sense. However, as we shall see, the uncertainty is a known quantity. Where the error is known we generally use the knowledge to correct our results. Usually the error, *i.e.* the "wrongness" of a result, is unknown.

of radioactive materials. Counting statistics will then give us information about the number of counts to be accumulated and the required counting time.

To understand how this is done we begin with the concept of the standard deviation. This is a measure of the uncertainty in a measurement. A suitable definition of the standard deviation is that if the measurement of the quantity under observation is repeated many times, 68 per cent of these measurements will deviate from their mean by an amount which is smaller than the standard deviation. An extension of this statement, which follows from elementary probability theory and which applies to nuclear counting, is that about 95 per cent of all observations will have deviations less than twice the standard deviation and over 99.7 per cent will have less than three times the standard deviation.

The random nature of radioactive decay, *i.e.* the independence of the decay of one nucleus from that of any other, allows the process to be described by the "Poisson Distribution." As a result of this, the standard deviation is easily expressed in terms of the number of observed events. If this number is N then σ, the standard deviation, is given by

$$\sigma = \sqrt{N} \qquad\qquad 15\text{---}(1)$$

Let us take as an example an experiment in which the counting rate is known to be roughly 5 counts per second. Suppose that we desire to determine the actual counting rate to an uncertainty of 3 per cent. How many counts must we obtain or for how long must we count to achieve this precision? If we assume tentatively that we want the standard deviation σ to be equal to 3 per cent of the accumulated total counts, N, we have the equation:

$$\sigma = \frac{3}{100} N$$

which expresses the stipulation that σ should be 3 per cent of N.

Substituting σ from (1) we get

$$\sqrt{N} = \frac{3}{100} N$$

and

$$N = \left(\frac{100}{3}\right)^2 = 1{,}111 \text{ counts}$$

This will take about 200 seconds, or only a little over three minutes. It is, however, very important to realize that a standard deviation of 3 per cent means only that our chances to obtain a value of N within 3 per cent of the presumably correct value every time we count for 200 seconds is about 2 to 1. This is certainly poor betting odds. If we want to have a value of N less likely to differ from the correct value by as much as 3 per cent, we have to recall that these chances increase as we reduce the value of the standard deviation.

If we make σ half the desired uncertainty of 3 per cent, that is

$$\sigma = \frac{1.5}{100} N$$

we get for the required N the value

$$N = 4{,}444$$

The chances now will be 20 to 1 that the observed N does not differ by more than 3 per cent from the correct value. And if σ is reduced to one-third of the required uncertainty of 3 per cent, we get

$$\sigma = \frac{1}{100} N$$

and

$$N = 10{,}000$$

In this case our chances of being within the 3 per cent limit of error are 370 to 1.

It is frequently convenient to express an uncertainty in per cent of the measured magnitude. The uncertainty corresponding to the standard deviation in per cent will be designated as V (this is called the coefficient of variation)

$$V = 100 \frac{\sigma}{N} \qquad\qquad 15\text{—}(2)$$

Since $\sigma = \sqrt{N}$, V can be expressed as

$$V = 100 \frac{\sqrt{N}}{N} \qquad \text{or}$$

$$V = \frac{100}{\sqrt{N}} \qquad\qquad 15\text{—}(3)$$

If we want to find the value of N, which assures a given coefficient of variation V, we get from (3)*:

$$N = \frac{10{,}000}{V^2} \qquad\qquad 15\text{—}(4)$$

The use of this per cent uncertainty or coefficient of variation has an advantage beyond mere convenience. Later the uncertainties in counting

* References to equations within this chapter are given in shortened form, *i.e.* (3) means Eq. 15–3.

rates will be discussed. If they are to be determined from the standard deviation, σ, of the total number of counts, N, some additional mathematical operations will be needed: the standard deviations of the total counts, N and of a counting rate R, are not the same, whereas the per cent uncertainty has the same value for both N and R, under certain conditions, which usually obtain.

From equation (4) the required number of counts can be calculated which are needed to have the actual per cent uncertainty within a given limit with a given confidence. *If this uncertainty is designated as P per cent*, then in order to have 2 out of 3 observations with an uncertainty not to exceed P, we have to make V = P; in order to have about 20 out of 21 such observations V should be = P/2 and to have 370 out of 371 observations within the limits, we need V = P/3.

This gives the rule for determining the required coefficient of variation to be used in equation (4) for a given per cent uncertainty:

Low reliability: $V = P$ 15—(5)

Medium reliability: $V = P/2$ 15—(6)

High reliability: $V = P/3$ 15—(7)

By substituting V in (4) we get the required number of counts:

Low reliability: $N = \dfrac{10,000}{P^2}$ 15—(5a)

Medium reliability: $N = \dfrac{40,000}{P^2}$ 15—(6a)

High reliability: $N = \dfrac{90,000}{P^2}$ 15—(7a)

It will be noted that increase in reliability is achieved at a considerable cost in time: almost 10 times as many counts and hence time is needed to achieve high as compared to low reliability!

This discussion demonstrates that after deciding on the required precision, we still have to make the further decision about the degree of assurance so that the limits of the selected uncertainty are not too frequently exceeded in the measurements. There is no hard and fast rule in this respect, and the only simplifications which can be given are some practical guides:

For preliminary information the standard deviation or coefficient of variation may be made equal to the desired uncertainty (low reliability).

In every day work, when a compromise has to be made between available time and the reliability of individual measurements, a standard deviation or coefficient of variation equal to half the accepted uncertainty is a reasonable compromise (medium reliability).

When the conditions of the observation are such that a high order of confidence is needed in keeping the uncertainties within the stipulated limit then the standard deviation or coefficient of variation should be made equal to one-third of that uncertainty (high reliability).

Different levels of reliability are described as "confidence limits." Confidence limit signifies the probability that an observation describes the true state to within the uncertainty limits. In other words, it is the fraction of such observations which actually will have errors less than or equal to these limits. We can express our descriptive terminology quantitatively:

Low reliability corresponds to confidence limit of 0.68

Medium "   "   "   "   "   " 0.95

High   "   "   "   "   "   " 0.997

Background. Whenever a radiation detector is used to measure a radioactive sample, it will receive, in addition to the radiation emitted by this sample, radiation coming from the outer space ("cosmic radiation") and from naturally occurring radioactive materials in the earth. To these two extraneous sources of radiation is added whatever may have been introduced in and around the laboratory, as for instance other samples in the vicinity, radioactive sources in storage, and x-ray machines. All these sources create a radiation background which affects a detector and is observed by a counting rate even when no sample is introduced into the measurement arrangement. This background, or background counting rate, can be reduced but not completely eliminated when an observation is made, so that whenever a sample is actually "counted," the sum of the sample counts and of the background counts is obtained. The background counting rate has to be determined separately and the counting rate of the sample itself can then be obtained by subtracting the background counting rate R_b from the combined or gross counting rate R_c. The sample or net counting rate R_s is therefore

$$R_s = R_c - R_b \qquad\qquad 15-(8)$$

This introduces a new complication to the statistical considerations discussed in the preceding section: the determination of the sample counting rate R_s depends actually on the determination of two distinct and separate magnitudes, that is, on the background as well as on the combined or gross counting rate.

This complication disappears if the background is negligibly small compared to the sample count; in this case gross and net counts are practically identical. But when the background is significant in comparison with the combined count, it will contribute to the uncertainty in the determination of the sample counting rate.

The statistical rule for the determination of the standard deviation σ_d of a sum or a difference of two other magnitudes which themselves have the standard deviations σ_1 and σ_2 is:

$$\sigma_d = \sqrt{\sigma_1{}^2 + \sigma_2{}^2} \qquad\qquad 15\text{—}(9)$$

In order to apply this equation to the calculation of the standard deviation of the net sample counting rate R_s, we have to know the standard deviations of the gross and background counting rates R_c and R_b.

From equation (1) we know that the standard deviations of the total accumulated gross counts N_c and the background counts N_b are $\sqrt{N_c}$ and $\sqrt{N_b}$ respectively. If the time to accumulate the gross counts is t_c, and the time for the background counts is t_b, then the counting rates are

$$R_c = \frac{N_c}{t_c} \qquad\qquad 15\text{—}(10)$$

$$R_b = \frac{N_b}{t_b} \qquad\qquad 15\text{—}(11)$$

From this it follows that

$$\sigma_c = \frac{\sqrt{N_c}}{t_c} \qquad\qquad 15\text{—}(12)$$

and

$$\sigma_b = \frac{\sqrt{N_b}}{t_b} \qquad\qquad 15\text{—}(13)$$

where σ_c and σ_b are the standard deviations of the gross and background *counting rates* respectively. Equation (9) can now be used and we get for the standard deviation σ_s of the net or sample counting rate

$$\sigma_s = \sqrt{\sigma_c{}^2 + \sigma_b{}^2} \qquad\qquad 15\text{—}(14)$$

and by substituting (12) and (13)

$$\sigma_s = \sqrt{\frac{N_c}{t_c{}^2} + \frac{N_b}{t_b{}^2}} \qquad\qquad 15\text{—}(15)$$

By substituting N_c and N_b from (10) and (11), equation (15) can be written also in the form:

$$\sigma_s = \sqrt{\frac{R_c}{t_c} + \frac{R_b}{t_b}} \qquad\qquad 15\text{—}(16)$$

which will be useful in a different connection, to be discussed later in this chapter.

Or finally by substituting t_c and t_b in (16) from (10) and (11):

$$\sigma_s = \sqrt{\frac{R_c{}^2}{N_c} + \frac{R_b{}^2}{N_b}} \qquad 15-(17)$$

The per cent standard deviation of the sample counting rate V_s is now, according to (2)

$$V_s = \frac{100\sigma_s}{R_s} \qquad 15-(18)$$

and σ_s is known from (14), (15), or (16). Equation (15) will permit calculation of the standard deviation of the sample counting rate, when the total counts and times of the gross and background measurements are known, but it still leaves open the answer to the following important problem: how many counts should one accumulate for gross and for background counting in order to achieve a desired precision, that is, a selected value of standard deviation? Expressing this problem in other terms, what fraction of the available time should be spent in counting background? The answer is too complex for a complete treatment here.

A rigorous solution of this problem was given by Loevinger and Berman*. Since the numerical calculations from their equations are somewhat lengthy and a graph of a family of curves is used, a simplified assumption will be used in the following presentation. The limitations of this simplification will be also discussed.

It can be seen from the equations (14) and (15) for σ_s that it is pointless to count background to a higher precision than the gross counts, since, however small the background uncertainties become, the final uncertainty in the sample counts will not be reduced below the uncertainty in the gross counts. The uncertainties in gross counts and background count should be balanced. The simplest approximation to such a balance is to make them equal, that is to have

$$\sigma_c = \sigma_b \qquad 15-(19)$$

On the basis of this approximation, it is possible to determine the number of counts to be accumulated for gross and for background counting, provided we know *approximately* these counting rates from a preliminary rough measurement. Let these approximate counting rates be R'_c and R'_b. We have from (12)

$$\sigma_c{}^2 = \frac{N_c}{t_c{}^2} \qquad 15-(20)$$

---

* See R. Loevinger and M. Berman: Efficiency Criteria in Radioactivity Counting Nucleonics **9**, 26–39, 1951. The graph and instructions for its use are now conveniently available in: "A Manual of Radioactivity Procedures," National Bureau of Standards Handbook 80, 1961. For sale by the Superintendent of Documents, Washington, D.C., 20025, price 50 cents.

and by substituting t_c from (10)

$$\sigma_c^2 = \frac{R_c'^2}{N_c} \qquad 15-(21)$$

and similarly from (13) and (11):

$$\sigma_b^2 = \frac{R_b'^2}{N_b} \qquad 15-(22)$$

Since we decided to use the assumption of equation (19), it follows from it and from (14) that

$$\sigma_s^2 = 2\sigma_c^2 \qquad 15-(23)$$

and also

$$\sigma_s^2 = 2\sigma_b^2 \qquad 15-(24)$$

Equations (23) and (21) give

$$\sigma_s^2 = 2 \frac{R_c'^2}{N_c} \qquad 15-(25)$$

and equations (24) and (22) give

$$\sigma_s^2 = 2 \frac{R_b'^2}{N_b} \qquad 15-(26)$$

Finally we can calculate the required number of counts to be accumulated in order to have a standard deviation σ_s of the net counting rate:
From (25) we get the gross counts

$$N_c = 2 \frac{R_c'^2}{\sigma_s^2} \qquad 15-(27)$$

and from (26) the background counts

$$N_b = 2 \frac{R_b'^2}{\sigma_s^2} \qquad 15-(28)$$

We decide on the value of σ_s on the basis of the per cent standard deviation which has been selected. Let this be V; we have then from (18)

$$V = \frac{100\sigma_s}{R_s}$$

$$\sigma_s = \frac{VR_s}{100}$$

R_s is known approximately from R_c' and R_b' as their difference. Hence

$$\sigma_s = \frac{V(R_c' - R_b')}{100} \qquad 15-(29)$$

We can express now the combined counts N_c and background counts N_b which must be accumulated in order to insure the coefficient of variation V, by substituting the values for σ_s from (29) in the equations (27) and (28):

$$N_c = 20{,}000 \left[\frac{R'_c}{V(R'_c - R'_b)} \right]^2 \qquad 15-(30)$$

and

$$N_b = 20{,}000 \left[\frac{R'_b}{V(R'_c - R'_b)} \right]^2 \qquad 15-(31)$$

The two equations (30) and (31) are useful when preset count technique is used. For preset time technique the counting times for combined and background counting t_c and t_b can be calculated by substituting $N_c = t_c R'_c$ in (30) and $N_b = t_b R'_b$ in (31). This gives

$$t_c = \frac{20{,}000\ R'_c}{[V(R'_c - R'_b)]^2} \qquad 15-(32)$$

and

$$t_b = \frac{20{,}000\ R'_b}{[V(R'_c - R'_b)]^2} \qquad 15-(33)$$

Equations (32) and (33) are also useful for estimating the time which will be required in order to obtain a given value of V. This total time is obviously $t_c + t_b$.

Whether preset time or preset count technique is used, it is essential to keep in mind that the preceding four equations are calculated from counting rates which have been determined only roughly from preliminary experiments. The standard deviation σ_s and the coefficient of variation V of the final determination of R_s will be only approximately of the desired magnitude. It is useful therefore to check their value on the basis of the finally observed t_c and t_b if N_c and N_b were preset, or on the basis of the observed N_c and N_b if t_c and t_b were preset. σ_s can be calculated from (15). V can be calculated by substituting in (18); σ_s from (15) and R_s from (8), (10) and (11):

$$R_s = \frac{N_c}{t_c} - \frac{N_b}{t_b}$$

$$V = 100\ \frac{\sqrt{\dfrac{N_c}{t_c^2} + \dfrac{N_b}{t_b^2}}}{\dfrac{N_c}{t_c} - \dfrac{N_b}{t_b}}$$

This can be simplified by algebraic manipulations to

$$V = 100 \frac{\sqrt{N_c t_b^2 + N_b t_c^2}}{N_c t_b - N_b t_c}.$$ 15—(34)

The use of the equations will be illustrated by an example in which the approximate gross counting rate is $R_c' = 150$ counts per minute and background counting rate is $R_b' = 100$ counts per minute; the required coefficient of variation is $V = 5\%$.

We obtain the needed total counts from (30) and (31)

$$N_c = 20,000 \left(\frac{150}{5 \times 50}\right)^2 = 7,200 \text{ counts}$$

$$N_b = 20,000 \left(\frac{100}{5 \times 50}\right)^2 = 3,200 \text{ counts}$$

and the counting times from (32) and (33)

$$t_c = \frac{20,000 \times 150}{(5 \times 50)^2} = 48 \text{ minutes}$$

$$t_b = \frac{20,000 \times 100}{(5 \times 50)^2} = 32 \text{ minutes}$$

The total counting time will be 80 minutes. If the finally observed counting rates should turn out to be exactly $R_c = 150$ and $R_b = 100$, then V will be necessarily 5 per cent. Should the observed counting rate differ from the approximately estimated values, the value of V obtained can be calculated from (34) and compared to the required value of $V = 5$. Should the actually obtained uncertainty be too large, it will indicate that R_c' and/or R_b' were too poor approximations. The calculations will have to be repeated using the newly obtained combined and background counting rates as R_c' and R_b' and the counting done again.

Let us compare the above result with the Loevinger-Berman method. The example given in Handbook 80 (see footnote page 227) corresponds to our example. The values obtained from the graph are in our notation:

$$N_c = 6,600 \text{ counts}$$

$$N_b = 3,600 \text{ counts}$$

The counting times would be

$$t_c = 44 \text{ minutes}$$

$$t_b = 36 \text{ minutes}$$

or the total of 80 minutes, identical with ours. This agreement is fortuitous and is due to small errors in reading the graph. The superiority of the Loevinger-Berman method should appear in a smaller uncertainty obtained in the same counting times. If the actually observed counting rates were identical to the assumed ones, the final uncertainties due to both methods could be calculated from (34), and it would show that the uncertainty is less than 5 per cent by a negligible amount.

A mathematical comparison of the two methods shows that the gain in time with the Loevinger-Berman method is negligible, when combined counting rate is less than twice background. The choice between the two methods may be left therefore to personal preference. When combined counting rate is greater, the time saving may become significant, though the counting times will be progressively shorter, so that absolute time saved will be significant only when many samples are to be counted. Under such conditions the examination of the data by the Loevinger-Berman method will be advisable.

If the background in the example discussed above were 0.1 count per minute, it is obvious that it could have been disregarded, gross counts considered equal to sample counts and the calculations simplified. The decision between disregarding and not disregarding the background may be difficult in a borderline situation, for instance if in the above example the background rate were two counts per minute. It is of course possible to calculate generally the error introduced by disregarding the background, but the resulting equations are of moderate practical use. A simple rule may be given instead: background can be disregarded when the background counting rate does not exceed one-fifth of the desired percentage uncertainty of the gross counting rate. If the desired coefficient of variation is V, then background may be disregarded when R_b is equal to or smaller than $\dfrac{V}{5} \times \dfrac{R_c}{100}$. If this rule is followed, disregarding the background will not introduce significant error into the determination. The suggested factor of one-fifth is somewhat arbitrary, one-third may be used for less critical work and one-tenth when greater reliability is required. The more stringent criterion will cost somewhat more in terms of time spent in counting.

The rule for neglecting background may be formulated as subject to the condition that

$$R_b \lessgtr \frac{R_c V}{500} \text{ counts per minute} \qquad 15\text{—}(35)$$

Let us apply this rule to the example with combined counting rate $R_c = 150$, required uncertainty $V = 5$ per cent.

$$\frac{R_c V}{500} = 1.5 \text{ counts per minute}$$

According to the rule of equation (35), background could be neglected in this example if it were 1.5 counts per minute or less.

The equations for required number of counts and for the counting time are very much simplified when background can be neglected. R_s becomes R_c; instead of (23) we have $\sigma_s = \sigma_c$, and not $\sigma_s^2 = 2\,\sigma_c^2$, so that the factor 2 becomes 1 in the following equations in which also σ_b, N_b and t_b vanish, and we return to (4) in the form

$$N_s = \frac{10,000}{V^2} \qquad\qquad 15\text{--}(36)$$

It will be noted that N_s is now independent of estimated counting rates, which cancel out in the modified equation (30). The required counting time is from the modified equation (32):

$$t_s = \frac{10,000}{V^2\,R_s'} \qquad\qquad 15\text{--}(37)$$

which is dependent on the preliminary determination of the approximate counting rate.

If the standard deviation σ_s of the observed counting rate R_s is needed, it follows from the definition of coefficient of variation and equation (3)

$$\sigma_s = \frac{R_s V}{100} = \frac{R_s}{\sqrt{N}}$$

σ_s can be expressed directly in terms of the observed counts and counting time, since $R_s = N_s'/t_s$

$$\sigma_s = \frac{\sqrt{N_s}}{t_s} \qquad\qquad 15\text{--}(38)$$

Preset Time and Preset Count Methods of Counting. After the discussion of the statistics of counting, the basic advantage of counting for a preset and therefore constant number of counts is obvious; by presetting the total number of counts to be observed and by measuring the time required for their accumulation, a constant counting uncertainty is maintained.

A disadvantage of present count technique is that the scheduling for counting a large number of samples is difficult. If it is important to have the counting of a given number of samples finished within a certain time, preset time technique is to be preferred at the expense of some non-uniformity of the experimental uncertainties.

Automatic sample changers with associated printers are sometimes used in the preset count mode to secure statistical constancy. The samples to be counted are assumed to all have roughly the same activity and therefore require about equal counting times. Occasionally a sample will have very much less than the expected activity and an undue amount of time will be spent on this sample. Such a time waste can be prevented by the use of an additional circuit which terminates the counting of a sample after a preselected maximum time interval. This method of counting can be termed preset count-preset time. The printer should record both the count and the time interval. The preselected time should exceed the expected time of count of a normal sample by a large enough factor to take care of statistical fluctuations, else the advantages of the preset count mode will be lost.

One potential pitfall of preset count technique should be mentioned, which sometimes occurs with high counting rates. Let us consider a sample which gives 100 counts per second, and a required uncertainty of 3 per cent. This will mean that a total of 1000 counts is needed. Time for this number of counts will be ten seconds. A timer, electrical or mechanical, is usually reliable at best to 0.2 seconds. Ten seconds will be measured therefore with an uncertainty of about 2 per cent, which will increase the "preset" statistical uncertainty. This means that the uncertainty in measurement of time cannot be neglected when the time intervals become short, and that we shall have to increase the preset count setting in such a way that this uncertainty becomes negligible. As a rule, it can be neglected when times of one minute or longer are measured. When the preset time method is used, it is possible that small time intervals of less than one minute or so may introduce timing uncertainties in addition to the statistical uncertainties determined by the number of counts accumulated during this interval.

Background Counting. The role of background in radiation measurements can now be summarized. Background counting rate, when it is of comparable magnitude to sample counting rate, increases the time required to make the determination with a desired precision. Under these conditions, precision of the sample measurement depends on the reliability and hence the constancy of the background. Attention must be directed therefore to the constancy of the background, unless it is so small in relation to the sample count, that it can be disregarded. The constancy of the background depends to a large degree on environmental conditions such as proximity of x-ray generating equipment which is turned on and off, radioactive sources which are moved around (patients with tracer and therapeutic amounts of radioactive material should not be overlooked), or sample containers which are used and may contain traces of previous radioactive samples. The shielding of counting devices by lead enclosures serves therefore a twofold purpose: to reduce the background due to cosmic and terrestrial radiation and to reduce fluctuations of this background produced by changing levels of radiation in the laboratory. Shielding will not affect variations of background due to contamination of sample containers; this can be accounted for only by checking the background with the empty individual containers and by either using this background as determined for each container, or by discarding or storing contaminated containers until they are either decontaminated or the radioactivity has decayed.

Background measurements should be made with sufficient frequency to avoid serious error. Even under ideal conditions of low and constant background an accident may occur, unbeknownst to the technician, which increases the background by a larger factor. A spill which contaminates the detector occurs all too frequently. Unauthorized movement of radioactive material in the laboratory is another common source of background count rate alteration. A regular and frequent schedule of background determination will not only detect such alterations but will also prevent an error from being continued for a prolonged period.

The Use of Rate Meters and Recorders. Counting rate meters and recorders have been mentioned in the section on scaling circuits. Since the evaluation of the statistical uncertainties and hence the reliability of observations with these instruments presents some special aspects, they must be discussed separately from ordinary scalers. On the first casual inspection of a rate meter, it will not be apparent how the general rule of statistics of random events can be applied to it. If such a meter is connected to a radiation detector and a radioactive source brought into its vicinity, it will be noticed that the deflection does not occur instantaneously but slowly until it reaches a final value around which the pointer of the instrument (or the line traced by a recorder) will oscillate. In most rate meters a selector switch will be found on the panel which permits variation in the response speed. This speed of response is a characteristic value of a rate meter; it is usually called its "time constant." The functional role of this time constant corresponds to the time interval selected in a scaling circuit, when it is used with preset time method of counting. To be more precise, the inherent "preset time" of a rate meter is equal to twice its "time constant." If the time constant of a rate meter is thirty seconds, for instance, and if the observed counting rate is 50 counts per second, a total of 3000 counts have been "collected" for this reading since the equivalent "preset time" is sixty seconds. The 3000 counts correspond to an uncertainty of about 2 per cent for the observation of a source of constant activity. When the radiation intensity changes, it will again take the instrument some time to reach the new deflection; this time will have a value between its response time and twice its response time, depending on the magnitude of the change.

Counting Statistics in Rate Meters and Recorders. In ordinary counting the operational controls on the scaling circuit are: 1. Manual, where a switch is operated to start and to stop the counting with a read-out for time and total counts. 2. Preset counts, with a read-out for elapsed time. 3. Preset time with a read-out for accumulated counts. The controls on a rate meter are different. There is a selector switch for "response time" and one or two switches or controls for "range" or "sensitivity." The read-out is either a meter or a strip chart recorder, with some scale or chart divisions, indicating the counting rate directly. The sensitivity or range control permit changing the calibration of the meter or recorder in the sense that the rate corresponding to a given deflection (for full scale or per division) may be made larger or smaller. This is a different way to present the results than in a scaling circuit. We shall designate range control(s) setting(s) as producing a *sensitivity of the instrument S, which we define as the change in counting rate which produces a deflection of one division.*

The statistical variations will appear as fluctuations of the pointer or of the record, superimposed on the actual changes of counting rate with changes of activity in the observed sample (organ or animal for instance). These fluctuations, as we actually observe them, are best described by the number of divisions over which they are spread. If we express the standard deviation in a rate meter as σ_d divisions, we shall know that one-third of the fluctuations will be larger and two-thirds smaller than $2\sigma_d$ since the errors will be $\pm \sigma_d$ from the mean deflection.

We shall express the fluctuations in term of scale divisions, since this is what we actually observe on the recording.

In the rate meter, background appears as a baseline deflection and cannot be subtracted except by reference to this baseline. All deflections are a measure of "combined" counting rate, which will be designated in the following paragraph simply as R. The response time will be designated as t_r. The equivalent preset time is then equal to $2t_r$.

The standard deviation of the counting rate R will be as in (12)

$$\sigma_R = \frac{\sqrt{N}}{2t_r}$$

and since $N = Rt = R \times 2t_r$:

$$\sigma_R = \sqrt{\frac{R}{2t_r}} \text{ counts per second} \qquad 15-(39)$$

or, since we want to know the standard deviation in scale divisions:

$$\sigma_d = \frac{1}{S} \sqrt{\frac{R}{2t_r}} \text{ divisions} \qquad 15-(40)$$

Figure 15–1 illustrates an example. The graph paper has 10 divisions, full scale deflection corresponds to 100 counts per second ($S = 10$) and response time is set to $\frac{1}{2}$ second. For a counting rate of 10 per second we get

$$\sigma_d = \frac{1}{10} \sqrt{\frac{10}{1}} = 0.3 \text{ divisions}$$

and when the counting rate goes up to 90 per second

$$\sigma_d = \frac{1}{10} \sqrt{\frac{90}{1}} = 0.9 \text{ divisions}$$

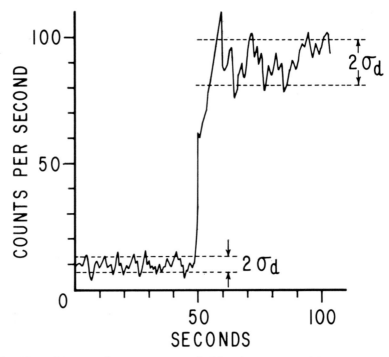

FIG. 15–1.   Diagram of a rate meter record with a time constant of $\frac{1}{2}$ second and a full scale range of 100 c/s (1 scale division = 10 c/s). In the beginning the counting rate is 10 c/s. After 50 seconds it rises suddenly to 90 c/s. σ_d calculated from equation (40). $2\sigma_d$ in the first half = 0.6 div; in the second half it is = 1.8 div.

Two characteristics of the rate record, which can be seen in the illustration, must be pointed out:

1. Standard deviation means that about one-third of the observations will deviate by more than this amount from the mean value.   The band which encloses fluctuation equal to or smaller than σ_d is $2\sigma_d$ wide (0.6 div for $R = 10$ and 1.8 div for $R = 90$.)

2. This band becomes wider, as the counting rate increases.

Figure 15–2 illustrates the same observation made with an increased response time $t_2 = 5$ seconds.   Here for $R = 10$:

$$\sigma_d = 0.1 \text{ div}$$

and $R = 90$

$$\sigma_d = 0.3 \text{ div}$$

It will be seen that the fluctuations have decreased in magnitude according to (40).   Due to the increased response time they also become less frequent, but the deflection to the higher counting rate takes longer.

Figure 15–3 shows the effect of reduced sensitivity to a full scale value of 1000 counts per second with $t_r = 5$, for the two rates used in Fig. 15–2 and

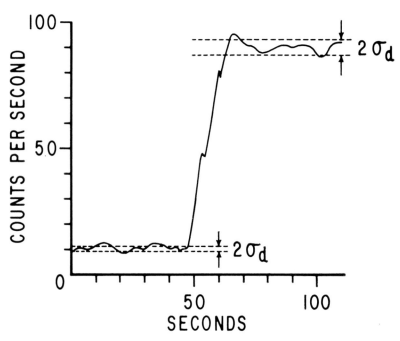

Fig. 15–2.   Same as in Figure 15–1 except that the time constant has been increased to 5 seconds. $2\sigma_d$ in the first half is now = 0.2 div, and in the second half it is = 0.6 div.

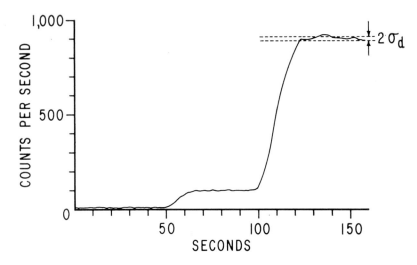

Fig. 15–3.   For the first 100 seconds this is the record of the same counting rates as in Figures 15–1 and 15–2.   The time constant is the same as in Figure 15–2, 5 seconds, but the scale has been changed so that full deflection corresponds to 1000 c/s (1 scale division = 100 c/s). $2\sigma_d$ during the first 50 seconds is now = 0.02 div and between 50 and 100 seconds it is = 0.06 div.   After 100 seconds the counting rate rises suddenly to 900 c/s; $2\sigma_d$ is here = 0.2 div, or one-third of what it was in Figure 15–2 when the deflection was also 9 divisions.

for R = 900. From (40) we calculate the expected fluctuations σ_d, considering that S is now equal to 100 c/s. We get ± 0.01; ± 0.03 and ± 0.1 respectively for σ_d at the three counting rates.

Equation (40) and the illustrations show that fluctuations are reduced when longer response times are used and when strong samples permit a less sensitive setting of the range. The experimental conditions determine here, as in all counting, the acceptable uncertainty, which appears as fluctuations in a rate meter: the changes to be observed must be larger than the fluctuations, since otherwise they would be masked by them. Increase in response time is limited by the experimental conditions also: if response time is longer than the time in which the relevant changes of counting rate take place, these changes will not be registered.

It may appear at first that a rate meter is an ideal substitute for a scaler, if preset time method of counting is desired. This is not quite true, because of one inherent technical limitation of electronic rate meters: the longest practical time constant is limited to not more than a few minutes, while no such limitation exists with an ordinary scaler. This limitation of time constant means a limitation of total counts determining a single reading, so that when the counting rate is low, precision is also quite low.

The use and the limitations of a rate meter can now be summarized: When the counting rate is high enough to give the required precision within the given time constants of the instruments, a rate meter is a useful and simple device. When the counting rate is too low to satisfy this requirement, a conventional circuit is preferable, although when a rate recorder is used, it is possible to recapture some of the lost precision by a graphical interpolation of the recorded wavy line; this corresponds to the taking of a mean of several readings made with low preset time on a scaler.

A recording meter is of very great usefulness when a rapidly changing source of radioactivity is under observation, as for instance in observing the circulation time with sodium-24 or another physiological mechanism with a rapid turnover. A printing counter, which prints either the time elapsed with a preset count circuit or counts accumulated with preset time mechanism, can also be used, but this will require a manual plotting of the data to obtain a graphic representation, whereas a rate recorder produces such a plot directly. Whenever a rate recorder is used, it must always be taken into consideration that on the one hand response time limits the precision of the reading or recording, if it is short compared to the counting rate, and that on the other hand, if the response time is long compared to the speed with which the observed physiological phenomena change, such changes will be masked by the slow response. A compromise will have to be made under many circumstances between the speed of response and the attainable precision. For a given time constant, the precision can be increased by increasing the counting rate, which can be achieved either by using a counting arrangement of higher sensitivity or by administering a higher dose of the radioactive material. When neither is possible, either some degree of precision has to be sacrificed, or a longer time constant must be used, although this may involve getting inherently less frequent readings; a smooth record may deceive one in this case; there are no more frequent readings ("points on the chart") than the response time offers, the smooth line is simply a form of electrical interpolation. If a time constant longer than a few minutes is acceptable and higher precision is required than can be attained with a rate meter, a printing scaler can be used instead of a recorder. Very special equipment utilizing multichannel analyzers (see page 220) in what is termed the "multichannel scaler" mode can offer another method of recording such data.

Evaluation of Equipment Performance Using Counting Statistics. Since nuclear events as seen by a properly functioning radiation detector are of purely random nature and as such subject only to the Poisson distribution, the proper function of a counting set-up can be tested by investigating whether the variations of observed counting rates follow the Poisson distribution or not.

A casual way of doing this test consists of taking two consecutive readings. As an example, let us consider a counting set-up with a given radioactive sample which gives 8000 gross counts in ten minutes (sample and background counts need not be considered separately in this connection) on the first observation and 8100 counts on the second observation in the same interval; the question is now whether this observation agrees with the theoretical expectation. The standard deviation should be $\sqrt{N}$ counts. The mean of the two observed counts is 8050, its square root is 90. The difference between this mean and the two counts is 50, smaller than what was expected. The statistical meaning of the standard deviation has to be recalled in this connection: this is the deviation which has the odds of 2 to 1 of not being exceeded. In other words, we should expect in 2 out of 3 observations to have a difference of 90 counts or less and in 1 out of 3 to observe a larger difference. If the equipment is working properly, we should expect in 2 out of 3 measurements to have the observed result. This is of course not very meaningful. If we had observed a difference of 270 counts between the two measurements and their mean, this would have meant that if the equipment were working properly, such a result might occur once in over 300 measurements, or would be quite unlikely; the conclusion would be that that instrument is *not* working well. This example shows that two observations alone will never reassure us that an instrument performs well, but can only indicate when it malfunctions rather badly. A test by two observations is only a very rough check.

A more reliable procedure is to repeat the observation about 10 times, to obtain for instance N_1, N_2, N_3, N_4, N_5, N_6, N_7, N_8, N_9, N_{10} counts for the same time interval t; to calculate the mean counts $N_{mean} = \dfrac{N_1 + N_2 .. + N_{10}}{10} = \dfrac{\Sigma N}{10}$, to obtain the deviation of the counts from this mean: $N_1 - N_{mean}$, $N_2 - N_{mean}$, $N_3 - N_{mean}$, etc. and to compare these deviations with the standard deviation $\sqrt{N_{mean}}$. Table 15–1 gives a numerical example. The expected deviation is $\sqrt{2992} = 55$; there are two deviations larger than this (#3 and #9) and eight which are smaller. The theoretical expectation is to find about three larger and seven smaller deviations. The observed result is not significantly different from the expected one and it is reasonable to assume that the apparatus is working properly. What result would indicate the opposite? A rigorous answer is not possible, but a practical guide may be given: if six or more of the observed deviations are larger than the expected value or if only one or none exceed it, one should question the performance and repeat the series of observations; if the second series gives the same result, something is probably wrong with the equipment.

Table 15–1. Counts Observed in 5-minute Intervals

#	N	Deviation
1	2940	− 52
2	3020	+ 28
3	3065	+ 73*
4	3010	+ 18
5	2980	− 12
6	2970	− 22
7	3025	+ 33
8	3030	+ 38
9	2890	−102*
10	2985	− 7

| Sum: | 29915 |
| Mean: | 2992 |

Expected standard deviation 55

* Observation with a deviation exceeding the standard value

It may be surprising to read the statement that something is wrong not only when deviations are larger than expected, but also when they are smaller than expected, since it is unusual to complain when variations are to small. It must be realized, however, that the "expected" deviations under discussion are not human or instrumental errors, but are inherent in the random nature of radioactive decay. As long as our observations reflect nuclear disintegrations only, they must fluctuate within the range of the Poisson distribution. If our observations have smaller or larger fluctuations, both can take place only if something other than nuclear disintegrations influences them: either can be due only to an artifact.

The given example was for preset time counting technique. For preset counts technique, the arithmetic is a little more involved, since the standard deviation is determined as always by the total number of counts accumulated, while the variable in this technique is the time required to accumulate

Table 15–2.   Time Required to Accumulate 6400 Counts

#	Time	Deviation
1	68.0	−0.3
2	68.9	+0.6
3	67.6	−0.7
4	68.8	+0.5
5	68.3	+0
6	69.2	+0.9*
7	67.3	−1*
8	69.1	+0.8
9	67.3	−1*
10	68.3	0

Sum:	682.8
Mean:	68.3

Expected standard deviation 0.85

* Observations with a deviation exceeding the standard value.

these counts. The difficulty is handled easily if we use the per cent standard deviation, since this applies equally to counts in a given interval or to time for a given number of counts.*   If we accumulate N counts, the per cent standard deviation is

$$V = \frac{100}{\sqrt{N}}$$

If the mean interval is t_{mean} and the expected standard deviation of the time intervals σ_t,

$$\sigma_t = \frac{t_{mean}\, V}{100} = \frac{t_{mean}}{\sqrt{N}} \qquad\qquad 15-(41)$$

Table 15–2 illustrates an example where time required to accumulate 6400 counts has been measured. The mean time $t_{mean} = 68.3$ (it is immaterial for this purpose whether it was measured in seconds or in minutes); the expected standard deviation in time is from (41) $\sigma_t = 0.85$. It can be seen that this value is exceeded in 3 out of the 10 observations (#6, #7 and #9). The conclusion is that the equipment works properly.

The described method of checking the randomness of results and hence of equipment testing is reasonably rigorous and is suitable in practice. It may leave a feeling of dissatisfaction in the reader, however, since it does not lead to a definite number expressing the probability that the equipment is performing properly or odds against such a conclusion. A way to obtain a numerical expression of this sort is indeed available in statistics as the chi square method. Its presentation in sufficient detail would go

* This statement has been occasionally questioned; rigorous proof will be found in Robley D. Evans: *The Atomic Nucleus*, New York, McGraw-Hill Book Co., 1955, pages 797–798.

beyond the scope of the present book. The interested reader is referred
to standard textbooks on statistics* for general description and to Evans†
for its application in nuclear counting. The more simple procedure discussed above will be found sufficient for most applications encountered in
clinical use of counting circuits.

When a statistical check of a counting set-up reveals that something is
wrong with the apparatus, it must be determined first whether the source of
trouble is in the radiation detector or in the electronic scaling circuit. For
this purpose there is frequently provision for the "calibration" of the scaler,
consisting of a switch which disconnects the detector and applies electrically
a uniform counting rate of 60 counts per second to the scaler. If the scaler
counts this incorrectly, the trouble is in the electronic circuit. A correct
counting rate indicates that the trouble is probably in the radiation
detector part of the apparatus.

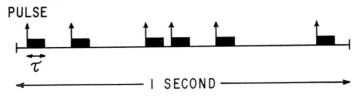

PULSE

— I SECOND —

Fig. 15–4.   The sequence of pulses and the ensuing "dead times" (resolving time) of
duration τ in a radiation detector.

Resolving Time.   In the discussion of the mechanism of counters, mention was made of a time interval immediately following the occurrence of
a pulse, during which a Geiger-Mueller counter is insensitive and does not
respond to ionizing events; this was called "dead time" of a counter. A
similar dead time exists also in scintillation counters. This is, however, very
much shorter, so short in fact that the response speed of the electrical or
electromechanical counting mechanisms may become the limiting factor.
Whatever the cause of the overall "dead time" of a counting set-up may be,
it will put an upper limit on the counting rate which can be measured
accurately. It will influence the observed counting rate when it is high
enough, and it is necessary to have information about this dead time, or
"resolving time."

In Figure 15–4 a time interval of one second is charted, with several pulses
occurring during this time. The dead time or resolving time is symbolized τ.
If a second pulse occurs within this time after a first pulse, it will not be
recorded; the counting set-up will "miss" it. If R counts per second have
been observed, some radiation bursts may have been missed. The true
counting rate R_t will be larger than the observed counting rate R_o by the

---

* For instance: M. Bancroft: *Introduction to Biostatistics*, New York, Hoeber-
Harper, 1957.

† See footnote, page 241.

number of counts which will have occurred during the dead time and there-fore been missed. The duration of the total dead time during each second will be $R_0\tau$. The number of counts missed will be the number of radiation events which actually occured during this time, that is $R_tR_0\tau$. Since by definition the number of counts missed is also $R_t - R_0$, we have the equation

$$R_t - R_0 = R_t\,R_0\tau \qquad\qquad 15-(42)$$

Solving for R_t we get

$$R_t = \frac{R_0}{1 - R_0\,\tau} \qquad\qquad 15-(43)$$

Since $R_0\tau$ is the total dead time per second, it is also obviously the frac-tion of the time during which the counting equipment will not respond. Calling this fraction F, equation (43) can be rewritten as

$$R_t = \frac{R_0}{1 - F} \qquad\qquad 15-(44)$$

In Figure 15–5 the ratio of the true counting rate to observed counting rate (R_t/R_0) is shown as a function of the fractional dead time, F. For reasons discussed below the use of a curve of this type to correct for count-ing loss above 20 per cent (F > 0.2) is not recommended.

The derivation of the formulas connecting the observed and true count-ing rates assumed that the resolving time was constant. Counting detectors and scaling circuits which behave according to this assumption are termed "nonparalyzing." This term implies that the observed counting rate ap-proaches a plateau value no matter how high the true counting rate may go. This requires that the system is affected in no way by a count which occurs during the dead time. Practically no counting system behaves in this fashion. Actually when a pulse occurs during a dead time interval, some-thing does happen in the counter or scaling circuit which prolongs the dead time. The extent of this prolongation depends on whether the new impulse occurs at the beginning or the end of the dead interval. While complex, this phenomenon can be treated mathematically. However, to do so is of little practical value as the relevant parameters are rarely known.

The result of this behavior, however, is extremely important. As the prolonged dead times merge into each other and encroach upon each other, counting stops and the counter shows no counts at all: it is blocked or jammed. It is "paralyzed." The dotted curve in Figure 15–6 illustrates this behavior. Also shown are the behavior of a zero resolving time counter (no dead time) and a non-paralyzing counter. Notice, at low counting rates all three curves merge and the true and observed counting rates are equal (negligibly small resolving time correction). With increasing counting rate the resolving time correction becomes appreciable and for a limited range the actual counter agrees with the hypothetical non-paralyzing one. As the

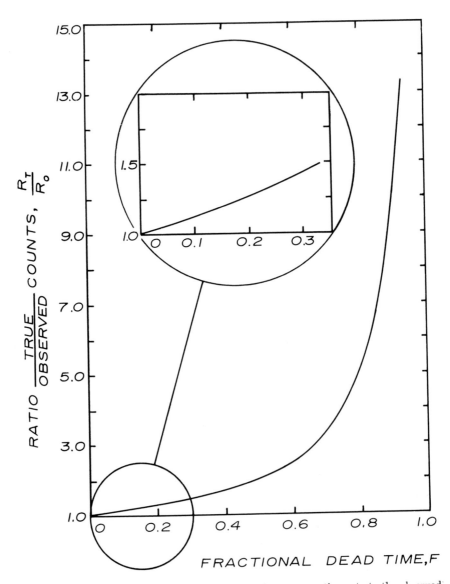

F<small>IG</small>. 15–5.   Relationship between the ratio of the true counting rate to the observed counting rate and the fractional dead time.   For values of F greater than 0.2 the curve seldom represents actual detector and circuit operation and should not be employed for correction purposes.   Insert shows lower F values in more magnified form.

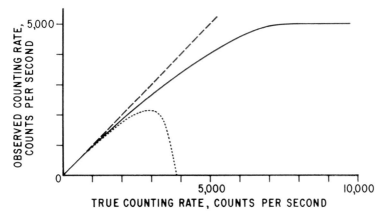

FIG. 15–6. Relationship between the observed and the true counting rate. Dashed line: no counting losses, resolving time is zero. Solid line: hypothetical, not paralyzing counter. Observed counting rate reaches asymptotically a maximum. Dotted line: actual counter, which shows paralysis at high counting rate. Note that near the origin all three lines coincide and that over a part of the range the solid and dotted lines coincide. Note also that for any observed counting rate in the range of the dotted curve there are two possible corresponding true counting rates; for any true counting rate above the intersection of the descending limb with the abscissa the observed counting rate is zero (jamming).

resolving time correction becomes greater than 20 per cent, the actual behavior deviates significantly from non-paralyzable and at slightly higher rates a maximum observed counting rate is reached. Following the maximum, the observed rate drops rapidly to zero as the counter jams completely.

In summary the important points of this discussion are:

1. Resolving time corrections should be made only to about 20 per cent. Above this the correction is unreliable. The product $R_o\tau = F$, the fractional dead time, determines the correction.

2. At very high true counting rates the counter may jam, not count at all, and behave as if no radiation were present. This can lead to grave errors. If this condition is suspected, slowly move the sample away from the detector, thereby reducing the true counting rate, and the counter will thereby resume counting.

Determination of Resolving Time. The experimental determination of resolving time for a given counter and circuit combination is done by using two sources of radiation which give sufficiently high counting rates to show observable counting losses between the sum of separately determined counting rates R_1 and R_2 for each of the two sources, and the counting rate for the two sources counted simultaneously, R_{12}. In other words, the counting rates should be such that $R_1 + R_2$ is appreciably larger than R_{12}. A quantitative evaluation is possible only if the separate and the simultaneous counts are done with the sources in identical positions with respect to the

17

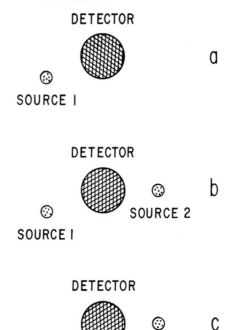

FIG. 15–7. Three successive arrangements a, b, and c, of two radioactive sources 1 and 2 for the determination of resolving time.

counter. A simple way to achieve this is shown in Figure 15–7. In addition to the three determinations illustrated, the background R_b has also to be determined.

The true net counting rate R_{t12} for the two sources counted together must be equal to the sum of the net counting rates R_{t1} and R_{t2} of the sources counted separately.

$$R_{t12} = R_{t1} + R_{t2}$$

Also, the counts observed with any source present result from the true counts of the source and the background combined. Thus with source 1 present from (43)

$$R_{t1} + R_b = \frac{R_1}{1 - R_1\tau}$$

and we have similar equations with source 2 and with both sources present. Subject to the assumption that the background counting rate is not affected by the dead time (practically always valid), we have a total of four equations and four unknowns (R_{t1}, R_{t2}, R_{t12} and τ). These can be solved for τ in terms of the observed counting rates. An approximate solution is

$$\tau = \frac{R_1 + R_2 - R_{12} - R_b}{R_{12}^2 + R_1^2 - R_2^2} \qquad 15-(45)$$

To obtain (45) terms of the magnitude of $(R\tau)^2$ were considered negligible compared to one. This introduces no more than a few per cent error in the value of τ at even the largest value of $R\tau$ (0.2) for which this analysis is valid. When this method is used to determine τ the sources should be chosen and positioned so that counting both of them does not give more than 20 per cent dead time. However, the dead time should not be very small or else the statistical uncertainties in the observed values may cause the calculated value of τ to be very inaccurate.

Efficiency and Sensitivity of Radiation Detectors. The terms efficiency and sensitivity as applied to nuclear measurements are sometimes confusing. Since they describe two different aspects of the response of a counter to radiation bursts accompanying the disintegration of radioactive samples, they are very useful indeed and the confusion has to be untangled.

Efficiency in the narrow sense of the word refers to the ratio of actually observed counts to the total number of radiation bursts *reaching the counter*, expressed in per cent. Not all gamma rays traversing a Geiger-Mueller counter interact with the counter walls and filling gas to produce a discharge, in fact usually less than 1 per cent of them do so. If one count is observed per 100 gamma rays traversing the counter, we say that the efficiency is 1 per cent. Beta rays interact much more frequently with the filling gas and produce counts, but they are much more easily absorbed by the walls and so prevented from interaction. For thin counter walls, beta efficiency is usually higher, but for walls which are thicker than the beta range, the efficiency may be close to zero (it will not be zero because of bremsstrahlung). Evidently the efficiency of any radiation detector depends on the energy of the measured radiation. The efficiency of any counter may be different for the softer gamma radiations from ^{131}I than for the harder radiation from radium; a counter with reasonably thin walls will be highly efficient for beta radiation from ^{32}P and it may have diminishingly small efficiency for ^{14}C beta radiation. Similar considerations apply to scintillation counters. For a NaI(Tl) detector the efficiency for gamma rays is much higher owing to the higher probability of interaction in the solid. However, because of the material surrounding the crystal the efficiency for low energy beta-ray emitters is close to zero. These considerations will be developed more completely in the next chapter.

Efficiency is also used in a wider sense of the word, applied not only to the number of counts observed per hundred *radiation events reaching the counter*, but also with reference to the number of counts observed per 100 disintegrations *occurring within a given radioactive sample*. Efficiency in this sense depends not only on the efficiency of the detector in the strict meaning of the word, but also on the overall counting set-up, that is, distance of the sample from the counter and a variety of other factors. Efficiency used in this second way always has a smaller value than the first. As an example let us consider a counter bombarded by the beta rays from a ^{32}P source. When 110,000 beta particles per second strike the counter, the counting rate is observed to be 60,000 counts per second; its efficiency in the narrow sense is 54 per cent. In a practical counting set-up the source will be at some distance from the detector so that many of the beta rays emitted will not strike the detector. The actual counting rate from a ^{32}P source emitting 110,000 beta particles per second will be much lower, say 5,000 counts per second. Thus, the efficiency in the second sense is only 4.5 per cent.

This second efficiency is closely related to the calibration of a counting set-up for a given radioactive nuclide. The unit used to express activity is the curie (abbreviated Ci), but for counting purposes the microcurie (μCi), one millionth of a curie, is a more convenient unit. One microcurie has 37,000 disintegrations per second. The sample in our example contains 3 microcuries. The counting set-up gives a counting rate of 5,000 counts per second for 3 microcuries. The calibration is then expressed by the calibration factor: 1670 counts per second for 1 microcurie. When a counting set-up is used for actual measurement, its calibration factor indicating the counting rate per microcurie is the basic and essential datum.

Knowledge of the efficiency provides some information on the ultimate possibility of improving the counting set-up by changing the physical arrangement or by substituting a more efficient for a less efficient counter. If the efficiency is around 1 per cent, a great deal may be done in improvement. When the efficiency reaches the neighborhood of 50 per cent, nothing will improve matters by better than a factor of 2, which would give the theoretical maximum of 100 per cent.

Efficiency and calibration factors also contain information on the sensitivity of a counting set-up, although discussion of sensitivity in nuclear measurements is complicated by the random nature of the events under observation. Let us compare this with an everyday measurement procedure, such as weighing with a balance. Here sensitivity is expressed simply in terms of the number of scale divisions the balance pointer deflects when the weight of 1 milligram is put on a balance pan. It may also be necessary to know the ultimate sensitivity, that is the precision, of a balance. This can be achieved by determining that weight which corresponds to the standard deviation in weighing, or that weight in milligrams which can be detected in about half the trial weighings and will be missed in another half (for a more precise definition of standard deviation, this ratio will be two-thirds and one-third). Since the weight equivalent to the standard deviation will frequently remain undetected, it is more appropriate to use not one but three standard deviations in describing sensitivity of nuclear counters. Such a quantity will be almost always detected. It might be compared with the weight on a balance which causes the deflection of one full scale division. Henceforth precision will be expressed as the activity which gives a counting rate equal to 3 standard deviations.

In nuclear counting we encounter some further complications. Let us consider a counting set-up with an efficiency of 50 per cent, that is a calibration factor of 18,500 (counts per second for 1 μCi). In analogy with the balance, we may equate sensitivity and calibration factor and say that this counting set-up has a sensitivity of 18,500 counts per second for 1 microcurie. This would correspond to a complete description of the sensitivity of a balance, but gives only partial information for a nuclear counter, since nothing has been said about the background. In our example we may have two different counters with different backgrounds, but with the same calibration factor, one with a background of 1 count per second and another with a background of 10,000 counts per second. The first counter should have been described as having a much higher precision than the second, since less time will be required to achieve a comparable uncertainty with the same sample, due to the lower background. The time element and its relation to background are essential in nuclear counting and cannot be disregarded if statements about sensitivity are to be of use in comparing different counting set-ups and in evaluation of their performances and limitations.

The application of the second method of describing the performance of a balance by indicating its ultimate sensitivity, its precision, appears more complicated, but it can be applied unequivocally to nuclear counters. Precision was defined as the magnitude equal to 3 standard deviations (the smallest "detectable" amount). In a nuclear counter it can be defined as 3 standard deviations in counting rate and it can be expressed in units of activity (microcuries for example). Let us examine equation (16) for standard deviation of net counting rate:

$$\sigma_s = \sqrt{\frac{R_c}{t_c} + \frac{R_b}{t_b}} .$$

Here σ_s is the standard deviation in counts per second. $3\sigma_s$ when expressed in microcuries, corresponds to precision as defined in the preceding paragraph.

$$\text{Precision} = \frac{3\sigma_s}{\text{calibration factor}} \mu\text{Ci.} \qquad 15\text{—}(46)$$

The usefulness of this concept of precision in nuclear counting becomes apparent when we consider that it depends not only on the calibration factor, but also on the background and on the time spent in counting ($t_c + t_b$). Since precision depends on counting time, some time interval must be agreed upon for intercomparison of counters. In the following, as a somewhat arbitrary compromise, the value of ten minutes ($t_c + t_b = 600$ seconds) will be used as total counting time for both sample and background; it will have to be remembered that high precision can be obtained by using longer counting times.

A precise calculation of the counting rate for the minimal detectable sample, which is equal to three standard deviations, leads to somewhat involved calculations. But the equation (16) for σ_s can be simplified. The value of R_c/t_c will differ little from R_b/t_b as both the counting rate and the time will be smaller in the second ratio. Thus to a close approximation we can substitute the second ratio for the first in (16) obtaining

$$\sigma_s = \sqrt{2\,\frac{R_b}{t_b}} \qquad\qquad 15\text{---}(47)$$

It was decided to use a total counting time of 600 seconds: $2t_b = 600$; $t_b = 300$. With this assumption we get

$$\sigma_s = \sqrt{\frac{2}{300}}\,R_b = 0.08\,\sqrt{R_b} \qquad\qquad 15\text{---}(48)$$

and an expression for precision, by substituting this in (46) and multiplying it by 3.

$$\text{precision} = \frac{0.24\,\sqrt{R_b}}{\text{calibration factor}} \qquad\qquad 15\text{---}(49)$$

Let us consider an example: a counting set-up with a calibration factor of 70 counts per second for 1 μCi and a background of 0.5 counts per second. The standard deviation when counting a very small sample for a total of ten minutes (combined and background counts) is, according to (48)

$$\sigma_s = 0.08\,\sqrt{0.5} = 0.058\ \text{c/s}$$

Therefore we have from (49)

$$\text{precision} = \frac{0.17}{70} = 0.0024\ \mu\text{Ci}$$

This indicates that we shall be able to detect the presence or absence of 0.0024 μCi = 2.4 nanocuries*, if ten minutes are spent for each observation. In a counter with the same calibration factor, but a background of 5 counts per second, the calculation will lead to a precision of 0.0075 μCi = 7.5 nCi, by using (49). With the higher background, the smallest detectable activity is considerably higher.

The great practical value of knowing the precision of a counter is that it tells the order of magnitude of the smallest sample that can be detected and makes it possible to estimate approximately, but rapidly, the size of sample needed for a measurement of given reliability. In the first example the precision was 0.0024 μCi. If a measurement with 10 per cent uncertainty has to be made, a sample of about ten times precision, that is 0.024 μCi will be needed with ten-minute counting. This sort of estimate is not possible with the calibration factor, which has of course its own use and importance. The calibration factor permits the interpretation of

* 1 nanocurie or 1 nCi = $\frac{1}{1000}$ μCi. From Greek "nanos," meaning, "dwarf."

observed counting rates in terms of activity. It also permits the estimation of the sample strength required to obtain desired counting rates, which is necessary in order to determine required counting times. The calibration factor can be used finally for the determination of the sample strength needed so that background can be disregarded.

In describing the characteristics of counters the concept of *background equivalent activity* is sometimes used. This is the activity of a radioactive material in μCi which will give a counting rate equal to the background.

$$\text{Background equivalent activity} = \frac{R_b}{\text{calibration factor}} \qquad 15-(50)$$

The various concepts presented above will be illustrated by the following example.

A sample of about 0.001 μCi is to be measured within about 10 per cent ($V = 10$). The following 3 counters are available, and the question is which counter should be selected for this measurement.

Counter 1: Calibration Factor 165 c/s for 1 μCi; $R_b = 0.4$ c/s
"   2:   "   "   1650 c/s " " " ; $R_b = 4$ c/s
"   3:   "   "   50 c/s " " " ; $R_b = 0.03$ c/s

Let us tabulate the smallest detectable amount (precision) from (49) and background equivalent from (50):

Counter	Precision μCi	Background Equivalent μCi
1	0.0009	0.025
2	0.0003	0.025
3	0.001	0.007

The selection of counters would be different, depending on the criterion used. Precision recommends counter 2. Background equivalent recommends counter 3 (it also appears to indicate that counters 1 and 2 are equal). We shall calculate the required total counting time for the given sample and for the required uncertainty with the three counters from (32) and (33):

Counter	$t_c + t_b$
1	2 hours
2	12 minutes
3	$2\frac{1}{2}$ hours

Counter 2 is unquestionably superior; counter 1 is almost as bad as counter 3. In this example it is obvious that precision is a good guide.

These considerations are valid, however, only when the background is constant. We are faced with an entirely different problem when background fluctuates and these fluctuations cannot be eliminated (this is frequently the case, for instance, in a clinical laboratory where treated patients come and go, and where there is a structural or economical limit to the weight of the lead shielding). Here there may be little advantage in the second counter. It may be necessary to use stronger samples than the one mentioned in the example to override the uncertainty of the fluctuating background.

The effect of background variations is of course eliminated when background may be neglected altogether under the condition of (35), assuming that the value assumed for background counting rate is near to the maximum background observed. By dividing this equation by the calibration factor we get:

Background equivalent $= \dfrac{V}{500} \times$ sample activity or in a more useful

form as the condition for neglecting background

$$\text{sample activity} \geqslant \frac{500}{V} \times \text{background equivalent}$$

This equation indicates what the smallest sample activity is for which the background can be neglected.

Following is a listing of this activity for the 3 counters:

Counter	Minimum sample activity for neglecting background for $V = 10$
1	1.25 μCi
2	1.25 μCi
3	0.35 μCi

It is seen that the background could be neglected for the smallest sample when using the third counter. This demonstrates the value and use of background equivalent activity in selecting a counter when the possibility of performing a measurement is not limitation in time but fluctuations of the background.

Since the terms introduced and discussed in this section will be used frequently in the following chapters, they will be recapitulated and summarized:

1. *Counting efficiency in the narrow sense of the word*: number of counts registered by the detector, per 100 ionizing events reaching the counter or entering its sensitive volume.

2. *Counting efficiency in the broader sense*: number of counts registered by the counting device, per 100 disintegrations occurring in the radioactive sample under observation.

3. *Calibration factor or sensitivity* (sometimes also called "response"): counting rate (counts per second or per minute) per unit of radioactive material (in millicuries or microcuries). The use of the term "sensitivity" for this factor may be misleading, since it does not contain consideration of background or counting time.

4. *Precision*: the smallest detectable amount of radioactive material, expressed in microcuries or other suitable conventional unit. It can be calculated from the calibration factor, background and an arbitrarily assigned total counting time (in this text this time has been assigned the value of ten minutes, for counting both sample and background).

5. *Background equivalent activity*: that amount of radioactive material which will give a net counting rate equal to background. In other words, that amount which will give a combined counting rate two times as large as background (background doubling activity).

Table 15–3. Formulas in Counting Statistics

No.	Purpose	Formula	Units	Equation # in text
	I. General			
1.	Standard deviation of accumulated counts (preset time)	$\sigma_N = \sqrt{N}$	counts	(1)
2.	Standard deviation of counting time (preset counts)	$\sigma_t = \dfrac{t}{\sqrt{N}}$	time	(41)
3.	Coefficient of variation	$V = \dfrac{100}{\sqrt{N}}$	%	(3)
4.	For an acceptable error of P% make the coefficient of variation:			
	For low reliability	$V = P$	%	(5)
	For medium reliability	$V = P/2$	%	(6)
	For high reliability	$V = P/3$	%	(7)
	II. Counting equations when background can be neglected			
5.	Background may be neglected when:	$R_b \lessgtr \dfrac{R_c V}{500}$	$\dfrac{\text{counts}}{\text{time}}$	(35)
6.	Counts to be accumulated	$N_s = \dfrac{10{,}000}{V^2}$	counts	(36)
7.	Counting time	$t_s = \dfrac{10{,}000}{R_s' V^2}$	time	(37)
8.	Coefficient of variation as in formula 3	$V_s = \dfrac{100}{\sqrt{N_s}}$	%	(3)
9.	Standard deviation of observed counting rate	$\sigma_s = \dfrac{\sqrt{N_s}}{t_s}$	$\dfrac{\text{counts}}{\text{time}}$	(38)
	III. Counting equations when background cannot be neglected			
10.	Background cannot be neglected when:	$R_b' > \dfrac{R_c'V}{500}$	$\dfrac{\text{counts}}{\text{time}}$	—
11.	Combined counts to be accumulated	$N_c = 20{,}000\left[\dfrac{R_c'}{V(R_c'-R_b')}\right]^2$	counts	(30)

Table 15–3.   Formulas in Counting Statistics (Continued)

No.	Purpose	Formula	Units	Equation # in text
12.	Background counts to be accumulated	$N_b = 20,000\left[\dfrac{R_b'}{V(R_c'-R_b')}\right]^2$	counts	(31)
13.	Combined counting time	$t_c = \dfrac{20,000\ R_c'}{[V(R_c'-R_b')]^2}$	time	(32)
14.	Background counting time	$t_b = \dfrac{20,000\ R_b'}{[V(R_c'-R_b')]^2}$	time	(33)
15.	Standard deviation of observed sample (net) counting rate	$\sigma_s = \sqrt{\dfrac{N_c}{t_c^2} + \dfrac{N_b}{t_b^2}}$	$\dfrac{counts}{time}$	(15)
16.	Coefficient of variation of observed sample (net) counting rate	$V_s = 100\ \dfrac{\sqrt{N_c t_b^2 + N_b t_c^2}}{N_c t_b - N_b t_c}$	%	(34)

IV. Correction for counting losses due to resolving time

17.	Corrected counting rate	$R_t = \dfrac{R_o}{1-R_o\tau}$	$\dfrac{counts}{time}$	(43)
18.	Condition for validity of 17	$R_o < \dfrac{0.2}{\tau}$	$\dfrac{counts}{time}$	

V. Rate meter fluctuations
two thirds of the fluctuations will be within a range of 2 standard deviations ($2\sigma_d$)

19.	Standard deviation of counting rate	$\sigma_d = \dfrac{1}{S}\sqrt{\dfrac{R}{2t_r}}$	divisions	(40)

VI. Measures of counter sensitivity

20.	Precision; smallest detectable activity	$= \dfrac{0.24\ \sqrt{R_b}}{\text{calibration factor}}$	μCi	(49)
21.	Background equivalent activity	$= \dfrac{R_b}{\text{calibration factor}}$	μCi	(50)

Explanation of symbols and of some terms used in Table 15–3.

Note: When a symbol has the sign′, as for instance in N'_c, it indicates that the value has been determined approximately only in a preliminary experiment.

N —accumulated counts in an observation over some time interval.

N_b —counts accumulated during time t_b in the measurement of background.

N_c —counts accumulated during time t_c in the measurement of background and sample combined.

N —counts accumulated during time t_s in the measurement of a sample (background neglected).

P —acceptable per cent uncertainty in a measurement.

R_b —background counting rate.

R_c —combined or gross counting rate observed when sample and background are measured together.

R_o —observed counting rate, which may be equal to or smaller than R_t, the true counting rate, due to counting losses.

R_s —counting rate due to sample alone (background subtracted from R_o or neglected) net counting rate.

R_t —true counting rate: the counting rate which would be observed if no counting losses due to the effect of dead time (resolving time) had occurred.

t_b —counting time when background is measured.

t_c —counting time when sample and background together are measured.

t_s —counting time when sample alone is measured (background neglected).

V —coefficient of variation (standard deviation in per cent). Determined on the basis of required P and required reliability (confidence limit)

V_s —coefficient of variation of a sample counting rate R_s, when R_c and R_b are determined experimentally by measuring N_c, N_b, t_c and t_b, or when it is determined by observing N_s and t_s by neglecting the background.

σ_N —standard deviation of the number of counts accumulated in preset time counting.

σ_s —standard deviation of a sample counting rate R_s when this counting rate is determined as described for V_s.

σ_t —standard deviation of time in preset count counting.

τ —dead time or resolving time determined for the assembly of a counter and the associated scaling circuit.

Background equivalent activity—activity in μCi or nCi which would give a net counting rate equal to the background ($R_s = R_b$).

Calibration factor (sensitivity, response)—sample counting rate R_s with a sample of unit activity: net counts per second obtained with a sample of 1 μCi. The dimension is sec^{-1} μCi^{-1} which is sometimes written as "counts/sec/μCi".

Precision, smallest detectable amount, minimum detectable activity—the activity of such a sample, the presence or absence of which will be almost always detected by counting when a set time is spent in counting sample and background (usually 10 minutes). It is calculated as three times the standard deviation for a vanishingly small sample, which is approximately equal to the standard deviation of the background.

16

Quantitative Measurements in Vitro

STANDARDIZATION OF RADIOACTIVE NUCLIDES

AT the present time, most of the clinically useful radioactive nuclides are available from responsible processing laboratories in a calibrated form, that is, under a label which not only identifies the nuclide, but also states how many millicuries the container held at a specified date. Nuclides are usually supplied in a solution, and the label states also the total volume, or millicuries per ml. Only rarely will the nuclide be available as the pure element. Usually it will be supplied either as an inorganic or organic compound, as for instance ^{131}I as sodium iodide, or ^{14}C as dextrose. If the particular compound contains only atoms of the radioactive nuclide, it is said to be carrier free. If it contains in addition identical chemical molecules with a stable isotope of the element, it is said to have a (stable) carrier. When a solid sample of a radioactive compound is considered, the amount of radioactive isotope, expressed in millicuries per gram of the total weight of the element in question, is called specific activity. This specific activity has then the dimension of mCi/gm. When the radioactive sample is obtained as a solution, specific activity is sometimes expressed also in terms of millicuries contained in a milliliter, and it has then the dimension of mCi/ml. A better word to describe this second meaning of the term "specific activity" would be *specific concentration*, but this has not found acceptance in the literature. This ambiguity of the term "specific activity," however, rarely leads to misunderstandings. The total amount of radio-activity in a given bottle or sample is called "absolute activity."

A few years ago, nuclides were not available in reliably precalibrated form and the determination of the radioactivity in a given shipment was the first step in its use. This absolute measurement or "standardization," sometimes called "assay," of the available sample is not a simple procedure, and in only a few laboratories is such standardization carried out at present. The methods involved, however, are still useful and their discussion is the best introduction to the measurement of samples *in vitro*, which embraces perhaps half of the work load of a radioactivity laboratory.

Handling of Radioactive Samples. A few preliminary remarks should be made at this point about the handling of radioactive samples. The first one refers to health protection. In a later chapter the physical measures to insure optimal health protection will be discussed (see also Chapters 11 and 12). The first encounter with maximal amounts of radioactive materials will occur when the shipment is received and opened, and when aliquots of this shipment are removed for assay and for use with patients or for preparation of dilutions. The monograph on *Safe Handling of Radioactive Materials*,* should be consulted before this work is attempted, with particular attention to the precautions against ingestion, inhalation and absorption of radioactive materials. External exposure of the body can be measured by instruments described in the appropriate chapter, but the material absorbed cannot be easily determined in the small amounts which are biologically effective over many years of possible exposure.

The next remarks refer to the precision in the quantitative techniques of weighing, pipetting and preparing dilutions. Careless working habits can introduce errors of 5 to 10 per cent at this point, and familiarity with the rudiments of techniques in preparing dilutions is essential (difference between blow-out and delivery pipettes for instance, etc.). There are also some specific pitfalls when handling carrier-free material. Since the gravimetric amounts are vanishingly small (minute fractions of a microgram), difficulties occur which are practically unknown in chemistry. Radioactive phosphorus will be adsorbed on the clean walls of glassware, unless this has been presoaked in a solution of stable phosphate. Salts of radioactive iodine may oxidize in solution, free iodine will be formed, which can volatilize. Sodium bisulfite should be added to the solution to prevent oxidation, and the solution should be kept alkaline by addition of sodium bicarbonate to give a pH of about 8, this will prevent volatilization of free iodine should it be present. The amounts of these chemicals are not critical. Fifty to 200 mg per liter solutions are about the required range. It must be remembered to add them also to water used in the preparation of the solution; otherwise they will be diluted beyond the effective concentration.

Such precautions are important because they affect the precision and reliability of measurements. Any radioactive contamination will increase the background in working areas and of counting equipment; the effect of background on sensitivity and precision has already been discussed at length. It is a matter of actual experience that the handling of a scintillation counter with hands only slightly contaminated with ^{131}I may put this counter out of commission for weeks. Contamination with other, longer-lived nuclides may require special cleaning or perhaps even demand that the counter be discarded.

Ionization Chambers. Ionization chambers are among the least sensitive but most reliable radiation measurement devices. In standardizing radioactive samples, sensitivity is of secondary and reliability of primary importance. In order to assay low activity samples an electrometer of high

---

* *Safe Handling of Radioactive Materials*, National Bureau of Standards, Handbook 92, 1964. Available from the Government Printing Office, Washington D. C., 20025, price 40 cents.

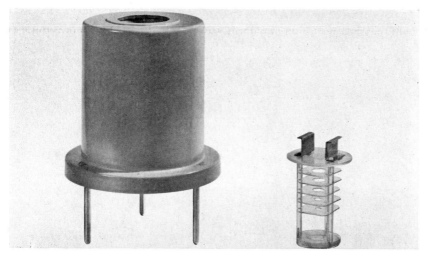

Fig. 16-1. Photograph of the Victoreen Radioassay Ionization Chamber (Courtesy of Victoreen Instrument Company).

Table 16-1. Calibration Factors for Victoreen Radioassay Ionization Chamber

Nuclide	Calibration Factors Picoamperes/millicurie*
^{22}Na	57
^{137}Cs	17
^{133}Ba	20
^{113}Sn	12
^{51}Cr	1.3
^{198}Au	20
^{57}Co	7.8
^{131}I	12
^{125}I	4.2

* 1 picoampere $= 10^{-12}$ amperes

sensitivity must be used with an ionization chamber. Transistor units of the required sensitivity and stability are available at reasonable cost.

Various ionization chambers have been designed for the measurement of activity of liquid samples inserted into the chamber in tubes or vials.* Figure 16-1 shows a photograph of a recently developed unit designed to permit low activity samples to be measured. Individual doses can be assayed rapidly prior to administration with such a unit. The device measures gamma emitters in a reentrant cylinder and beta emitters in a parallel plate chamber. Table 16-1 gives the sensitivity for several nuclides.

* Descriptions are available in Handbook 80. See footnote page 227.

One great advantage of the ionization chamber is that it can be checked reliably against a radium standard. Ionization due to 1 mCi of radium is of course not equal to that due to 1 mCi of another radioactive material, but any changes in the chamber, air density and electrometer will remain proportional within practically relevant limits, unless the ionization chamber is severely, and usually obviously, damaged. When using an ionization chamber, as when using other radioactivity measuring instruments, the background has to be determined and taken into account whenever it has a significant value.

Proportional, Geiger-Mueller and Scintillation Counters. There are two basic differences between a counting device and an ionization chamber. Counters usually have much higher sensitivity (a determination can be done within the same time and precision on a sample of considerably smaller activity) but their performance is less stable on a long term basis. This lower stability makes it practically impossible to obtain a counter or a counting set-up which has been "precalibrated" for various nuclides. Every counting device has to be calibrated by the user himself, and this calibration rechecked at every standardization.

Standardization can take two forms. In the first the calibration is performed in terms of the actual activity, i.e. the number of mCi or μCi present. This is called absolute standardization. In the second the calibration is measured in terms of a "standard" sample. This may be no more than one aliquot of a stock solution. Other samples can then be expressed in terms of fractions of this standard. Uptake measurements are typical of those in which this latter calibration suffices. Of course, some knowledge of the actual activity is always required to insure that an appropriate dose is administered to the patient. The first type of calibration includes all precautions required for the second plus knowledge of the true activity of the standard sample. Thus, our discussion can be confined to this first type of standardization.

In order to perform an absolute calibration it is necessary to have available a standardized sample of the nuclide to be used. These are generally available from commercial laboratories referenced to activity determinations by the National Bureau of Standards. Standardized samples of most radioactive nuclides in clinical use are available from such sources with a guaranteed accuracy of about 3 per cent. When such a sample is obtained, an aliquot of it is counted in the given set-up and a calibration factor (net counts per second or per minute for one microcurie) is obtained. A calibration sample of each nuclide used in the laboratory has to be obtained and the counter calibrated for each separately: the calibration factors will be different for every nuclide.*

Calibration standards (standardized samples) are usually obtained only

---

* W. B. Mann and H. H. Seliger. Preparation, Maintenance and Application of Standards of Radioactivity. NBS Circular 594, June 11, 1958. U.S. Government Printing Office, 35c. Also Handbook 80 (see footnote page 227).

a few times a year by clinical laboratories. Most nuclides have a short half-life, and a standard will decay to below a useful activity before a new one becomes available. Thus, a laboratory may be without a useful calibration standard for several months. This creates a problem which can be solved in two ways.

A stronger reference sample is prepared, which is calibrated against the original standard sample, and when the original standard begins to become too weak by decay, the reference standard is used. This can be done repeatedly, but the errors in each preparation will add up; it must be expected that a fifth derived standard may have an activity error of more than 25 per cent.

The second solution is to use a sample of some long-lived radioactive material such as radium, ^{60}Co or ^{137}Cs as a *performance standard*. Such a standard is not as reliable as a *calibration standard* of the particular short-lived nuclide, but it will permit detection of gross changes in the performance of a counter. Let us assume that a given ^{32}P calibration standard gave 107 counts per second for 1 μCi, and that a performance standard of a few μCi of radium sealed in some container gave 155 counts per second; as long as the same radium standard continues to give the same 155 counts per second, there is *some* assurance that 1μCi of ^{32}P will continue to give 107 counts per second. This assurance is not very great however, since it is possible that sensitivity to ^{32}P beta radiation may change without a change in the sensitivity to the gamma radiation of the radium standard. For this reason every standardization set-up should be recalibrated with standard samples at least twice a year. This applies to every radiation detector when absolute accuracy is important. Between the times when recalibration is possible, a performance standard should be used daily.

These remarks assume the use of a discriminator in the electronic counting circuitry. In the example considered, *i.e.* beta ray measurements, this would generally apply; always with a Geiger-Mueller counter. However, the use of a scintillation counter in conjunction with a single channel analyzer complicates the check-out process. With such equipment, performance standards must be carefully chosen to have radiation whose energy falls within the acceptance range of the analyzer. This radiation should, when possible, be emitted by the performance standard nuclide directly and not obtained by radiation energy degradation in a scatterer. Thus, the choice of a nuclide for this service is very limited and may at times be insoluble. When accurate absolute activity determination is required no substitute for the calibration standard is possible and arrangements must be made to obtain new ones at intervals, such that derived standards will not have an unacceptable error.

For use with ^{131}I, a performance standard is available which has a gamma ray spectrum so closely approximating the spectrum of ^{131}I that it may be used also as a calibration standard, provided that all beta radiation of the ^{131}I sample to be measured is filtered out. (This is usually achieved by the

18

wall of the scintillation counter or can be accomplished with a 1 mm aluminum filter when using a Geiger-Mueller counter). This "mock-iodine" standard is a mixture of ^{133}Ba and ^{137}Cs. The two nuclides have different half-lives and their relative proportion changes with decay; the similarity of the spectrum of the mixture to ^{131}I remains adequate for about ten years; the half-life is also approximately ten years. It must be emphasized that "mock-iodine" is useful as a calibration standard only for gamma ray measurements; when a counting set-up is used which is sensitive to ^{131}I betas, it is no better than any other performance standard.

The specific counting techniques in standardization work are basically the same as for any sample counting *in vitro*, which will be treated below. The only special requirement is a high order of reliability. An uncertainty of 5 per cent should not be exceeded, which means the use of equation 15—(7); for a 5 per cent uncertainty, a minimum of 3600 counts must be collected when counting rate is high relative to background. Scintillation counters are generally employed for standardization although Geiger-Mueller counters are still sometimes used, particularly with beta-ray emitters. Both will give good results, and the accuracy depends more on the care of sample preparations and the calibration than on the choice of one particular instrument.

SELECTION OF ELECTRONIC CIRCUITS AND CONTROL SETTINGS

The electronic equipment available for counting purposes varies widely in its sophistication. The nature of the measurement to be made will determine the type of detector to be used and, in large measure, the associated circuitry required. Of course, a general rule to follow is the simpler the better. The Geiger-Mueller counter is the simplest, and whenever its properties suffice it should be chosen, particularly for high energy beta-ray measurements where no energy discrimination is required. If energy discrimination is necessary, then a proportional or scintillation counter is demanded.

Gamma-ray measurements are also practical with a Geiger-Mueller counter provided high sensitivity is not required. Efficiency of a Geiger-Mueller counter to gamma radiation can be increased by coating the counter walls with a high atomic number material, such as bismuth, or by inserting metal baffles in the counting volume; this increases the production of secondary electrons and is particularly useful in ^{131}I measurements. However, the scintillation counter offers a higher sensitivity and is to be preferred.

Along with the detector choice the degree of complexity of the electronic circuits to be employed must also be determined. The Geiger-Mueller counter requires a high voltage supply with easily attained regulation, an amplifier with little overall amplification and a simple discriminator. The scintillation or proportional counter requires a more complex voltage supply and more amplification. To utilize their properties fully, some form of pulse height analysis must also be performed, requiring still more sophisticated circuitry. In exchange for this complexity, of course, we obtain more information, greater sensitivity, etc.

These electronic circuits contain controls which must be properly adjusted to obtain the optimum in performance. Particulars of these adjustments will vary, of course, and therefore cannot be discussed here. The manufacturer's manual usually provides this type of information. However, there are some general remarks on circuit adjustments applicable to each kind of detector. These are appropriate in work of this kind and are given below for each of the detectors.

Geiger-Mueller Counters. Beyond a discriminator setting which is generally an internal adjustment best left to service personnel, equipment designed specifically for Geiger-Mueller counters provides only a counter high-voltage adjustment. The fundamental role of the high voltage applied to a Geiger-Mueller counter has been discussed in considerable detail (p. 190ff). It will be recalled that the Geiger-Mueller region is defined as that range of applied voltage where every ionizing event reaching the counter produces an electrical pulse of equal amplitude independent of ionization intensity of the event. In this region the total number of pulses (or counts in reference to a scaling circuit) observed from a source with a constant disintegration rate is independent of the voltage, or largely so. Below this range the pulse amplitude is too small to activate the counting circuit. Above it spurious pulses occur due to a variety of causes which are inherent in the detector itself and are not due to ionizing events reaching it. Reliable information on this useful range of voltages and its limitation is essential for the operation of a radiation detector. The curve representing this information is called the *"Voltage Characteristic"* of a counter.

If a Geiger-Mueller counter is connected to a scaling circuit and a suitable source of radioactive material is placed near it, no counts will be observed until the voltage reaches a certain value. If the voltage is gradually increased, occasional counts will be observed at a certain value called the *starting voltage*, as indicated in Figure 16–2. It should be noted that the ordinates in Figure 16–2 represents counting rate, and are different from the ordinates in Figure 13–4, where they represent pulse height or amplitude.

As the voltage is increased, the counting rate will at first also increase and then level off. The voltage range where the counting rate levels off is called the *threshold voltage* or simply "threshold." It will be noted that this threshold does not have a precise value, since there is no sharp kink in the voltage characteristic; nevertheless a value can be assigned to it within about ± 10 volts.

Further increase of voltage will not produce marked changes in the counting rate in a well-functioning counter for a few hundred volts. This region is called the *plateau*.

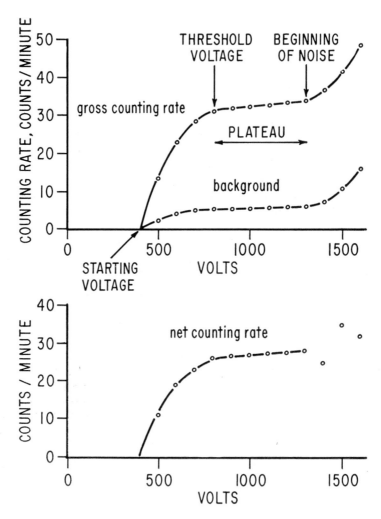

FIG. 16–2. Voltage characteristic of a Geiger-Mueller counter. The bottom curve of the net counting rate was obtained as difference of the two curves in the top graph; note that it is difficult to find the beginning of noise in this curve.

The end of the plateau occurs at a voltage where the counting rate begins to increase at first slowly and then quite rapidly. This increase is due to spontaneous discharges produced in the Geiger-Mueller counter by the excessive voltage, and is called *noise*. The excessive voltage in this region can easily damage the counter, therefore it should be approached slowly in determining the voltage characteristic. Readings should not be taken beyond the voltage at which the counting rate is about two times that in the plateau region.

The whole voltage characteristic can be determined and plotted with a radioactive sample giving a few thousand counts per minute. The higher the counting rate (within the limits of resolving time, see Chapter 15), the easier it is to observe starting and threshold voltage and the less time it will take to get data of desired precision. A high counting rate, however, may mask the beginning of noise, and a low counting rate (preferably background alone) will permit a more precise determination of noise voltage. When a radioactive sample is used for the plateau determination, the gross counting rate must be plotted; if the net counting rate is used for plotting, the noise may become completely masked or it may appear at a misleadingly high voltage.

Three basic data about a counter can be derived from the voltage characteristic: length and slope of the plateau and correct operating voltage.

The *length of the plateau* is simply the difference between noise voltage and threshold voltage. It is usually a few hundred volts. A counter with a plateau less than 100 volts long is considered, as a rule, unsatisfactory, unless it has some other especially desirable properties. The plateau length becomes shorter as a counter ages; usually the noise appears at lower voltage, but the threshold may also go up on occasion. Periodic determination of the plateau and its length is the best way to anticipate a counter breakdown. As a general rule, a counter should be replaced when its plateau reaches 100 volts.

The *operating voltage* is the voltage at which the counter is used. It may be placed anywhere on the plateau, but for optimal reliability a few rules should be followed. Since noise voltage goes down with aging, it is poor practice to operate a counter close to the upper limit. It may be used nearer to the threshold voltage, but not too near either, since this also may shift. For these reasons the best operating voltage is close, but not too close to the threshold, and as far below noise voltage as this recommendation permits. To give a specific rule: when plateau length is less than 200 volts operate the counter at the voltage corresponding to the center of the plateau; if the plateau is 200 volts or longer, use as operating voltage the threshold plus 100 volts.

The *slope of the plateau* is a measure of the independence of the counting rate from changes and fluctuations in the high voltage supply. It is generally expressed as per cent increase in counting rate per hundred volt increase and has values of between 1 and 5 per cent. In most modern scaling circuits the high voltage is stabilized to a degree which makes changes in counting rate from this cause negligible except in case of circuit failure. However, such failure is generally catastrophic, *i.e.* total failure of the stabilizing circuit with an accompanying large change in output voltage, and is therefore easily noticed.

As has been stated the voltage characteristic of a Geiger-Mueller counter is independent of the nature and energy of the primary ionizing event. Thus, if the voltage characteristic of such a counter has been determined with one radioactive nuclide, or even on background alone, the same plateau length, slope, operating voltage, etc. will be observed with any other nuclide.

Proportional Counters. The height of the pulse from a proportional counter, unlike that from a Geiger-Mueller counter, does depend upon the energy of the primary ionizing event. The proportionality permits extremely sophisticated measurements to be made with the proportional counter. Such measurements may require advanced electronic circuitry with correspondingly complex adjustment procedures. Measurements of this kind are rarely encountered in the medical-biological area where the proportional counter is generally employed in a manner similar to a Geiger-Mueller counter. At most, the proportional counter is used to distinguish gross differences in energy deposition. An example of this kind of use occurs in the counting of a mixture of an alpha-and a beta-ray source. Here, the counter can be used to determine the separate activity of each.

The effect of the counter voltage on the height of the pulses emanating from a proportional counter was shown in Figure 13–3. It is obvious from this figure that a very large increase in pulse height is produced by a relatively small increase in counter voltage. However, the effect of this increase in pulse height on the observed counting rate is not obvious, and in fact depends upon the distribution of primary ionizations by particles traversing the counter. This, in turn, depends upon the nature of the particle (*i.e.*, alpha, beta), its energy, and its path length in the counter. While this can result in a highly complex distribution, fortunately the situation is often relatively simple.

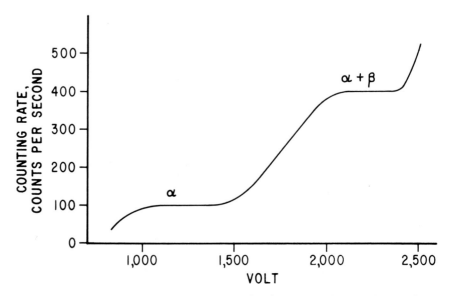

Fig. 16–3. Voltage characteristic of a proportional counter with a sample of Radium D plus E. The first plateau is due to α radiation. The second plateau is due to $\alpha + \beta$ radiation.

Figure 16–3 shows how the observed counting rate of a commercial proportional counter varies with the voltage applied. The source here is a nuclide which produces both α and β particles. There are two distinct plateaus. The α particles have a much higher linear ionization density than do the β particles and will produce much larger counter pulses. These override the discriminator threshold at relatively low counter voltage, before any of the beta particles are counted, and produce the lower voltage plateau marked α on the figure. The second, higher voltage plateau marked $\alpha + \beta$, occurs when almost all the β particles, as well as all the α particles, are counted. It is obvious from the figure how to determine the count rate from alpha particles alone. Subtracting this from the count rate on the second plateau yields the count rate for beta particles.

In some equipment the amount of electronic pulse amplification can be varied by means of front panel controls. These controls may be stepwise, continuous, or both. Their function is similar to that of high voltage control. The difference between the two is in the location of the amplification change. Increasing the high voltage applied to a proportional counter increases the amount of gas amplification within the counter. Change of the amplifier controls varies the amount of external, electronic amplification. In contrast with the high voltage changes, the change in amplification by amplifier control variation is a quantity known from the control markings. Precise knowledge of the change in amplification can be useful in some measurements.

Scintillation Counters. The scintillation counter also yields a pulse whose size is proportional to the energy deposited in the detector by the ionizing radiation. This proportionality, along with the high probability for the gamma rays to interact with the crystal, makes the scintillation counter a widely used detector and employed in conjunction with a great variety of electronic equipment. To aid in understanding the action of the various controls, we begin with a discussion of the pulse height spectrum from a scintillation counter, which is a plot of the number of pulses as a function of their height.

Figure 16–4 shows such a spectrum from a thallium-activated sodium iodide scintillation counter irradiated by the gamma rays of ^{60}Co. The ordinate is the count rate (pulses/time), and the abscissa is the pulse height or, in the units chosen here, the energy which the height represents. The origin of this spectrum is explained from the interaction processes between gamma rays and matter as described in Chapter 7. We begin with the two peaks at the right side of the figure. They are produced by gamma rays whose energy is completely absorbed in the crystal and are called photopeaks. There are two gamma rays emitted by ^{60}Co; one has an energy of 1.17 MeV and the other an energy of 1.33 MeV. Because the photopeaks represent complete gamma energy absorption, the abscissa values of these peaks are 1.17 MeV and 1.33 MeV respectively. The term photopeak is indicative of the total absorption of the gamma ray energy

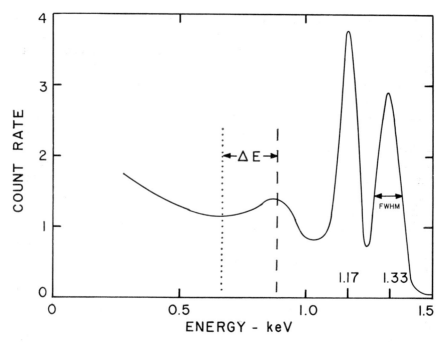

Fig. 16–4. Pulse height spectrum of ^{60}Co for a NaI (Tl) counter. The full width at half maximum of the upper peak is shown. The resolution for this peak is 6.9 per cent (see text).

because a gamma ray absorbed by the *photoelectric* process transfers its entire energy. However, all the totally absorbed gamma rays are not absorbed photoelectrically. Multiple processes, involving Compton interactions, also occur.

Above (to the right of) the photopeaks very few counts are observed because no single gamma ray interaction can deposit this much energy in the scintillation crystal. Immediately below (to the left of) the peaks there is a sharp drop in the number of counts. This is indicative of the impossibility of transferring this amount of energy to the crystal in a single interaction. Only through multiple processes can the crystal absorb energy in this region. Such multiple interactions are not very probable, so few pulses are observed.

The number of observed pulses is seen to increase at still lower energies. Counts in this region result from single Compton interactions within the scintillation crystal.

Another nuclide will yield a different pulse height spectrum. The general features remain constant, however. Each gamma ray will produce a photopeak. The position of the peak is proportional to the gamma-ray energy. The height of the peak depends upon a number of factors which include the gamma energy, the size of the crystal and the frequency of emission of the gamma ray by the nuclide. The details of any pulse height spectrum are easily explained in terms of the decay scheme of the nuclide and the interaction processes of the gamma rays with the scintillation crystal.

One question might well be answered at this point. Why is a photopeak, representing as it does the absorption of a fixed gamma-ray energy, not a very sharp spike in the pulse height spectrum? The answer to the question involves all the processes which occur in a scintillation detector when energy is deposited. These include the production of light (the scintillation), the transfer of this light to the cathode of the photomultiplier tube, the formation of photoelectrons at the cathode and the multiplication of these electrons. The efficiency of each process varies from pulse to pulse resulting in a distribution in the height of the pulses out of the photomultiplier. This distribution is displayed as the spread of the photopeak.

For some applications, particularly gamma-ray spectroscopy, this spread should be as small as possible. Generally in the medical field, the magnitude of the spread is not very important. It is specified by the *resolution* of the detector, which is usually stated in terms of the full width at half maximum (FWHM). The FWHM is the width of the photopeak at a count value equal to one half the count at the peak of the curve. It is indicated in Figure 16–4 for the higher energy photopeak. The resolution is generally given as a percentage and is equal to one hundred times the ratio of the FWHM divided by the abscissa value at the peak, *i.e.* the energy of the gamma ray.

The resolution of a detector depends on the gamma ray energy, decreasing as the energy increases. Most manufacturers specify the resolution of their detectors in terms of the ^{137}Cs photopeak (0.662 MeV). The lowest value attainable with NaI(Tl) scintillation counters is about 7 per cent. Frequently, the resolution is much higher than this figure, particularly with well scintillation counters. Fortunately this is not of great consequence for most applications.

Let us now examine the effects of electronic control adjustments on the counting rate observed from a scintillation counter and explain them in terms of this pulse height spectrum. We begin with a system which has adjustable high voltage, electronic amplification, and discriminator level. As with the proportional counter, the high voltage and the amplifier controls have a similar effect. In terms of Figure 16–4 an increase in high voltage or amplification results in stretching the abscissa proportionately to the right. The only difference in function between these controls lies in the location of the amplification increase. The high voltage increases the amplification in the photomultiplier tube while the amplifier control changes the external amplification.

When we count pulses using a discriminator between the amplifier and scaler, we count only those pulses whose height exceeds the value determined by the setting of the discriminator control. One such setting is shown by the dotted vertical line in Figure 16–4. The scaler will count all those pulses of higher energy than the dotted line, *i.e.* all pulses to the right of that line. If we change the discriminator setting to count smaller pulses (lower energy), the count rate increases. Reduction of the discriminator level corresponds to moving our dotted line in the figure to the left. Increasing the discriminator level will reduce the count rate. Again, this is equivalent to moving the dotted line, but this time to the right. If we now plot the count rate as a function of the discriminator setting, we obtain the curve shown in Figure 16–5. In this figure we have plotted the discriminator level in MeV so that it can be directly related to the pulse height spectrum (Fig. 16–4). Notice the two regions where the count rate changes little with discriminator setting. These are observed at settings immediately below the photopeaks, i.e. in a region where relatively few counts occur. For routine applications a discriminator setting on the lower energy "plateau" is used. This setting is indicated by an arrow in the figure.

A similar, but more frequently encountered curve is a plot of the count rate against the high voltage to the scintillation counter with the discriminator level fixed. Such a plot is shown in Figure 16–6. This curve is anal-

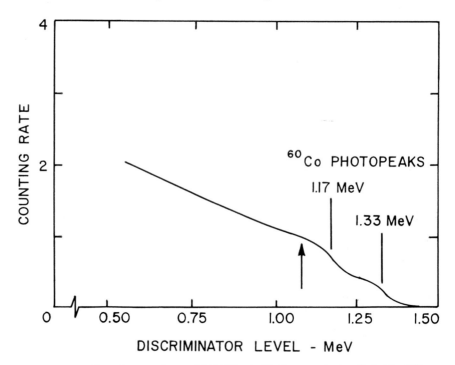

FIG. 16–5. Counting rate from a NaI (Tl) scintillation counter irradiated by ⁶⁰Co as a function of discriminator level. The positions of the two photopeaks are indicated. Their influence is demonstrated by the two regions of lowered slope below the peaks. The arrow indicates an operating point chosen for stable operation.

ogous to the voltage characteristic curve for the Geiger-Mueller counter, but results from quite different processes, *i.e.* those related to the pulse height spectrum of the scintillation counter. As we have remarked, all pulses to the right of the discriminator setting are counted (see Fig. 16–4). When the high voltage is increased, the height of all pulses is increased because the amplification of the photomultiplier tube is increased. The count rate, in turn, increases because more pulses are to the right of the discriminator level. The net result is the curve of Figure 16–6.

The two regions indicated by arrows on the figure are termed "plateaus" in analogy with the voltage characteristic curve of the Geiger-Mueller counter. These regions are also the result of the lowered counting rate immediately below each of the photopeaks. The term plateau is not very applicable however. They are very short, *i.e.* not spread over a wide voltage range, because of the rapid change of photomultiplier tube amplification with applied voltage. Some nuclides produce a plateau which is nearer to that of Geiger-Mueller tube but in general the scintillation counter plateau is short and has a steep slope.

The results of using a single channel analyzer instead of a discriminator can also be understood in terms of Figure 16–4. (The analyzer is discussed

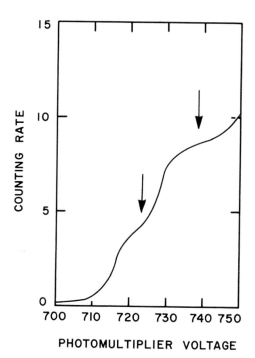

PHOTOMULTIPLIER VOLTAGE

Fig. 16–6. Counting rate as a function of photomultiplier voltage for a NaI (Tl) scintillation counter irradiated by ^{60}Co. The influence of the two photopeaks is demonstrated by the flattening of the curve in the regions indicated by the arrows. The arrow at higher voltage also indicates a commonly used operating point on this "plateau."

on pages 217ff.) We will now consider the dotted line in the figure as the base line discriminator setting of the analyzer. Also shown in the figure is a dashed line drawn at a pulse height $\triangle h$ (or energy $\triangle E$) above the base line. This represents the window setting of the analyzer. As was discussed in Chapter 13, the analyzer passes only those pulses which lie above the base line and which do not exceed the window setting. Thus, only pulses which lie between the dotted and the dashed lines in the figure will be counted. As the base line control is varied, the window is moved over the entire pulse height spectrum. When the window is narrow, a plot of the count rate against base line setting will yield the pulse height spectrum itself. With wider windows the spectrum will be "smeared." Narrowness here is to be judged in terms of detector resolution. A window width-base line ratio which is small compared to the detector resolution defines a narrow window.

From the above description it is relatively easy to choose the appropriate settings for the several controls. When only a discriminator is used, a choice of high voltage and discriminator setting to operate on the plateau is usually made. Such a choice renders the system reasonably free from error due to small drifts in either the discriminator level or the high voltage. Use of a single-channel analyzer can require different settings which depend on the function the analyzer is to perform. Often such equipment is used for background reduction and a more complete discussion of this subject is given below. In routine counting the base line is set below the photo-peak(s) and the window chosen to have sufficient width to encompass the peak(s). Use of a wide window promotes freedom from errors due to small equipmental drifts. Most nuclides have one principal peak and the control settings are made for this peak. If the analyzer is to be used to determine the pulse height spectrum, a narrow window is required to limit spectral smearing.

Another frequent use of a single-channel analyzer is counting one nuclide in the presence of another. The function of the analyzer here is to separate, as far as is practicable, the counts from the two nuclides. This procedure is discussed more fully at a later point in this chapter.

SAMPLE MEASUREMENTS IN VITRO

Gamma Ray Counting. Because of the high penetrating power of gamma radiation, there is a considerable freedom in arranging a counting set-up.

When a sample is at some distance from the counter, as illustrated in Figure 16–7a, only a small fraction of the total rays emitted by the sample impinges on the counter. In Figure 16–7b, the sample is very close and a much larger share of the emitted rays will reach the detector. The sensitivity will be even higher if the sample surrounds the counter as in Figure 16–7c. The highest sensitivity is achieved in an arrangement as in Figure

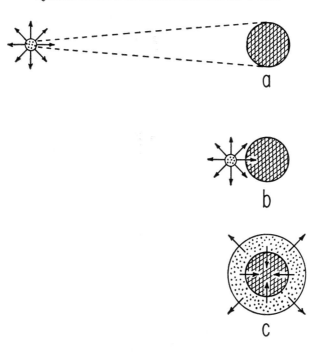

FIG. 16–7.   Four typical counting geometries: (*a*) sample at a distance from detector, (*b*) sample in close proximity to the detector, (*c*) sample surrounding the detector, (*d*) detector surrounding the sample.

16–7*d*, where the counter surrounds the sample and practically all radiation from the sample goes through the detector.

This relative arrangement of counter and sample is called the "geometry" of a set-up.   The differences in calibration factor, etc. are listed in Table 16–2, to be discussed in detail presently.   When sample and counter are close to each other, no exact rules about the expected change of the calibration factor with change in position can be given; when the distance between the two is greater than about 10 times the physical size of either (height or length, whichever is greater), the inverse square rule gives a good approximation.

The inverse square rule can be formulated as follows: If at a distance d_1 of the sample from the counter a counting rate R_1 is observed, and the counting rate R_2 at a new distance d_2 is to be estimated, we have the relationship

Table 16-2. Approximate Sensitivity in Gamma Counting for Various Methods of Some Selected Nuclides

Method	Nuclide	Sample Form	Background c/s	Data for Activity — Calibration Factor c/s for 1 μCi	Data for Activity — Precision nCi	Data for Specific Activity — Calibration Factor c/s for 1 μCi/ml	Data for Specific Activity — Precision nCi/ml
NaI(Tl) well counter 1 3/4" diameter × 2" high crystal with 21/32" diameter × 1 35/64" deep well	^{51}Cr	Solution 5 ml	1.7	1,000	0.3		
	^{59}Fe	Solution 5 ml	0.5	2,200	0.08		
	^{60}Co	Solution 5 ml	0.3	3,000	0.04	27,000	0.008
	^{60}Co	Point Source in plastic	0.3	4,000	0.03		
	^{85}Sr	Solution 5 ml	1.2	4,000	0.07		
	^{99m}Tc	Solution 5 ml	2.7	13,600	0.03		
	^{131}I	Solution 5 ml	1.2	6,000	0.04	30,000	0.009
	^{131}I	Solution 250 ml on top of crystal	2.7	400	1.0	100,000	0.004
	^{137}Cs	Solution 5 ml	1.0	2,600	0.09		
	^{137}Cs	Point Source in plastic	1.0	4,300	0.06		
Plastic phosphor well counter 5" diameter, 6" high*	^{60}Co	Solution 100 ml	7	9,000	0.06	900,000	0.0006
Marinelli Beaker Geiger-Mueller counter†	^{131}I	Solution 150 ml	0.25	4.5	27	675	0.2

* Data from G. J. Hine and A. Miller: Large Plastic Well Makes Efficient Gamma Counter, Nucleonics 10, No. 10, 78 (1956).
† Data from The Thyroid, edited by Sidney C. Werner, New York, Hoeber-Harper, 1955, page 188.

$$\frac{R_1}{R_2} = \frac{d_2^2}{d_1^2} \qquad\qquad 16-(1)$$

or

$$R_2 = R_1 \left(\frac{d_1}{d_2}\right)^2 \qquad\qquad 16-(1a)$$

The use of increased distance is sometimes useful when samples have too high activity and resolving time correction becomes excessive, or when a sample has large volume, as for instance in counting of stool specimens, and where the use of an aliquot fraction is inadvisable because of the inhomogeneity, or for some other reasons. In increasing the distance it is necessary to guard against two sources of error. (1) When the sample is at a distance from the counter, shielding of the sample-counter assembly becomes difficult and the background may increase and become variable. (2) The sample may come close to some objects which contribute to scatter; this does not interfere with counting, provided calibration was done with the same objects (tabletops, sample support, shielding materials) in the same position as when the samples are counted. One such scattering object is easily overlooked, and that is the observer himself, who can contribute 10 to 20 per cent of the counting rate if he is accessible to the radiation emitted by the sample and is "visible" to the counter.

Biological samples are usually in the form of liquids (blood, urine), semisolids (stool), or tissues of comparable density, approximately equal to water. The differences in absorption of gamma radiation by such samples can therefore be neglected, particularly if the calibration standard is homogeneously mixed with similar material. The radioactivity in the samples is practically always due to the administration of a tracer or a therapeutic amount of the particular nuclide previous to the withdrawal of the sample. This simplifies considerably the calibration of the counter, since an aliquot of the original dose can be retained, dissolved in a volume of water similar to that of the samples to be measured and used as a comparison standard. The results are then expressed as fractions of this comparison standard. This method is an example of the second standardization technique discussed above. Frequently the sample activity is only a small fraction of the original dose; the comparison sample should then be suitably diluted. This procedure does not insure absolute accuracy in terms of microcuries, but it permits the reliable and comparatively simple determination of the *ratio* between the activity in the sample and the administered amount. A long-lived performance standard should still be used, since the reliability, even in the determination of ratios, may suffer when a counter begins to fail; this can frequently be detected in time if the use of a performance standard is a part of daily laboratory routine.

In any given sample there is, as a rule, a given specific activity, that is, an activity per unit of volume. The total activity presented to a counter depends, therefore, on the volume. The smallest specific activity which can be measured can therefore be decreased by using a larger sample volume. This is limited only by the amount of sample available and by the counting geometry.

Limitations of available sample volume are determined by the biological condition, for it is rarely possible to obtain more than a few ml of blood, while urine may be available in liters.

Limitations of sample volume which can be used in a given counting geometry depend on the physical size and type of counter. In the case of Figure 16–7a and b, there is practically no limitation in this respect, but distance of sample from counter reduces the sensitivity. A better arrangement in this respect is offered by Figure 16–7. This is called the Marinelli set-up. A beaker as shown in Figure 16–8 is generally used as sample container. The radiation detector is usually a Geiger-Mueller counter and the beaker is put over the counter. Table 16–2 lists the data for the Marinelli type counter and the other counter arrangements to be discussed in the following pages.

In this and in other tables with data on counters, the column labeled "precision" is calculated from equation 15—(49) on page 250, where this term is defined.

Geometry similar to that of the Marinelli beaker can also be obtained with the "dip" counter. Here the Geiger-Mueller tube is placed directly into the radioactive solution. The wall of the counter is fabricated from stainless steel or other easily decontaminated material so that it may be cleaned between measurements. It is important when using dip counter devices to maintain constant geometry and to check background after each cleaning. Very large volumes can be handled with dip counters.

The Marinelli beaker or dip counter arrangement are among the best devices for urine counting, since a large beaker can hold several hundred

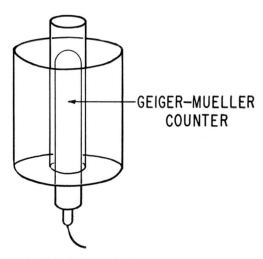

Fig. 16–8.   Marinelli beaker counting arrangement (geometry c of Fig. 16–7).

ml, so that errors in pipetting are reduced. A small volume Marinelli beaker with a suitably smaller Geiger-Mueller counter has also been used successfully, but better sensitivity can be obtained for smaller sample volumes by using the arrangement of Figure 16–7d.

This arrangement, with the counter surrounding the sample, is used with some special purpose Geiger-Mueller counters. Among these is the so-called "flow-through" counter where a radioactive solution flows through a helical tube mounted inside the counter volume. Such counters have been used as detectors in liquid chromatography.

By far the widest use of the arrangement of Figure 16–7d is the *well-type thallium activated-sodium iodide scintillation counter.* A fairly large crystal has a hole drilled into it axially so that it is able to contain a standard test tube. Typical dimensions for the crystal are $1\frac{3}{4}$ inches in diameter and 2 inches thick with the hole $\frac{3}{4}$ inch in diameter and $1\frac{1}{2}$ inches deep. Such crystals are encased in an aluminum housing with reflective material surrounding the crystal and a window at the end opposite the well. This window is optically coupled to a phototube. A well counter is illustrated diagrammatically in Figure 16–9. It is also quite usual today for the crystal and photomultiplier to be encased in a common container by the

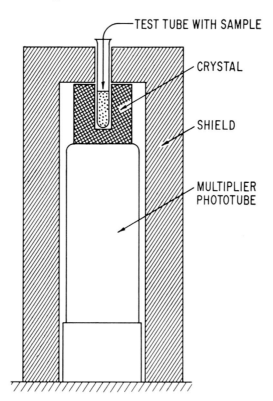

Fig. 16–9.   Well type scintillation counter (geometry of Fig. 16–7d).

manufacturer. These "integral" detectors have a distinct advantage in reliability of the optical coupling between the crystal and the phototube. However, phototube replacement is obviously more difficult and costly, and requires the unit to be repaired by the manufacturer.

When the test tube contains a liquid volume up to 5 ml, the whole of the liquid is within the crystal well and there is little difference in sensitivity with volume. In Table 16–2 are listed the data for a typical NaI well-type crystal.

The test tube may be filled with a sample of larger volume than 5 ml; the liquid column is then partly outside the counter, the well geometry of Figure 16–7d is combined with the geometry of Figure 16–7b and the sensitivity drops. Still a gain in the determination of a given specific activity may be achieved by using volumes greater than 5 ml within certain limits (see Fig. 16–10). For the particular crystal and shielding illustrated there, the optimum volume is 7 ml; there is negligible gain with a larger sample.

When larger sample volumes must be used, a larger well and a larger counter are needed. This may be of advantage when only very low specific activity is present, or where it is difficult or undesirable to use a portion of the sample, as in counting stool specimens. Large crystals are prohibitive in cost for most routine uses; large well-type Geiger-Mueller counters have been made, but are not generally available. On occasion an attempt has been made to imitate a well-type geometry by arranging several Geiger-Mueller counters on the periphery of a circle; the sample is positioned in the middle and a scaling circuit is adapted in such a way that the counts of all counters are registered and counted together. A more practical solution is to change over from well-type geometry to the arrangement of Figure 16–7b, by using a large crystal (the well crystal can be easily adapted for this) and positioning a large sample over the crystal. An example of

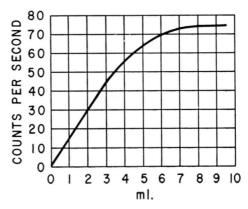

FIG. 16–10. Increase of counting rate with increasing sample volume of constant specific activity in a well type scintillation counter with a well capacity of 5 ml.

such a use with ^{131}I is listed in Table 16–2. It can be seen that the calibration factor for total sample activity and for specific activity becomes very small, but that due to the large sample, a much smaller activity per ml can be detected. Similar results will be obtained with most other gamma-emitting nuclides.

When comparing the sensitivity and calibration factors for scintillation counters with the discussion given earlier, what appears to be a discrepancy will be noted. It was stated that a larger pulse results from the absorption of a higher energy gamma ray. This makes the detection of higher energy photons easier provided they are absorbed in the crystal. On the other hand, the higher the photon energy the smaller the probability of their being absorbed. More of them will pass through the crystal without interacting with it, *i.e.* the efficiency becomes smaller. In examining efficiency data or sensitivity factors it is also necessary to consider the decay scheme of the nuclides being compared. For example, ^{60}Co and ^{137}Cs may appear to have about equal sensitivity although the gamma rays from ^{60}Co are above one MeV in energy while those from ^{137}Cs are primarily 662 keV. This equality of the sensitivity arises from the fact that only 92 per cent of the ^{137}Cs decays produce the 662 keV gamma ray while two gamma rays are emitted for each ^{60}Co disintegration.

Well scintillation counters for large samples can be fabricated from plastic phosphors at a reasonable cost. Data for a phosphor 5 inches in diameter, 6 inches high, with a well holding 100 ml samples, are included in Table 16–2.

It is perhaps of interest to mention the largest type of well counter currently in use. It is designed to accept a human body. The scintillating material is a liquid phosphor which is viewed by an array of photomultiplier tubes. The first of this type of well counter was built at Los Alamos to investigate body burdens of radioactive material in humans. A number of other institutions now also use this type of "whole body counter."

The geometry in which a sample is at some distance from the radiation detector (Fig. 16–7a) is used generally for *in vivo* counting, but it is useful in some *in vitro* counting problems, when the activity of the sample is too great for use with another arrangement or when the sample is too bulky and at the same time has sufficient activity for measurement in this set-up.

When the specific activity in a liquid sample is too small for counting with any of the mentioned set-ups, it is frequently possible to concentrate it by evaporation. Whenever this procedure is used, it is necessary to guard against loss of activity during evaporation; when this evaporation is carried out to dryness, a correction for self-absorption may have to be done. This will be discussed in the next section on beta counting.

Beta Particle Counting. While one of the problems of optimal sensitivity in gamma counting is to achieve maximum absorption of this penetrating radiation within the radiation detector, the difficulty with beta counting is the opposite. Beta rays are easily absorbed; once they reach the sensitive volume of the counter (gas in a Geiger-Mueller counter, crystal in the scintillation counter) their efficiency is very high, close to 100 per cent. But because of this ease of absorption, they are as readily absorbed in the walls of a counter and may not reach the sensitive volume at all. Counter walls must be made as thin as possible.

Geiger-Mueller counters have been made of rather thin aluminum which permits the penetration of higher energy beta particles; such counters are quite fragile, since the thin walls have to withstand the difference between atmospheric pressure and the reduced pressure in the counter. For the same reason, thin-walled counters of glass are not in general use. In order to compromise between strength and need for thinness, counters for beta radiation are usually made of a strong material (glass, metal) except for a thin window at one end: *end-window counters*. The preferred material for

Table 16-3.

Relative Counting Rate

Window thickness in mg/cm²	^{32}P	^{198}Au	^{131}I	^{60}Co	^{45}Ca	^{35}S	^{14}C
0	100	100	100	100	100	100	100
1	99	98	96	92	89	81	78
2	99	96	92	84	78	66	60
3	98	94	88	77	69	53	46
4	97	92	84	70	62	43	35
5	96	90	81	65	54	35	27
6	96	89	78	60	48	28	21
7	95	87	75	54	43	23	16

the window is a natural mineral, mica, which can be split into very thin but strong sheets. Mica windows are available in thicknesses down to about 1.5 mg per square centimeter. Very thin window counters are both expensive and fragile; they are used for the measurement of soft beta-emitters such as ^{14}C and ^{35}S. For higher energy betas, as with ^{32}P for instance, thicker and stronger windows of about 3 to 4 mg/cm² are preferred. Table 16–3 lists the reduction of counts with increasing window thickness for several typical nuclides, after deduction of the counting rates due to gamma radiation of those nuclides which have both gamma and beta rays.* It will be seen that a window thickness of a few mg/cm² causes a negligible reduction of counting rate for ^{32}P, ^{198}Au, ^{131}I and ^{60}Co, this rate is halved by 5 mg/cm² for ^{45}Ca, by 3 mg for ^{35}S and by only 2.5 mg for ^{14}C.

There is less variation possible in the position of the sample and counter for beta than for gamma counting. The counting geometry is in practice always of the type illustrated in Figure 16–7a and 16–7b when using Geiger-Mueller counters. Liquid scintillation counters (see p. 285) use the

* A. I. Gleason, J. D. Taylor and D. L. Tabern: Absolute Beta Counting at Defined Geometries. Nucleonics, 1951, *8*, No. 5, page 18.

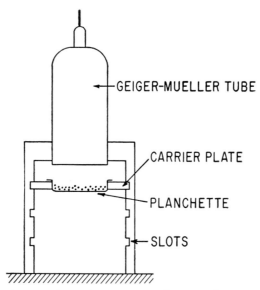

GEIGER-MUELLER TUBE

CARRIER PLATE

PLANCHETTE

SLOTS

FIG. 16–11.   An example for the use of an end window Geiger-Mueller counter
(geometry *b* of Fig. 16–7).

geometry of Figure 16–7*d*. With the other geometries large distances are
neither necessary nor practical, since bulky samples of large volume are
useless for beta counting due to self-absorption. This will be discussed in
detail presently.

The typical set-up is illustrated in Figure 16–11. The sample is contained
on a metal planchette; the planchette fits into a plate which can be inserted;
and removed by sliding it in and out of slots in a stand; the stand has sometimes several slots in order to change the distance of the sample from the
counter (the purpose is to vary the sensitivity by changing sample distance).

The efficiency of a counter for beta radiation is close to 100 per cent,
that is, most beta particles once they get inside will produce a count. The
actual sensitivity is considerably smaller. It depends on the window absorption, and it is also reduced by the distance of the sample from the
counter, and by the fact that only half of the beta rays leave the surface of
the sample and go towards the counter, while the other half impinges on the
planchette supporting the sample where they are either absorbed or scattered back towards the counter. Absorption of beta rays by the sample
itself can be disregarded in most standardization measurements when the
sample contains nothing but the radioactive nuclide and a negligible
amount of carrier and impurities and when dry samples are used.

For beta counting under these conditions, dry samples are used almost
exclusively; solvents increase absorption and reduce sensitivity and also
introduce an erratic erorr due to slow evaporation.

A fraction of the beta radiation which is scattered from the planchette may reach the counter. Not all beta particles, therefore, which go in a direction away from the counter, are lost as a source of counting events. The same occurs with beta rays hitting the supporting structures.

Assuming no absorption in the window and an inherent 100 per cent efficiency of the counter it might be expected that the counting efficiency with a sample on a planchette would be never greater than 50 per cent. Due to backscatter, however, it may exceed this figure significantly. It is important to realize that the amount of energy of this backscatter depends on the atomic number of the scattering material. It is essential, therefore, to use identical planchettes for a series of measurements and the associated calibration. A recalibration is always necessary when planchette types are switched (steel to plated iron or to aluminum) or when the support or enclosure is replaced, even when the identical counter is used and the dimensions are exactly reproduced.

When beta counters are used for the purpose of standardization, it is advisable to use a standardized sample of the identical nuclide. ^{32}P can be standardized by bremsstrahlung counting in a scintillation counter, as described under the heading of "Specialized Methods" page 291f. Long lived, low energy, pure beta emitters such as ^{45}Ca, ^{35}S and ^{14}C, are of prime interest, and for these standardized samples are useful over long periods

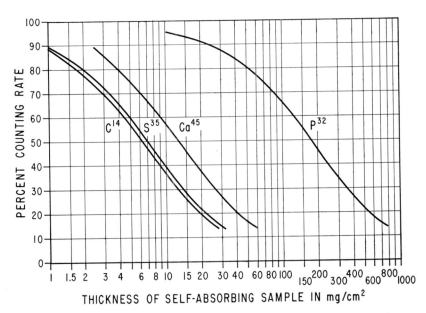

Fig. 16–12.   Decrease of counting rate due to self-absorption, when the counting rate of the *total* activity in the sample without absorption (weightless samples) is 100. (When the absorbing material has intermediate or high atomic number there is some initial increase of counting rate in thin samples due to selfscattering; this effect is disregarded in the illustration).

after they have been obtained. Performance standards are therefore of secondary interest with beta counters. Radium D + E, deposited on a metal planchette, may be used for general checking, but even a gamma-emitter (radium, ^{60}Co) might be used; it must be realized in this case that the position of the gamma-ray standard is quite critical and provision must be made so that it can be easily and securely placed in the same position for every check (a holder which is screwed to the counter housing and into which the standard container fits snugly is the simplest solution).

Self-absorption. When biological samples are prepared for beta counting, they usually contain, even when dried, a significant amount of material (inorganic salts in urine, proteins in blood, etc.) which will absorb a fraction of the beta radiation. The fraction absorbed will depend on the sample thickness which is expressed best in mg/cm.^{2} The graph in Figure 16–12 permits estimation of the expected counting rate for several nuclides if the calibration factor for a "weightless" sample, expected activity in the given sample, and its mg/cm^2 are known. This graph applies to samples which contain the same *total* activity. So long as the sample thickness does not exceed the beta-ray range of the nuclide the counting rate will *increase* for thicker samples of the same *specific* activity.

This graph, however, can be used only for a rough evaluation. For reliable measurements it is essential to determine the correction for self-absorption for any particular experiment. This can be done by preparing a duplicate sample; a known amount of the carrier free nuclide, q μCi, is added to the second sample. Both samples are processed (dried, etc.) in the identical fashion, and counted. Let the two observed counting rates be R_1 and R_2. The calibration factor f for the given sample is then given by the increased counts for the sample with the added activity $R_2 - R_1$, divided by the added activity:

$$f = \frac{R_2 - R_1}{q} \qquad 16-(2)$$

and this factor can be used to calculate the unknown activity A:

$$A = \frac{R_1}{f} \qquad 16-(3)$$

Although no improvement in sensitivity is possible by increasing sample size beyond the thickness corresponding to the range, an advantage of a different type is gained. When such "thick" samples are used, the counting rate becomes independent of sample thickness, since no beta particles reach the counter from material behind the range layer (this applies for pure beta-emitters only and when bremsstrahlung can be disregarded). A calibration of the counting set-up under these conditions can be made in terms of specific activity (counts per second for 1 μCi per mg). The sample preparation, particularly the amount of material used, becomes then less critical. The expected calibration factor can be evaluated from Figure 16–12.

As an example, the estimated calibration factor in a given counter for ^{32}P will be calculated. Let us assume that a calibration without self-absorption gives 20 c/s for 1 nanocurie total activity. The planchette area (1″ diameter) is 5 cm². A blood sample of a given volume is estimated to contain 7 nanocuries and to weigh, when dried on the planchette, 0.62 gm. The thickness is then 125 mg/cm². The counting rate without self-absorption would be 140 counts per second. This will be reduced for this sample thickness (curve for ^{32}P in Figure 16–12) to 60 per cent; the estimated counting rate will be, therefore, about 80 counts per second. Now let us consider a "thick" sample (exceeding the beta range); the same sensitivity will be assumed as before without self-absorption (20 counts per second for 1 nanocurie). It will be further assumed that 0.02 nanocuries per mg dry residue are present on the planchette. The thickness of the layer corresponding to ^{32}P beta range is 900 mg/cm². The total weight of this layer on the planchette is 900 × 5 = 4500 mg. This will contain altogether 4500 × 0.02 = 90 nanocuries. Figure 16–12 indicates that the counting rate drops to 14 per cent for distribution in beta-range-layer thickness. A weightless sample of 90 nanocuries will give a counting rate of 90 × 20 = 1800 counts per second. With self-absorption, 14 per cent of this counting rate will be observed or 250 counts per second. To generalize for this case: 0.02 nanocuries/mg will give 250 counts per second; 1 nanocurie/mg therefore will give 12,500 counts per second. This calibration factor for specific activity (per unit weight of sample) is now independent of the sample thickness, provided of course this thickness exceeds the beta range.

If liquid samples are to be counted it is practically essential that they be counted as thick samples. The calibration factor for thick samples as deduced above will apply to such samples, i.e. the specific concentration is determined by such a measurement.

A few specific suggestions on problems in the preparation of dry samples should be given. Weightless samples (carrier-free) may dry unevenly, cause erratic geometry and produce, therefore, errors in calibration and counting. This unevenness can be reduced by cleaning the planchettes well, to make sure that no oily film is present, by adding some wetting agent to the sample before drying, or by using a piece of thin filter paper (dripolator coffee filters are the only source of really thin filter paper known to the writer!) in the planchette. A check for self-absorption is necessary, if the latter device is used. When samples with significant dry residue are prepared, the deposit may lack uniformity; this can be reduced by slow drying (heater lamps at sufficient distance). Such samples are sometimes powdery and flaky, and some of the material may be lost and even contaminate the counter. A thin film of collodion solution (a fraction of 1 per cent concentration) or a carefully placed disc of thin plastic foil may reduce this. In this case, the absorption by the protective layers has to be checked in addition to the self-absorption.

Most beta measurements need not be absolute in reference to a standard precisely known in terms of mCi, but only relative with reference to an administered tracer dose. Calibrations may be done therefore by using a suitable portion of the tracer dose used. This method can be used also for calibration with self-absorption as discussed in connection with equation 16—(2).

Very Low Energy Beta-Ray Counting. Almost any counter window is sufficiently thick to absorb completely the beta particles from emitters such as ^{3}H (18.6 keV maximum energy). In addition, it is extremely difficult to estimate appropriate source thickness corrections for such nuclides, and a truly thin source is unobtainable. However, a liquid scintillation counter can be employed for very low energy beta-ray counting. This device requires no source thickness corrections and is windowless.

In the liquid scintillation counter the radioactive material and the scintillator are dissolved in an organic solvent. Organic scintillators are used exclusively. The vessel containing this mixture is placed in a light-tight chamber where it is viewed by two photomultiplier tubes. Because the radioactive material is uniformly disbursed throughout the scintillating liquid, there is no self-absorption in the source and no counter window to stop the beta rays.

Low energy beta rays are difficult to detect with a scintillation counter because of the noise from the photomultiplier tube. This noise can be greatly reduced by decreasing the temperature of the tube and so liquid scintillation counter systems include a refrigerator to cool the tubes and the sample. The effect of the remaining noise is further reduced by the use of the two photomultipliers in a coincidence circuit (see page 215). A single beta particle will cause light to be given off in all directions in the scintillator, and this light will strike both phototubes simultaneously. Thus, beta produced pulses are in coincidence in the phototubes. Noise pulses in the two tubes are random and independent in each and therefore seldom in coincidence. By counting only the coincident events, most of the beta pulses and few of the noise pulses are detected.

The efficiency of the liquid scintillation counter is very high because the source is distributed in the scintillating liquid. Were it not for the noise, which despite the use of refrigeration and coincidence circuitry becomes considerable at very low discriminator settings, the efficiency would approach 100 per cent. Efficiency in a liquid scintillation counter is the same in a broad sense as it is in the narrow, because all disintegrations occur in the scintillating solution. Despite the noise, the efficiency for ^{3}H (a particularly difficult nuclide to count) is better than 30 per cent and for ^{14}C approaches 80 per cent.

The liquid scintillation counter, like all scintillation counters, produces pulses whose height is proportional to the energy deposited. This permits them to be used with pulse height discrimination circuitry for application such as the determination of the separate activities of each of two nuclides in a mixture. A frequently encountered mixture is one containing ^{14}C and ^{3}H. The double nuclide technique will be described in a later section of this chapter.

Liquid scintillators do suffer from a problem analogous to source absorption. This is quenching, a reduction in the light output of the liquid due to presence of impurities in the solution. A very common quenching agent is water. To obtain a precise measurement, the calibrating source must have the same impurities as does the unknown. Elimination of quenching agents from the unknown is desirable although not always possible and at times even the amount of quenching agent in the sample is not well known. In such a case the precision obtainable is reduced. A determination of the amount of quenching as a function of the concentration of the agent must be made. From this information and the possible range of agent concentration in the unknown the precision of a measurement can be determined.

Shielding of Counting Set-Ups. Every nuclear counting set-up must be shielded to reduce the amount and variability of the background. The shielding requirements depend on the sensitivity of the counter to gamma and beta radiation.

A scintillation counter requires considerable shielding because of its relatively high efficiency to penetrating cosmic radiation. A well crystal for instance needs an enclosure of at least 2 inches of lead. Suitable lead shields are supplied by the counter manufacturers, but they can be easily assembled by the user with "lead bricks" which usually measure $2 \times 4 \times 8$ inches. Lead bricks can be either bought from suppliers of nuclear equip-

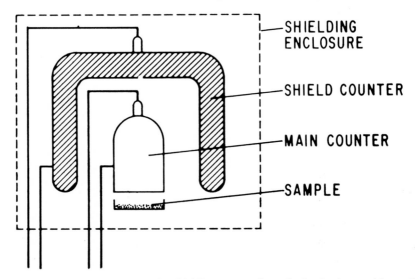

SHIELDING ENCLOSURE

SHIELD COUNTER

MAIN COUNTER

SAMPLE

Fig. 16–13. Assembly for use of a shielding counter for reducing background by anti-coincidence counting.

ment, or can be cast by a local lead foundry, sometimes at a considerable saving.

Geiger-Mueller counters need less shielding and 1 inch of lead is frequently sufficient.

The sensitivity of beta counters to external background radiation may be equal to that of Geiger-Mueller counters used for gamma counting, but it is frequently smaller and therefore less shielding may be needed. One potential difficulty with beta-counter shielding should be pointed out: lead occasionally contains natural radioactive elements, usually alpha and beta emitters. In such cases the lead enclosure has to be lined with a suitable material (brass, steel or plastic), to shield the counter from this soft radiation.

Effective shielding is heavy and expensive, particularly when it is thick enough to reduce significantly the background due to very energetic cosmic radiation. An arrangement illustrated in Figure 16–13 reduces the effect of this background for β counting without excessive shielding. The main counter and sample are surrounded by a second bell-shaped counter. This second counter is shielded from β radiation of the sample by the sample holder and the housing of the main counter. The two counters are connected to an anticoincidence circuit of Figure 14–6, the main counter as Detector A and the shielding counter as Detector B. When a β ray from the sample causes the main counter to operate, a count will be registered in the counting circuit. When, however, a photon penetrates the shield in such a way that both counters operate, no counts will be registered, due to the operation of the anticoincidence mechanism. Should the photon operate only the shielding counter, also no counts will be registered since the circuit B is only passive: it can only close a contact, but cannot pass any pulses. Therefore such photons will not be counted at all. Some background, however, will remain. It will be due to ionizing events which bypass the shielding counter, either because they did not interact or because they came through the opening of this counter. An assembly of this sort can reduce the background by a factor of 10. Sensitivity as expressed by the smallest detectable amount is proportional to $\sqrt{R_b}$, according to equation 15—(49). A background reduction to one-tenth will, therefore, reduce the smallest detectable amount to about one-third.

Use of Pulse Height Discrimination for Background Reduction. With a detector such as a scintillation counter the pulse height spectrum from background is quite different from the spectrum due to a nuclide. This difference can be used to advantage in the reduction of background by pulse height discrimination.

Raising the discriminator level (or its equivalent, reducing the high voltage) will, of course, reduce the counting rate due to background, but will also reduce the counting rate due to the nuclide. A change of discriminator level can only be useful if, by such a change, the precision, *i.e.* the minimum detectable activity, is decreased. The precision (Equation

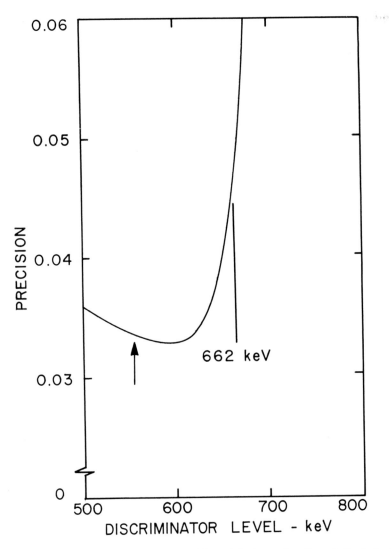

Fɪɢ. 16–14. Precision (minimum detectable activity) as a function of discriminator setting for a NaI (Tl) scintillation counter irradiated by [137]Cs. The photopeak position is indicated. Arrow shows the discriminator setting chosen for stable operation.

15—[49]) depends upon the ratio of the square root of the background counting rate to the calibration factor. Figure 16–14 shows a plot of the precision as a function of discriminator level for a NaI(Tl) scintillation counter irradiated by [137]Cs. The discriminator level is plotted in keV and the position of the ^{137}Cs photopeak (662 keV) is noted on the figure. Notice the minimum of the precision curve occurs somewhat below this value, in fact at a point which is close to the beginning of the plateau for this

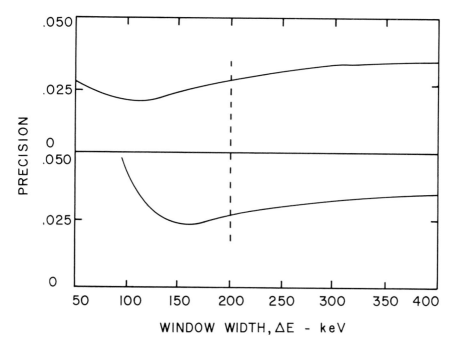

Fig. 16–15. Precision (minimum detectable activity) as a function of window width for a NaI (Tl) scintillation counter irradiated with [137]Cs. Upper curve is for a window centered about the photopeak while the lower curve is taken with the lower edge of the window set at the trough below the photopeak. The dashed line indicates a window of sufficient width to encompass the entire peak.

nuclide. In the discussion of control settings (see pages 267ff) for reasons of stability, it was recommended that the discriminator be set at a point only slightly lower than the minimum precision point. The precision at this point is little different from the minimum. Thus, the choice of the operating point (either discriminator level at fixed high voltage or high voltage at fixed discriminator level) made on the basis of independence from difficulties due to equipmental drift yields a good selection in terms of minimum precision, *i.e.* minimum detectable activity.

A single channel pulse height analyzer reduces background to a lower level than does a single discriminator. To see the effect of the use of an analyzer on the precision we plot (Fig. 16–15) the precision against window width for [137]Cs. The data for the upper curve are taken with the window centered at the photopeak, while those for the lower curve are taken with the lower edge of the window at the trough below the photopeak. When the window is at the peak, the precision can be improved slightly (decreased) by the use of a narrow window, *i.e.* one which encompasses only part of the peak. However, this improvement is gained by operating with a window so narrow as to make the calibration factor very sensitive to equipmental drift. This can induce sizable errors into activity determinations and is therefore not advisable for routine usage.

When the lower edge of the window is held fixed, the precision increases when the window becomes wider than the photopeak (lower curve). In fact the increase begins somewhat before the widow is wide enough to encompass the entire upper side of the peak. Again, for reasons of stability of calibration, it is advisable to sacrifice some precision and to use a slightly wider window. Thus, when the desirability for stable operation is considered along with the need for minimum activity detection, the control settings which accept pulses from the entire photopeak are found to be the best compromise.

This discussion has been based on the pulse height spectrum of ^{137}Cs which was chosen for its simplicity, $i.e.$ a single peak. The conclusions, however, are general, although the spectrum for a different nuclide may alter them to a minor extent. For example, with ^{60}Co the desirable analyzer settings are those which include both photopeaks. When choosing control settings for routine work, stability should have first preference over precision. Precision can always be improved by counting for a longer time.

Identification of Nuclides in a Sample. There are many occasions in the work with radioactive nuclides when it becomes necessary to identify the unknown radioactive material in a sample. The range of possibilities is usually small, since only a few of the available nuclides are handled in a given laboratory.

If the possibilities are limited to a pure beta emitter and a gamma emitter, the decision is easily made by using over the sample an absorber exceeding the beta range (see Table 16–4). If the counting rate drops close to background, the sample contains the beta emitter. It must be remembered that, due to bremsstrahlung, some net counting rate will be observed even with a beta counter; a strong sample of a high energy beta emitter (^{32}P) will show a considerable counting rate with a gamma counter even when its walls exceed the beta range. The higher the atomic number of the absorber the more bremsstrahlung produced. For this reason, plastic or aluminum absorbers are to be preferred over those of heavier metals.

A more positive identification can be made by plotting the absorption curves for the nuclides which are being handled. Plastic films and sheets are a suitable material for low energy beta emitters; aluminum is more convenient for higher energies, and lead or steel for gamma emitters.

Such absorption curves must be plotted for every counting set-up used, since window thickness and geometry may cause changes from the theoretical curve. From such plots the absorber which reduces the counting rate to half ("half value layer") may be selected for a quick decision among several possible materials. $Approximate$ values of such absorber thicknesses for several common pure beta emitters are listed in Table 16–4.

A similar technique can be used for identification of gamma emitters, except that they do not have a limited range, but a continued exponential

**Table 16-4. Energy, Range and Half Value Layers for
Several Nuclides having Pure Beta Emission**

Nuclide	Max. Energy MeV	Range mg/cm²	Half Value Absorber mg/cm²
^{14}C	0.155	29	4
^{35}S	0.167	32	4.5
^{45}Ca	0.256	59	8
^{32}P	1.70	790	100

absorption. In order to avoid confusion by the faster absorption of beta radiation present in some gamma emitters, one should be sure that all betas are filtered out before the gamma absorption is plotted; usually the counter walls of a gamma counter are thick enough to accomplish this. The half value layers in lead are listed for some nuclides in Table 11–1, page 163. Here again this is only a general guide and measurements with actual counters must be performed. As with beta emitters, it is convenient to select a filter corresponding to the half value layer of every nuclide in use for ease in routine identification.

With gamma emitters it is possible to make a more precise identification by gamma-ray spectrometry. We employ a scintillation counter and a pulse height analyzer, single or multi-channel. The pulse height spectrum obtained with the unknown sample can be compared to spectra obtained from samples of known nuclides for identification. Spectrometry, especially with single channel analyzers, requires the expenditure of a good deal of time but is the most positive technique available.

Specialized Methods. Several methods of beta counting will be described in the following pages. These methods are specialized in the sense that they are not routinely used for clinical counting applications. However, an acquaintance with such methods is desirable as they can provide solutions to problems which are difficult to solve by more conventional techniques.

The development of counting gas mixtures which can be used at atmospheric pressure, made it possible to use windowless counters where the dry sample is introduced directly inside of the counter. Whenever a sample is changed, the counting gas becomes contaminated by air which has to be flushed out. These *"Flow-Gas Counters"* are, therefore, always connected to a pressure cylinder containing the counter gas, which must flow through the counter for a definite short period after each sample change. The gain in sensitivity is due not only to the absence of window absorption, but also to improved geometry (the sample is directly adjacent to the counting gas). For samples without self-absorption, the efficiency is close to 50 per cent. A disadvantage of windowless counters is the ease with which they are contaminated by dry sample material which dusts off the planchettes. Some flow-gas counters have been built, therefore, with exceedingly thin windows (0.1 mg/cm²), which is possible since the counting gas is at atmospheric pressure. Such counters need no flushing between the insertions of samples; only a small gas flow needs to be maintained, to replace gas which decomposes during the counting process. Flow counters can be used either as Geiger-Mueller or as proportional counters depending upon the gas mixture employed. As proportional counters they are useful, though less so, than liquid scintillation counters, for double tracer studies with ^{14}C and ^{3}H.

Solid scintillation counters can also be used for beta counting; special provisions for sample positioning are needed to exclude extraneous light. The crystal housing must be very thin so as not to absorb too large a fraction of beta rays. There is no need to have thick crystals, wafers of thickness corresponding to the largest used beta range are adequate; this reduces considerably background due to ambient gamma radiation.

Several techniques have been developed to overcome self-absorption in a source. In addition to the liquid scintillation counter which we have already described (page 285) these include:

1. *Chemical purification.* This can eliminate a considerable portion of inert material which contributes to self-absorption. The suitable methods will depend on the chemical compounds involved and no general directions are therefore possible. When the nuclide can be removed from a solution by electroplating, as with iron for instance, relatively simple techniques can be worked out.

2. *Gas Counting.* The radioactive compound can be converted into a gas, as for instance into CO_2 with ^{14}C and this is added to the counting gas with which a Geiger-Mueller counter is filled. This method means of course that the counter has to be filled every time a new sample is counted, and that the samples must be prepared and handled as a gas. The advantage is, however, complete absence of self-absorption and efficiency approaching 100 per cent namely 37,000 counts per μCi. This method is particularly useful for ^{3}H and has even a higher sensitivity than the liquid scintillation counter. It is not satisfactory for double tracer techniques.

3. *Bremsstrahlung Counting.* Self-absorption difficulties can be practically eliminated also in counting higher energy β-emitting nuclides like ^{32}P, not by observing interaction of β particles with the radiation detector directly, but by counting x-ray quanta produced by bremsstrahlung, when β radiation is absorbed in the sample itself and in surrounding matter. The high efficiency in a well-type scintillation counter makes this practical, and the increased sample size which can be used makes the sensitivity of this method approach the sensitivity of direct β-counting. The liquid sample is used in a test tube as in γ-counting, so that sample preparation is simplified.

An example for such counting in a well type crystal for ^{32}P in blood samples gives a calibration factor of 0.3 counts per second for 1 nanocurie sample. Background is 4 c/s. The smallest detectable amount in absolute activity measurement is 1.6 nanocuries and for specific activity 0.3 nanocuries per ml (5 ml well capacity). (See page 249.)

This method is useful also for other nuclides. With ^{90}Y the efficiency will be greater than for ^{32}P and for ^{90}Sr it will be considerably smaller except for ^{90}Sr in equilibrium with its ^{90}Y daughter.

Radiochromatography. It is frequently of interest to examine to which particular protein fraction some tagged material belongs or becomes associated with during metabolic processes. This can be done by chromatographic or electrophoretic separation of protein fractions and by determining in which fraction or fractions the radioactive material is located.

After the paper strip with separated proteins is obtained, there are several methods available to determine the location of the radioactive tracer.

The simplest method is to cut up the strip of paper in narrow pieces normal to the migration direction and to count each piece like a sample with any suitable detector. The disadvantage is that the original strip is cut up and that the correlation of the observed activity with the migration pattern becomes difficult.

The other method uses a radiation detector equipped with a cap of a material which will absorb most of the radiations emitted by the radioactive nuclide used for tagging. A slit is made in this cap, and the paper strip is moved across it at a constant speed by means of a mechanical drive. The radiation detector is connected to a counting-rate recorder. As the paper strip moves in front of the slit, the counting-rate record plots the activity distribution over the strip.

If the speed of the recorder chart is the same as the travel speed of the paper strip, a simple and direct comparison between the chromatogram and the radioactivity distribution can be made, as illustrated in Figure 16–16. Tracing B indicates that the radioactive tracer migrated with β globulin and albumin.

In addition to the location of the activity on the strip it is sometimes required to know the total activity in various protein fractions. This can be obtained by integrating the areas under the rate record, for instance with a planimeter. This integrated counting rate can be, however, rather simply recorded directly, since the total activity is simply proportional to the accumulated counts. Electronic circuitry in the rate meter can provide an output current which is proportional to the total counts and a second pen can be used to record this current on the chart.

Such a paper-strip scanning device will have the following controls: 1, speed control for the motion of the chromatographic paper strip, 2, response time control for the rate meter, 3, calibration adjustment for the rate-recorder pen, and perhaps 4, calibration adjustment for the integrating recorder pen.

In selecting the speed of the chromatographic strip movement it should be considered that the counting rate will be independent of the speed with which a given spot on the paper passes under the counter slit, but that if it moves too quickly, the response time of the recording circuit may be too slow and the meter will not respond. The paper travel speed must be,

20

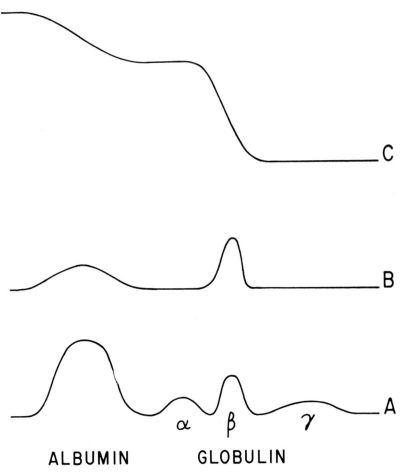

ALBUMIN   GLOBULIN

Fig. 16–16.   Chromatographic Strip with Tagged Proteins.   Curve A: optical density of the strip with protein fractions stained by a chemical reaction.   Curve B: record of scanning with a rate-meter (radioactivity is present in β globulin and in albumin). Curve C: integrated record of curve B (the first plateau from the right represents the total activity in β globulin; the second plateau represents the total activity present in the strip; the difference between the two represents the activity in albumin).

therefore, matched to response time: the optimal setting is that for which the time it takes a point on the paper to pass under the slit of the counter is about equal to twice the response time.   If faster scanning is desired, a shorter response time should be selected.   The limitations for the response time are of course due to statistical fluctuations, so that weak samples require long response time and slow paper travel.

The deflection on the integrating record is inversely proportional to the paper travel speed.   After this speed and the corresponding response time of the rate-recorder have been selected, the calibration adjustment for the integrating recorder must be set in such a way that the pen does not deflect off scale. This usually has to be done in a preliminary test run.

Double Nuclide Technique. When two different nuclides are present in the sample, it is not possible to determine their activities by simple counting. This can be achieved in three ways, depending on the nature of the nuclides present.

1. *Pulse Height Analysis.* The discussion which follows is based on the use of a scintillation counter with gamma-ray emitters. The technique is also applicable for beta-ray emitters using either a proportional or a liquid scintillation counter. The principle of the method is to count the sample twice using different control settings of a single channel analyzer for each count. (Some equipment is available which incorporates two single channel analyzers and scalers so both can be done simultaneously.) Control settings are used such that one nuclide contributes heavily at one setting and lightly at the other. This is accomplished by adjusting the analyzer to measure the photopeak of one nuclide in the first measurement and that of the other in the second. With nuclides whose photopeaks are well separated such as ^{51}Cr and ^{59}Fe this is easily done. In other cases they may not be so easily separable. Though only photopeaks are counted it must be remembered that the lower energy nuclide may contribute to counting at the photopeak of the high energy nuclide and vice versa. Calibration factors for each of the two nuclides have to be determined, therefore, at each control setting.

Let us assume that the calibration factors for the two regions of the spectrum of one nuclide are c_1 and c_2, and of the other nuclide f_1 and f_2. The counting rates for the sample, observed for the two regions, are R_1 and R_2. The unknown activities are A_c and A_f. We have then two equations: The observed counting rate R_1 in the first spectral region, due to the activities of both nuclides A_c and A_f is

$$R_1 = c_1 A_c + f_1 A_f \qquad 16-(4)$$

and for the other spectral region

$$R_2 = c_2 A_c + f_2 A_f \qquad 16-(5)$$

These equations are solved for the unknown activities A_c and A_f:

$$A_c = \frac{f_2 R_1 - f_1 R_2}{c_1 f_2 - c_2 f_1} \qquad 16-(6)$$

and

$$A_f = \frac{c_1 R_2 - c_2 R_1}{c_1 f_2 - c_2 f_1} \qquad 16-(7)$$

The simultaneous determination of the activities of the two nuclides will be impossible if the ratios of calibration factors in the two regions are the same. Let us call this ratio for one nuclide Q_c and for the other nuclide Q_f, so that:

$$Q_c = \frac{c_1}{c_2} \qquad\qquad 16-(8)$$

and

$$Q_f = \frac{f_1}{f_2} \qquad\qquad 16-(9)$$

No determination is possible if

$$Q_c = Q_f$$

Equations $16-(6)$ and $16-(7)$ can be expressed by substituting $16-(8)$ and $16-(9)$ after some transformation as:

$$A_c = \frac{1}{c_2} \times \frac{R_1 - Q_f R_2}{Q_c - Q_f} \qquad\qquad 16-(10)$$

$$A_f = \frac{1}{f_2} \times \frac{Q_c R_2 - R_1}{Q_c - Q_f} \qquad\qquad 16-(11)$$

For $Q_c = Q_f$ both the denominator and numerator become zero and A_c and A_f are indeterminate.*

The condition for the ability to separate the two nuclides is therefore that Q_c is different from Q_f; the larger the difference the better the method.

The analyzer settings for regions 1 and 2 must therefore be selected so as to give the greatest difference between Q_f and Q_c. It also must be considered that if the counting rates are low, counting times for acceptable uncertainties will be high. This means that narrow windows are undesirable; the windows must be selected as wide as it is possible to make them, provided the difference between Q_f and Q_c remains sufficiently high.   A

---

* It is not easy to see why the numerator becomes zero. It is equal to $R_1 - Q_f R_2$. From $16-(4)$ and $16-(5)$ it follows that

$$\frac{R_1}{R_2} = \frac{c_1 A_c + f_1 A_f}{c_2 A_c + f_2 A_f} = \frac{f_1}{f_2} \times \frac{\dfrac{c_1}{f_1} A_c + A_f}{\dfrac{c_2}{f_2} A_c + A_f}$$

Since $Q_c = Q_f$ it follows that $\dfrac{c_1}{c_2} = \dfrac{f_1}{f_2}$ and also $\dfrac{f_1}{c_1} = \dfrac{f_2}{c_2}$ so that the second fraction becomes unity and $\dfrac{R_1}{R_2} = \dfrac{f_1}{f_2} = Q_f$ and $R_1 = Q_f R_2$. By substituting this value for R_1 in the expression for the numerator $R_1 - Q_f R_2$, this numerator becomes zero.

guide to such a selection of suitable window setting is usually found by inspection of the scintillation spectra of the two nuclides of interest.

2. *Nuclides of Different Half-life.* If one nuclide has a much shorter half-life than the other, the sample is first counted while there is significant activity of both nuclides present and again later, when the short-lived nuclide has decayed. The second count will measure the activity of the long-lived nuclide; after correcting for decay, the counting rate corresponding to this nuclide is subtracted from the first count. The difference is then due to the first nuclide and its activity can be calculated from the appropriate calibration factor (these factors will be different for the two nuclides).

When the short half-life is too long to wait for essentially complete decay, it is still possible to determine the activities by using equations $16-(6)$ and $16-(9)$ and considering that the mathematical situation is identical if we say "at different times" instead of "at different analyzer settings." If the time elapsed between the two measurements is t, then what we called efficiencies of the two nuclides c_2 and f_2 will become

$$c_2 = c_1 e^{-0.693t/T_c}$$

and

$$f_2 = f_1 e^{-.0693t/T_f}$$

where T_c and T_f are the two half-lives, and c_1 and f_1, are the calibration factors. We have then by substituting in $16-(6)$ and $16-(7)$

$$A_c = \frac{f_1 R_1 e^{-0.693t/T_f} - f_1 R_2}{c_1 f_1 e^{-0.693t/T_f} - c_1 f_1 e^{-0.693t/T_c}} = \frac{R_1 e^{-0.693t/T_f} - R_2}{c_1 \left(e^{-0.693t/T_f} - e^{-0.693t/T_c} \right)}$$

$$16-(12)$$

and similarly:

$$A_f = \frac{R_1 - R_2 e^{-0.693t/T_c}}{f_1 \left(e^{-0.693t/T_f} - e^{-0.693t/T_c} \right)} \qquad 16-(13)$$

3. *One of the Two Nuclides is a Pure Beta-Emitter.* The calibration factors are determined for the second nuclide, which is also a gamma-emitter, in the usual way and also with an absorbing filter over the sample, in an end-window counter. The filter must be thick enough to absorb all beta radiation from the first nuclide. The sample is counted with this filter and without. The calibration factor with filter and the associated counting rate permit calculation of the activity of the second nuclide. The counting

rate due to this nuclide is then calculated from the no-filter calibration factor of this nuclide and subtracted from the counting rate of the sample observed without filter. The difference is the counting rate due to the first, beta-emitting, nuclide.

This method can be extended to two pure β-emitters or pure γ-emitters by measuring them first without and then with some suitable filter, which reduces the calibration factors for the two nuclides by a different factor. To do this, the calibration factors for the two nuclides will have to be determined first without the filter (c_1 and f_1) and then with the filter (c_2 and f_2). From the counting rates of the unknown mixture without the filter (R_1) and with the filter (R_2), the activities of the two components can be determined from 16—(6) and 16—(7). This method will be found useful on rare occasions only, but it is a way to use double nuclide techniques when no analyzer is available.

17

Quantitative Measurements in Vivo

THERE are no basic differences in the determination of the activity of a radioactive deposit within the body of a patient and of the activity in a sample *in vitro*. The practical differences, however, are considerable. They are due to the circumstance that it is not possible to manipulate the deposit of radioactive material at will with reference to the counter as is possible with a separate isolated sample. Distance of the counter from the radioactive source, size of the source, absorption and backscatter vary with the anatomical variation of the organ of interest. The conditions discussed for reliable measurements *in vitro* cannot be rigidly maintained, therefore, and the influence of their variability on the measurements has to be considered and minimized by suitable design of the experimental arrangements.

A representative example of the quantitative determination of a radioactive deposit in the body is the measurement of radioactive iodine uptake by the thyroid gland. This will be discussed, therefore, first and in detail, both as a guide for this particular procedure and as a typical example of the difficulties involved and of the methods available to overcome them.

Measurement of Thyroidal Uptake. The determination of the fraction of an administered tracer dose of radioactive iodine taken up by the thyroid gland is one of the most frequent nuclear measurements encountered in clinical use. This determination is performed on a "sample" which cannot be removed from the body; the measurement has to be done on the gland which is in the patient's neck, with a variety of uncertainties from patient to patient, due to differences in size, location and background. Different techniques proposed and in use have the common aim of minimizing the dependence of the results on these variations.

The requirements for the reproducibility of the measurements are determined by the physiological range of uptake variations between euthyroid and hyperthyroid patients. If it is assumed for the purpose of discussion that the overlap between the two conditions ranges from 55 per cent to 65 per cent uptake by the thyroid gland of the total administered test dose, it is only necessary to be able to determine whether the uptake is less than 55 per cent or more than 65 per cent. Should we accept an uncertainty of 10 per cent in the uptake, the practical requirements would be met.

The requirements in counting precision can be illustrated by an example. With a tracer dose of 10 μCi a diagnostically equivocal uptake would be between 5.5 and 6.5 μCi. A range of 1 μCi in 6 μCi (mean of the range) corresponds to a variation of 17 per cent, which determines the minimum precision needed in counting. This seems to be a very modest requirement, and a smaller error should be easily attainable. A survey on measurements with a mannequin-type phantom in a number of laboratories in this country has shown, however, that actual errors frequently exceed either of the above criteria by a considerable margin.

Although some of the difficulties in uptake measurements are inter-related, it is best to discuss the uncertainty factors involved, and the methods of minimizing their effects separately, and later to summarize this in the form of some recommended procedures.

The *size of the thyroid* gland is an uncertainty which is easily handled. The only problem in this connection is created by the necessity of shielding the radiation detector from the general body background, which is due to the fraction of the tracer dose in tissues and circulating blood. Shielding for this purpose will have to restrict the field of view of the counter. The size of this field is determined by the shield construction and by the working distance. The smaller this field, the less is the measured body background, but if the field is made too small, the counter may fail to "see," that is to detect, the radiation from parts of the thyroid outside of this field. The result would be a false low reading. The field of view there-fore must be large enough to contain the largest thyroid gland which may be encountered, taking also into account possible errors in "aiming" the de-tector in the right direction, preferably toward the center of the gland. Such a shielding is illustrated in Figure 17–1. The necessary condition is usually satisfied when the field of view is about 8 inches in diameter or an 8 × 8 inch square. This can be checked by using a small source of ^{131}I, placing it on a flat surface at the working distance from the counter and counting it in various locations on the surface. The area in which the counts are constant within say 5 to 10 per cent represents the field of view; outside of this field of view the counting rate will drop, depending on the effectiveness of the shield. A sharp drop is desirable, but a practical compromise between weight of the shield and degree of shielding has to be made. Such a com-promise results in lead wall thickness of about 1 inch. The suggested field of 8 inches diameter may not include a substernal extension of the thyroid gland. Clinical examination and scanning methods will indicate this con-dition; a larger than normal working distance will solve the problem after suitable recalibration.

The *variations in the location of the thyroid gland within the neck* are perhaps the greatest obstacle to precise uptake measurements. The effect of location and size of the gland cannot be separated completely, since a large gland not only occupies more space than a small gland in the field of view of a counter, but has also different dimensions in depth and there-fore a different average or effective distance. The thyroid gland is im-bedded in the neck; this affects the radiation intensity reaching the counter

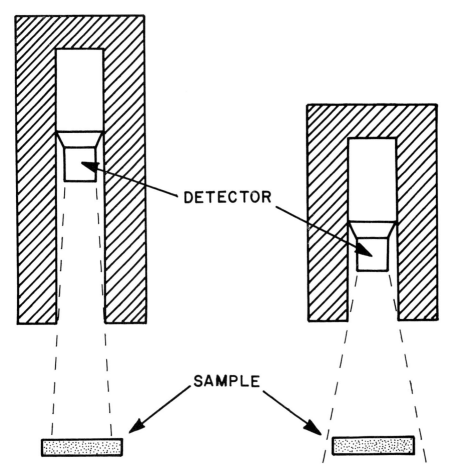

Fig. 17–1. Shielding of an uptake counter. *A*: excessive collimation, observed counting rate will be too low; *B*: suitable shielding, all of the organ contributes to the observed countung rate.

in several ways: 1. Distance of radioactive material from the counter, 2. Absorption by the gland itself (corresponding to self-absorption in a sample) and by the overlying tissues, and 3. Scatter by the tissues of the neck. It is a simple matter to adjust the counter to a given distance from the skin of the neck, but the average depth of the gland below the skin may vary by as much as 2 to 3 centimeters. This uncertainty in distance can be minimized by using such a long working distance that a few centimeters error would be negligible even within the range of inverse square relationship between counting rate and distance. Such a working distance necessary to achieve the desired effect would have to be a meter or more; this is impractical for several reasons. The sensitivity of the counter would be reduced by more than 10 times compared to conventional distances, the collimation requirement for the shield to keep the field of view to 8 inches becomes excessive, and the aiming of such a collimator is critcal and difficult. Short working distances increase the uncertainties due to the variations of gland position so that it is impractical to increase sensitivity in this way. The working distance selected in practice is a compromise between sensitivity and the possible error due to the uncertainty of the gland location. There appears to be general agreement that this compromise leads to a working distance of between 20 and 30 cm. The effects of absorption of radiation by the overlying tissues of the neck are normally more or less obscured by scatter. The effect of absorption alone can be studied when the scatter contribution to the counting rate is eliminated by a gamma-ray spectrometer or by suitable adjustment of the discriminator setting in a scintillation counter. This makes the radiation detector selectively sensitive to essentially only the primary ^{131}I energies. When measuring in suitable phantoms under these conditions, it is found that the counting rate decreases by about 10 per cent for each centimeter increase of thyroid depth below the skin. If the range of thyroid location below the skin is assumed to be within 2 cm only, the overall uncertainty due to absorption will amount to about 20 per cent.

When a spectrometer is not employed and the level of the discriminator lowered, the scatter by the neck increases the observed counting rate because some of the primary radiant energy which diverges from the field will be seen by the counter. When the counter is sensitive to the scatter, the observed counting rate is about 25 per cent* greater for an ^{131}I source 1 cm below the surface of a water phantom than for the same source suspended in air. This indicates that the increase of counting rate by scatter more than compensates for the loss due to absorption at this depth. This increase is cancelled by absorption only when the iodine source is about 5 cm or more below the phantom surface. It is therefore to be expected that scatter has considerable effect on the change in counting rate with change in thyroid depth. It should be realized that the scatter is proportional to the amount of radiation impinging on scattering material, so that when the thyroid gland is at the surface, only about half of all the radiation emitted within the gland impinges on neck tissues and produces backscatter, and that when the thyroid gland is deep within the neck, all radiation from the source hits neck tissues and contributes to scatter (backscatter *and* forward-scatter). The overall radiation intensity from the neck due to radioactivity in the gland is influenced therefore by two opposing factors: (1) absorption is increased with greater thyroid depth, which reduces the observed counting rate, (this is also reduced by the increased distance from the counter); (2) scatter is increased with increased depth (this effect is particularly pronounced within the first few centimeters under the skin), which increases the counting rate. These two effects tend to cancel each other, so that the

* The actual value will depend on the counter and on the discrimination setting.

dependence of the uptake measurement on the thyroid depth in the neck is minimized. Under these conditions, the change of counting rate due to change of thyroid depth by 2 cm is reduced from 20 per cent when scatter effect is eliminated, to about 10 per cent when the counter is sensitive to scattered radiation.

The next problem to be considered is the calibration of an uptake counter. This may appear to be quite simple at first. The most convenient source for such calibration is a duplicate of a tracer dose, identical to the tracer given to the patient. This has several advantages: the aliquot solution is readily available, the decay of the reference source and of the tracer material in the patient is the same, so that checking against such a reference source at the time of uptake measurement corrects automatically for decay. There are some disadvantages, however: this reference source may be a liquid requiring precautions against spillage, and errors of pipetting may occur in its preparation. This disadvantage does not exist when doses in individual capsules are used. In many laboratories "mock-iodine" sources have been found useful. They have been described under performance and reference standards.

The reasons for the difficulties in the calibration of a thyroid uptake counter become apparent with the consideration of scatter, absorption and uncertainty of thyroid location.

When a counter which is sensitive to scatter is used, the calibration must be performed with the reference source in a suitable phantom. It will be recalled that an error of about 25 per cent is introduced if the reference source is measured in air and compared to the counting rate of the source in a phantom and hence in the neck. A suitable phantom, however, is easily made. A cylindrical water container made of plastic, not less than 6 inches in diameter and about 10 inches high can be used, with the reference source positioned about 1 cm behind the front surface (the source can be a 20- to 50-cc volumetric flask or some other container of similar dimensions). The disadvantage of a water phantom is that it can be usually employed only in a vertical position. A plastic phantom, or a phantom made of masonite, can be handled more conveniently. There are only a few critical considerations: the phantom should not be too small; no significant errors are introduced if it is made larger than the neck; the reference source should be under the surface facing the counter, and between $\frac{1}{2}$ and $1\frac{1}{2}$ cm deep in the phantom material. Satisfactory phantoms are available from commercial suppliers. While the use of a phantom for calibration is a simple device which increases the reliability of uptake measurements under all circumstances, many laboratories still work without a phantom (calibrating with the reference source in air) or with an inadequate phantom. Under these circumstances the errors of calibration can be reduced by reducing the sensitivity of the counter to scattered radiation. The price of the simplification of the calibration set-up is the reduction of sensitivity by a factor of two or more, due to restricting the energy range of the accepted gamma rays and an increase of possible errors due to the uncertainty in the location of the thyroid gland.

The measurement of the patient takes usually two to ten minutes, and it is of course essential that the patient does not change position during this interval. Perhaps the easiest way to achieve this is to have the uptake set-up arranged so that the patient lies down; in a sitting patient, suitable immobilization of head and neck has to be provided.

One specific counter arrangement should be mentioned in this connection since it potentially not only eliminates the dependence of uptake measurements on the position of the patient but also reduces to some degree the influence of the thyroid gland location within the neck: this is a ring counter set-up where four counters are arranged around the neck of the patient so that he sits approximately in the middle of the counter array. The four counters are connected to a scaling circuit so that all counts are added and registered. The purpose of this arrangement is that if the source (or patient) moves and goes farther away from one or two of the counters, it comes closer to one or two of the other ones. In this way, the effects of changes in position on the observed counting rate tend to cancel out. This arrangement is rather expensive, and it appears that with some care, equally reliable uptake measurements are obtained with the simpler set-up using a single counter.

The sensitivity of an uptake set-up determines the tracer dose required for the measurement. A small ($1''\times1''$) sodium iodide scintillation counter can be satisfactorily employed with patient doses smaller than one microcurie. Typical operating data with ^{131}I for such a counter are a background count rate of 12 counts per second and, at a distance of 20 cm, a calibration factor of 40 counts per second per microcurie giving a precision (see Eq. 15—49)) of about .02 μCi. Larger crystals can provide greater sensitivity of course, but at a greater expense which is probably not justified for this purpose.

A problem closely related to the determination of the radioactive iodine uptake by the thyroid gland is the measurement of the uptake in a functioning metastasis of thyroid cancer. The difference is only the location of the deposit. The uncertainty about the size and location can be greater than with the thyroid gland. When x-ray films offer a guide in this respect, it is sometimes possible to construct a phantom (water or masonite) to obtain an approximate value for the combined absorption and scatter. As a rule, a lower reliability is acceptable for this purpose, and a simple correction for distance of the lesion from the skin is found satisfactory.

However complex the discussed uptake measurements may appear, one complicating factor has still been neglected, the radiation due to the presence of radioactive material in the other parts of the body and particularly in the circulating blood. This complication may be ignored when uptake measurements are done twenty-four hours after the administration of the tracer dose, since after that time, no significant activity is present outside of the gland. When measurements have to be done earlier, it may be necessary to use additional shielding of the counter from the rest of the body and to take into account the activity in the blood within the field of view of the counter.

A quite effective device to account for the contribution to the observed counting rate by the radioactivity from the body is to measure this contribution by shielding the organ under investigation with a few inches of lead. This will cut out most of the radiation from the organ itself, and the remaining counting rate is total background (conventional background plus contribution from the rest of the body). When this total background is subtracted from the observed gross counts without the added shield, a more nearly correct net counting rate is obtained.

It is more difficult to establish the contribution of the radioactivity in the circulating blood in the tissues surrounding the observed organ and also within the organ itself. The solution can be found by observing the activity in another part of the body which itself has no biochemical uptake of the particular element or compound used. This measurement gives a counting rate which is proportional to the blood level of the radioactive material, and if the ratio between blood volume in this part of the body (the thigh for instance) and the region under investigation (the thyroid gland and the neck for instance) is known, the contribution due to blood can be calculated and deducted from the measurement over the organ. This ratio can be established by using a compound which is not taken up by the examined organ (for the thyroid gland, iodinated serum protein may be used, or the uptake of iodine in the gland can be blocked by Lugol's solution). An average value for the ratio can be obtained by studying a few individuals in the manner described.

The need for the quantitative determination of deposit of other radioactive nuclides within other organs in the body is not frequent. When it is, the approach is similar to the measurement of iodine uptake in the thyroid gland.

A special problem is the uptake of ^{32}P in eye tumors. Due to the short range of the beta radiation and the small size of the organ, small thin-window or thin-wall Geiger-Mueller counters can be used without additional shielding. The quantitative reliability of the results is low, but the information required is actually only presence or absence of a significant increase in counting rate over the tumor, as compared to normal areas, so that the relatively crude results are of sufficient diagnostic value.

High energy β-emitting nuclides, like ^{32}P and ^{90}Y can be counted also *in vivo* by bremsstrahlung with a scintillation counter. Since the photon energy of bremsstrahlung has a very wide range and depends on the atomic number of the absorbing material, it is not easy to calibrate reliably a counting arrangement for this purpose. Careful construction of suitable phantoms is essential.

In vivo counting is basically identical to *in vitro* counting, when the amount of activity in the whole body ("body burden") has to be measured. The only difference is the size of the sample, which presents two distinct specific problems.

1. The counting assembly becomes large. This has the consequence that a simple well-type counter cannot be constructed from a solid crystal. Liquid scintillators have been used in a hollow metal cylinder large enough for a human subject to be placed in the center. A large number of photo-tubes must be used with such a cylinder in a complex mixing circuit. A single detector at a distance from the body can also be used. In order to reduce the effect of varying distance of different parts of the body, such a crystal has to be placed fairly far away from the body and the body must be given a curved position to approximate its shape to the segment of a circle with the detector as center. Since counting efficiency becomes smaller with increased distance, a large crystal with a correspondingly large photo-multiplier tube must be used to compensate for this. The shielding must enclose patient and detector, so that the necessary shield has the size of a small room. All these factors combined make a whole-body counter a very expensive instrument.

2. Self-absorption was neglected in γ-counting for *in vitro* samples. Due to the large sample size in whole-body counting, self-absorption is significant. It can amount to a 25% correction in a large dog and will be even higher in man.

Whole-body counters can be made sufficiently sensitive to measure the activity of naturally occurring radioactive nuclides. In order to utilize such high sensitivity in tracer work, γ-ray spectrometers must be used to separate the tracer from radioactive materials not normally present in the human body (whether naturally occurring or from fall-out). In such use the solid crystals are preferable to liquid scintillators, since they have a better spectrometric resolution.

18

Observation of the Time Factor in Physiological Processes by Radioactive Tracers

The measurements discussed so far were concerned with the determination of radioactivity at a certain instant. The samples were obtained in some way and at a given time, and the deposits within the body were observed under the tacit assumption that they did not change during the period of observation. Physiological processes, however, are not static but are subject to change with time, and this change is frequently a significant parameter in their understanding and in the evaluation of whether they are normal or disturbed by disease.

As a rule the biochemical processes are in a state of dynamic equilibrium; metabolic utilization and breakdown of any given compound, however simple or complex, is continuously counteracted by reconstruction from materials taken into the body, so that whatever is eliminated is replenished to insure the *status quo*. When a compound which plays a role in this metabolic equilibrium is tagged by a radioactive tracer, its passage through the phases of the dynamic equilibrium becomes detectable and the continuous changes which constitute the complex metabolic equilibrium become accessible to observation.

This possibility of observing the time sequence in metabolic processes is one of the valuable potentialities of radioactive tracers, and therefore the techniques in the observation of radioactivity within the body, as it changes with time, are of great importance.

In addition to metabolic and biochemical processes, there are other processes within the body which are characterized by their dynamic parameters; some are quite complex, as for instance formation of blood cells; some are relatively simple, as for instance cardiac action and blood circulation, or resorptive processes in and from various tissues and organs.

The particular techniques which are most suitable for a given problem are best classified by the speed of the physiological changes to be observed; a practical division for the purpose of discussion is (1) Slow changes occurring over periods of days, (2) Changes of intermediate speed, occurring over a period of hours, and (3) Rapid changes reaching an equilibrium value in seconds and minutes.

1. *Slow Changes*. When the changes under observation occur over a period of days, the techniques are for practical purposes identical with the quantitative *in vitro* or *in vivo* measurements. Let us take as an example the determination of the effective half life of ^{32}P in the body. If the administered dose is known, the easiest method is the daily collection of excreta and their measurement by a suitable *in vitro* method. When the daily value for the total dose administered minus total excretion up to that day is plotted, enough points will be obtained to evaluate the curve quantitatively. If correction for physical decay is made, a curve for biological decay will be obtained. If the collections and measurements were made each in weekly intervals, some significant characteristics of the phosphorus behavior would have been lost, since the excretion is faster during the first few days than later; this initial phase could have been overlooked in weekly measurements. This points up the necessity of determining the required frequency of measurements by the physiological characteristics of the phenomenon under observation.

Another example may illustrate this. Let us consider the determination of the effective half life of ^{131}I in the thyroid gland. The uptake phase is over about twenty-four hours after the administration of a dose. The elimination has an effective half life which varies between three and six days. Daily measurements are adequate and they will give the necessary number of points. The required technique will be, therefore, simply daily "uptake" measurements. When the problem is not only the determination of elimination of iodine by the thyroid gland, but also the speed of uptake or build-up, measurements will have to be done more frequently, at least every hour. More frequent observations would be also necessary, if instead of ^{131}I an iodine isotope of shorter half life such as ^{132}I were used. If the problem is limited only to the question of when the maximum uptake occurs, the measurements will have to be repeated every few hours or oftener. If the question is the shape of the initial rapid phase of the uptake curve (a problem relevant in some clinical diagnostic tests), the measurements have to be done every few minutes, and techniques other than simple uptake measurements become necessary. Figure 18–1 illustrates graphically the differences in handling these questions in our example.

The build-up of protein bound iodine in the blood is a slow process, occurring over a period of days. Simple collection of samples once or twice daily and their assay by a suitable *in vitro* method gives enough data for a complete evaluation of the time sequence.

2. *Intermediate Speeds*. For the observation of the build-up of iodine in the thyroid gland it is necessary to make measurements at least several times during the first hour. While this is possible by ordinary uptake measurements with a scaling circuit, it becomes quite a laborious procedure when it is necessary to start the scaler, watch for it to finish the counting for the preset number of counts or the preset time, take down the reading and restart the scaler again without loss of time. The same situation

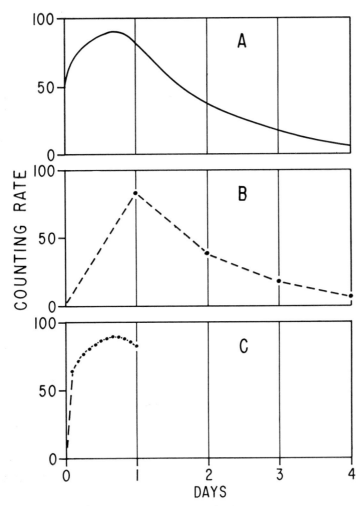

Fig. 18–1.   The effect of the interval between observations on the recognition of the shape of uptake and clearance curves. A: actual curve; B: daily observation represents well the elimination, but the uptake curve is distorted and the maximum seems to occur later than it actually does; C: hourly observations show correctly the time of maximum uptake, but the rapid initial rise appears to be slower than it is actually.

obtains in a variety of tests, as for instance in liver function studies with iodine-tagged Rose Bengal.   The use of an ordinary scaler with conventional reading methods is too arduous if such work is done frequently.

A good and reasonably inexpensive solution of this problem is a printing counter or a printing timer connected to an available scaling circuit, as described on page 213ff.

The speed of printing devices is limited, and the numerals do not follow the counts faster than about 10 per second.   Electronic scaling stages of

21

the circuit can be used to slow down the operation of the counter, but the intermediary counts are lost: if for instance a scaling factor of 100 is used, the numerals of the printer will jump every 100 counts and it can respond to counting rates up to 1000 per second. But if the printed result is inspected and is for instance 72, it is not known whether this means that a total of 7,200 or say 7,292 counts have accrued (92 counts will have appeared on the read-out lights, which do not enter the printer, since the mechanical printer was set to a scaling factor 100). It may seem therefore at first that no gain in statistical accuracy is achieved by using scaling factors in the counting circuit preceding the printer. This is not quite true, however, since circuit scaling "regularizes" the counts. What is meant will become clearer by an example. Let us assume a counting rate of 100 counts per second and a scaling factor of 64. We shall use a printing interval of one minute ("preset time"). The total counts accumulated for each "print" after each minute will be around 6,000 within statistical variations, and the statistical per cent uncertainty will be according to equation 15—(3) (p. 223) $V = 1.3\%$. The printer will show probably one of the three numbers: 93, 94, or 95. The "correct" number which corresponds to 6000 counts is 94 ($94 \times 64 = 6016$). The uncertainty here is ± 64 counts, or a possible error in printing of about 1 per cent. This will combine with the statistical uncertainty to an overall uncertainty of about 1.6 per cent. We could have used the printing counter also without the counting rate reduction in the scaling circuit by reducing the sensitivity of the detector (for instance by using a longer distance from the body or by a lead filter). If we reduce the rate by these means to 10 counts per second and even neglect the resolving time of the printer at this speed, we shall accumulate 600 total counts each minute with a per cent uncertainty, $V = 4\%$, or a considerably higher possible error than was obtained by using scaling factors. Still the speed of printers is a limiting factor, and measurements at intervals shorter than a minute lose reliability regardless of the actual counting rate.

Time printers, which print continuously the elapsed time for a preset number of accumulated counts, are potentially somewhat faster. Their printing speed is also about one-tenth of a second, which means that in a ten-second interval, a timing uncertainty of 1 per cent is reached. This is usually satisfactory and the actual limits of accuracy will be set more frequently by the statistical uncertainties in counts observed in this interval than by timing uncertainties.

In spite of the advantage of the shorter time intervals which can be used with time printers and the constant statistical uncertainty inherent in the preset count methods, count printers with preset time intervals are generally preferred in observations of changes in time. This has to do with the necessity of plotting the results obtained by any print method on graph paper. With preset time, say one minute, the observed counts can be plotted easily as ordinates against one-minute divisions on the abscissa.

For time printers with preset counts it is not only necessary to calculate the counting rate for each printed reading, but the abscissa for each point must be obtained by adding the total time elapsed since the beginning of the experiment; this procedure may become extremely tedious.

3. *Rapid Changes.* Some of the limitations of the printing methods have been pointed out above. They can be summarized as, (*a*) Manual plotting of the data is required to obtain a graph; (*b*) The response speed is limited, and not more than a few readings per minute can be obtained. Both limitations are overcome when a recording rate-meter is used; this consists of a rate-meter (see page 214) which is connected to a strip chart recorder, on which the observed counting rates are plotted automatically as a curve.

The accuracy of a counting-rate recorder depends on counting statistics. It will be recalled that a rate-meter is basically a "preset time" device, where the preset time equivalent is twice the response time. The accuracy is therefore determined by the selected response time and the observed counting rate.

Although the recorded curve may appear smooth, it does not contain inherently more "points" than those corresponding to the response time. The response time must therefore be selected with reference to the speed of the changes in the physiological phenomenon. If the whole change occurs within say ten seconds, and at least 20 points must be available for interpretation, a response time of one-half second is required. As the next step, it has to be ascertained whether during this half-second enough counts will be observed to assure the required precision; this is a straightforward problem using equation 15—(3). Let us assume that during the relevant period the counting rate is 200 counts per second; then 100 counts will be accumulated during each half-second interval and the uncertainty will be $V = 10\%$. This statistical uncertainty usually determines the shortest possible response time and therefore the fastest changes which can be recorded. The practical limitation in speed with rate recorders is not in the instrument itself but in counting statistics. This can be generally summarized by the statement that for the observation of rapid changes, high counting rates are needed which can be achieved by using high sensitivity detectors or large tracer doses, or both.

The convenience of having an instrument which performs by itself the plotting of the required curve brings up the question of why rate-meters and recorders are not used for observation of changes of activity of intermediate speeds. The answer to this lies partly in the technical characteristics of rate-meters and partly in counting statistics. Rate-meters have a response time which is limited in duration. Beyond a response time of a few minutes, electric components become less reliable, so that in practical instruments response times much longer than that cannot be achieved. If the counting rate is high enough so that sufficient counts can be observed within the maximum available response time, this limitation is of no significance. But for observing slow changes, nuclides of relatively longer half life have to be used, the total dose is more limited, counting rates usually become much lower and statistical fluctuation during the available response time too great. When this condition occurs, larger counting intervals are needed and printing timers or counters have to be used.

The decision between the selection of a printing device or of a rate recorder depends therefore on the expected counting rate and the needed frequency of readings (points on the curve). When more than a few readings per minute are required, a counting-rate recorder must be used. For the required frequency of readings, a sufficient counting rate is needed to keep the statistical uncertainties within the required value. The counting-rate recorder can be used also for observation of slowly changing processes, if the counting rate is high enough so that a significant number of counts are accumulated within the longest response time available in the rate-meter. If the counting rate for this interval is not high enough, printing devices have to be used which do not have this limitation.

A technical property of recording devices must be considered in the evaluation of the records obtained. Some recording instruments have a pen which deflects over an arc on the chart paper. This makes it very difficult to evaluate the slopes of the obtained curves. For this purpose, a rectilinear recording device is preferable, in which the deflection is perpendicular to the chart edge and linearly proportional to the observed magnitude. Such rectilinear recorders are available. When the physiological problem is less exacting, particularly if the essential information is simply at what time a maximum activity has occurred, as for instance in the determination of circulation time, the simpler non-rectilinear recorders are satisfactory.

Quite frequently the physiological changes observed by a tracer technique have an exponential build-up or clearance (decay) phase. In such cases the curves have to be replotted on semilogarithmic paper. This replotting can be eliminated if special amplifiers are used between the rate-meter and recorder which have a "logarithmic" response, and which therefore produce a deflection on the recorder not directly proportional to the counting rate but to its logarithm. In this way a curve is directly obtained which corresponds to a plot on semilogarithmic paper and "half lives" or their biological equivalents can be obtained by simply using a straight-edge.

Shielding in Radiation Measurements for the Observation of Changes with Time. One of the examples discussed in this section was the build-up of iodine in thyroid uptake and its clearance or elimination. It was mentioned that any uptake set-up can be used for this purpose with suitable counting apparatus. In some procedures for build-up and clearance measurements, it is neither necessary nor even desirable to have a radiation detector which "sees" the whole organ under examination, but it is sufficient when it sees only a sample or some fractional volume of this organ. This may have considerable advantages from the point of view of shielding. The field of view of the detector can be made narrower, so that the background is reduced and the measurements made more reliable and less dependent on the activity present in the circulating blood of surrounding tissues. The advantages of this arrangement become clear if, as an example, liver function tests with radioactive tracers are considered. A shielded enclosure seeing the whole of the liver would be not only extremely heavy, but also of such dimensions that the heart itself could not be wholly excluded. Valid rate observations can be performed better without sacrificing any physiologically relevant factors when the detector sees only a small part of the liver and excludes other organs in the vicinity. The necessary narrowing of the field of view of the detector can be achieved by a collimating shield, which will be discussed in detail in the next chapter. The suitability of a particular collimator is determined by the physiological conditions of the experiment. In the case of liver tests just mentioned, a narrow collimator, provided it has adequate sensitivity, is desirable. When observing the clearance rate of a deposit of radioactive sodium from the tissues, it must be made sure that the collimator sees all of this original deposit and is not so directional that small movements of the patient take the deposit outside the field of view of the counter and so simulate a misleadingly fast clearance rate.

19

Determination of the Distribution of Radioactive Material within the Body

BIOCHEMICAL affinity of some organs and tumors for some specific elements or their compounds leads to the concentration and deposition of these materials within such tissues. When radioactive elements are used for tagging these compounds, a deposit of higher concentration is found at such sites than elsewhere in the body. The ratio between the specific activity found in the organ or tissues under investigation and the specific activity elsewhere is called differential uptake. In preceding chapters, the determination of the amount of radioactivity in the body or the time sequence of its accumulation was discussed. In this chapter a different use of the radioactivity detectable in these deposits will be presented, namely the determination of their location and shape since this anatomical information is of as great potential use as the functional information discussed so far.

A radioactive deposit can be compared to a luminous body within a semitransparent, absorbing and diffusing medium; ionizing radiation is partially absorbed and scattered, but it also penetrates body tissues. Its presence cannot be detected by the eye, but it can be observed by radiation detectors.

In using such a detector to find a discrete source of radioactive material inside the body or in any accessible position, the first step is a direct application of the inverse square rule. That is, the closer a detector is to a source of radiation, the greater is the radiation intensity impinging on the detector and the higher the counting rate. This permits the location of lost or misplaced radium, for instance in a room or even in a building, and is one of the basic methods in prospecting for radioactive minerals. The detector must have two properties: it must be easily movable and the change of counting rate must be made conveniently and rapidly detectable. Precision requirements are low (presence or absence of a change is all the information needed), but sensitivity requirements are high.

When a large area (room or building) has to be explored, it is necessary that the whole detector and accessory circuits be portable; battery-powered instruments are extensively used for this purpose. When the task is the exploration of radioactivity in the human body or in an organ, only the detector proper has to be mobile, and a detector "probe," connected to the stationary circuit by a flexible cable is a convenient instrument.

Ease of observing an increase or decrease of the radiation level as the detector is moved can be achieved in several ways. A rate-meter shows changes on a scale; a neon bulb which flashes at every count gives a rough but frequently adequate indication of counting-rate changes. Visual indicators have a disadvantage; the eye must shift from watching the position of the detector probe to the indicating instrument and back. An audible signal, such as clicks in a loudspeaker or a headphone, overcomes this disadvantage. Audible signals are preferable to visual ones also because the ear can follow a higher rate of clicks than the eye can of flashes. For occasional use, an ordinary scaling circuit which contains an electromagnetic digital counter can be adapted to auditory indication, since the electromagnetic counters give audible clicks when they operate. All that is necessary is to select a scaling factor in such a way that the highest counting rate encountered does not exceed the resolving time of the register and block it. This improvised arrangement does not take advantage of the great frequency range of the human ear since the speed of the mechanical register is a limiting factor. It can also lead to mistakes in localization; if the detector comes suddenly close to a radioactive source, the counting rate may exceed the resolving time of the register so quickly that it becomes blocked before the transition to the higher counting rate can be noticed; when this occurs, the radioactive deposit will be missed. When this arrangement is used, the detector must be moved slowly while exploring an area, so that blocking can be anticipated.

Probe detectors of this type have been made and are used during surgical exploration for brain tumors and occasionally to check completeness of a thyroidectomy. Geiger-Mueller counters about $\frac{1}{8}$ inch in diameter and a few inches long, with thin stainless steel walls, have been constructed, which are sensitive to ^{32}P beta radiation. Scintillation counters are also constructed as probe detectors, by using a small crystal connected optically to a phototube by a plastic light-pipe; this permits having the crystal several inches away from the phototube with a sufficiently thin and long probe. Other solid state detectors have also been satisfactory for this service.

Collimation. Localization by "inverse square" has serious limitations. It is restricted practically to the rough localization of a single deposit. If there are two sources of radiation not far apart, within the body, it is usually impossible to distinguish them, and a more refined technique is needed.

The ideal solution is to obtain a complete image of the "luminescent" radioactive deposit, as is possible in photography with visible light by using an optical system. The only optical system useful with gamma rays is the pinhole camera. It will be briefly discussed later in this chapter.

A practical solution is to enclose a radiation detector in a tube with thick and heavy walls. Radiation emitted by a radioactive source can reach such a shielded detector only when it is located in the axis of the tube; when the source is sufficiently far off this axis, the shielding walls will absorb the radiation and no counts will be observed. Figure 19–1 illustrates

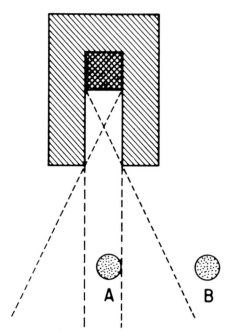

FIG. 19–1.   Directional sensitivity of a collimated radiation detector. Source B is shielded from the detector and the counting rate is small compared to that due to source A, assuming they have the same activity.

this. Such a collimated detector sees radiation sources only when they are within a limited field of view, which is determined by the geometry of the counter and collimator and the absorption by the shield material of the particular energy of radiation. Source A will be seen *in toto* by the detector in the illustration. Source B will be seen only so far as its radiation penetrates the collimating shield.

A collimated counter of this construction therefore has directional properties, and can be used to localize a single radioactive deposit even if there are several in a region, provided that they are sufficiently far apart so as not to appear together within the viewing angle of the detector.

When a collimated detector is used to search out a relatively small radioactive deposit in the body, collimation and the inverse square rule have important functions: that is, it is sensitive predominantly within its viewing angle and the counting rate increases with decreasing distance from the source. A small detector of this sort with a lead shield and an opening of $\frac{1}{2}$ to 1 inch can be made weighing a few pounds. It can be used freehand, without a stand, to search for thyroid metastases after a tracer dose of a few hundred microcuries of radioactive iodine has been given, and it is a valuable tool for preliminary orientation. Its precision in the localization of a deposit and in the determination of its shape is low because of its poor resolving power.

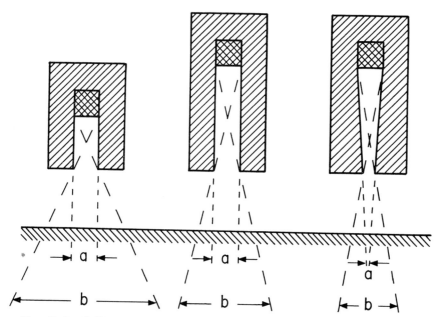

Fig. 19–2.   Collimated detector.   Maximum sensitivity is in the region a (umbra); reduced sensitivity is in the region b (penumbra); minimum sensitivity outside of region b. For straight holes region a is determined by the size of the collimating hole.   For tapered holes it depends upon hole size and taper.   Region b is largest on the left demonstrating the dependence upon the depth of the hole and smallest on the right because of the taper.

The resolving power of a collimated detector may be defined as the distance at which two small sources of radiation can be separated from each other, that is, detected as distinct deposits.   When their distance apart is less than this "resolving power," they will be seen as a single source.

In Figure 19–1, let us investigate whether or not the sources A and B will be distinguished separately with the illustrated arrangement.   To discuss this question, the viewing angle of the detector must be examined in more detail.

In Figure 19–2 a collimated detector "looks" at a plane surface.   By examining the area designated as "a" in this figure in relation to the detector itself, it will be realized that any small source of radiation within this area will be seen by any point within the detector, so that movement of a source along the plane within this field will not change the counting rate.   This, in analogy with optical terminology, is called the region of umbra.   If the source is positioned somewhere outside "a," but within the area "b," only part of the detector will see it, and other parts will be shielded from the source by the collimating shield.   Region "b" is called the penumbra region.   The farther the source is from the area "a," the greater will this shielding be, and the smaller the counting rate.   When finally the source is moved beyond the area "b," no radiation will reach the detector except that which actually passes through the collimating shield.

When the left and center diagrams of Figure 19–2 are compared, it is seen that the extent of the umbra region "*a*" is determined only by the diameter of the collimating hole but that of the penumbra region "*b*" depends not only on the diameter of the collimating hole, but also on the depth of the detector within the collimator and the distance of the detector from the source. If the collimator comes closer to the surface of the sources, the extent of the umbra remains unchanged, but the penumbra will be reduced; the overall angle of view of the collimator will become smaller and the resolving power better.

The response of the tapered hole shown at the right side of Figure 19–2 is quite different. The umbra varies with distance from source surface to collimator. The penumbra is narrower than that of a straight hole of equal depth. The resolving power of the tapered collimator is better, provided the source is located nearer to the collimator than the point at which the umbra vanishes. A tapered hole collimator is usually used with sources located closer than this point. The resolving power of the tapered hole varies less with the distance between source and collimator than does the straight hole.

While it is an easy matter to calculate the size of the umbra and penumbra, the value of the resolving power is not directly obtainable from these

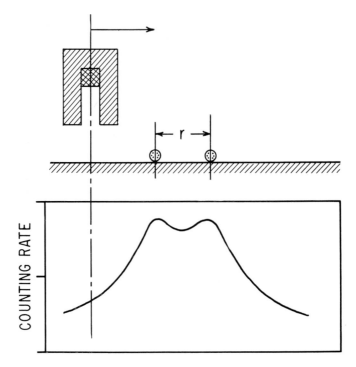

Fig. 19–3.   Linear scan with a collimated detector of two sources spaced 2 cm from each other, at a given distance between the plane of the sources and the collimator.

sizes, and, in fact, is difficult to calculate. It is possible to perform an experiment, such as is illustrated in Figure 19–3, to determine the resolving power experimentally. Two small radioactive sources are placed on a surface at a distance r from each other and a collimated counter suspended at a fixed distance over them in such a manner that it can be moved in desired increments along the line defined by the two sources. The distance by which the counter is moved at each step should be of the same order of magnitude as the diameter of the umbra (a practical figure is half this diameter for each step). The counting rate is determined for each position of the counter as it scans step by step along the line of motion and the counting rates are plotted as ordinates against the counter positions as abscissae.

Figure 19–4 gives three such plots for different distances r of the sources from each other. At first inspection the conclusion will be that when the

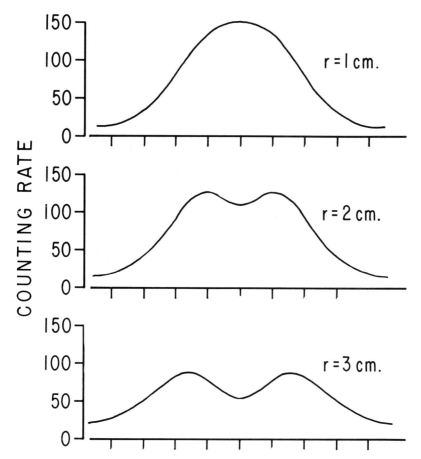

FIG. 19–4.   Linear scan of two sources spaced 1, 2, and 3 cm. apart. Resolving power of the collimated detector appears to be about 2 cm.

sources are 2 cm apart they are detectable as separate, and that at 1 cm they seem to fuse into a single source, hence the resolving power is 2 cm. This conclusion may be misleading, however, since we have to consider whether the observed dip in the curve is statistically significant or not; if it is not, its occurrence may be accidental and it may not appear when the experiment is repeated. The standard deviation of the counting rate at the adjoining peaks has to be evaluated, therefore, and the dip in the curve can be accepted as valid only if it exceeds the standard deviation.

This consideration is of considerable practical consequence. The per cent standard deviation decreases with the total number of counts accumulated; this number is greater, the longer the time used for counting and the higher the observed counting rate. The smaller the per cent uncertainty, the greater is the significance of a relatively small dip in the curve when two sources are being studied, hence the greater the resolution of the counter. The resolution of a given collimating counter thus depends not only on its construction but also on the time used for counting, on the tracer dose used, and on the sensitivity of the counter. These three factors are closely inter-related.

In an actual situation, *i.e.* counting radiation received from a patient, the surroundings of the sources are themselves radioactive and contribute to the counting rate. This provides a background counting rate which depends upon the dose given the patient and which markedly alters the observed resolving power.

To add the final complication to the discussion of this problem, let us consider what happens when the attempt is made to increase the resolving power by using smaller and deeper holes in the collimator. As a rule, we do not have within the body deposits of radioactive materials of very small dimensions. A collimator with a large hole sees a larger volume and therefore a larger fraction of the total radioactivity than when the angle of view is restricted by the size and depth of the hole. With smaller holes, low counting rates and larger statistical uncertainties result; the effective resolving power is reduced, so that the geometrical gain may be lost, unless high tracer doses or long counting times are used.

Since consideration of radiation damage to the patient as a rule limits the tracer dose which can be used, a practical compromise in the construction of a collimating detector and in the counting statistics has to be reached.

Maximal resolution is not always a desirable property. In a preliminary manual survey for radioactive deposits, particularly for thyroid metastases, it is easy to miss a small lesion when collimation is too good: the rise in counting rate may occur and disappear too quickly to be noticed under these conditions. It is advisable therefore to use moderate collimation ($\frac{3}{4}$ to 1 inch hole) for a preliminary survey, and maximal collimation for a careful examination of the active deposit, which has been roughly localized by the coarser method. If two different counters with suitable collimation are not available, it is possible to have a counter with different collimating adapters which can be readily interchanged. The assembly will be too heavy to be moved by hand, but flexible stands are available which support the detector and shield and permit moving the assembly with sufficient ease.

SCANNING

To determine the distribution of radioactive deposits within a sizable portion of the body, a technique of systematic external counting called scanning is employed. This consists of observing the counting rate as a function of the position of the counter over the surface area of interest. Such observations can be made either by moving one or a few counters over the surface or by the use of a large array of detectors which are placed over the area. The radiation detected in external counting is entirely photons, usually gamma rays emitted by the internal radioactive material.

General Remarks. It should be realized that the limiting factor in all scanning procedures is the statistical fluctuations in the data. These fluctuations distort the data so as to make it impossible to obtain as detailed a picture as desired in a fixed time interval.

We have seen the effect of fluctuations in sample counting as a limit to the level of activity which can be detected. These fluctuations depend not only on the sample counting rate, but also upon the background rate. In scanning, source and background counting rates have a somewhat different meaning. The display from a scan should show the relative concentration of radioactive material over the area of the scan. The activity which is just detectable above background in sample counting becomes for a scan the activity in a region which is just detectable above the activity of the adjacent regions. As this quantity depends upon the rates obtained over both the region of interest and its surroundings, and in no simple manner, "just detectable" is for a scan a somewhat complex concept.

Time enters into a scan in a fashion analogous to its role in sample counting. In both "just detectable" activity becomes smaller, the longer the time spent in counting. In scanning equal time is usually spent over equal areas, so that scanning procedures correspond to preset time rather than preset count methods.

It is obvious from the above that an increase in the amount of activity present will improve a scan. The increased activity can be used to reduce the relative statistical fluctuations, and thereby obtain a decrease in the concentration difference required for a "just detectable" level, or we can reduce the time of the scan and have the same level of fluctuations. Of course, giving more activity to the patient will increase his dose, so great care must be exercised to insure that the information to be gained is worth the risk to the patient.

In diagnostic procedures we desire a scan which demonstrates abnormalities rather than yielding a good picture of the activity distribution. For example, if a tumor has a large uptake of the radioactive material, all our scan need show is regions which have a higher than normal count rate. Unfortunately surrounding such a tumor and simultaneously viewed will be a large mass of normal tissue which also will have an activity concentration which differs from that of the tumor only by the differential uptake in the tumor. This differential uptake in a small tumor may not be sufficient to "override" the larger mass of normal tissue which surrounds it. It may also be hidden by activity in the circulating blood.

The time after administration of the radioactive material at which a scan is performed is an important consideration. First, we must have a quasi-static distribution during the time of the scan if we are using a system which views the scanned area piece by piece (*i.e.* moving detector systems —see below). Second, it is desirable to scan at a time when the differential activity distribution is most advantageous for our purpose. In our tumor example above, the tumor activity concentration may decrease very slowly compared to that in the circulating blood. Thus, by scanning a day or more post administration of the activity, a better picture can be obtained. A thyroid scan with radioactive iodine is best after about twenty-four hours for a similar reason, *i.e.* the circulating activity is eliminated and the gland still contains the bulk of its activity. In other cases scanning immediately after administering the activity may produce the best results. Each situation must be separately investigated to determine the optimum time. Also, the tagged chemical used can influence the optimum time. Several scans taken at different times post administration can, by the changes in the distribution from scan to scan, aid in diagnosis.

The activity distribution as determined by a scan represents a distorted view of the distribution of the activity in the volume beneath the surface scanned. The distortion is in part instrumental. For example, the collimator "views" this volume in a particular fashion which depends upon its design. It permits passage of gamma rays from a rather wide area of the surface with varying efficiencies. Also, the efficiency of passage changes with depth below the surface. The storage and display of the data also produce additional distortion. At times this distortion is intentional and serves to emphasize abnormalities, but most scanning systems have additional, unintentional distortions which cause loss of scan information. We shall discuss these points more fully below.

Finally, there is a fundamental limit to the information which a scan can supply about a volume activity distribution. The data obtained are surface counting rates and it is obvious that no single set of such data can completely specify a volume distribution. Fortunately such complete specification is usually unnecessary. A diagnosis only requires comparison with a "normal" distribution and for this purpose scan data can be adequate.

Instrumentation.   The actual instrumentation used in scanning can vary widely. The collimated detector with circuitry to provide an audible signal when moved systematically over the area of interest forms a simple scanning system. Such a device of course provides only qualitative information. At the other extreme, the scanner may be a matrix of scintillation crystals observed by an array of photomultiplier tubes which are, in turn, connected to a digital computer. Despite the differences all scanners have a common set of component parts. The variation in scanners depends upon the complexity of these individual parts.

Figure 19–5 shows a block diagram of a scanner in terms of these component parts. First is the collimator which restricts the view of the detector to a limited region. The detector signals the absorption of the gamma rays passing through the collimator. Electronic circuitry amplifies and analyzes the detector pulses as required, and in turn signals the storage section which records the number of events. This storage section must also be capable of simultaneously noting the origin of these events in terms of position of the detector over the scanned area. Finally, the information so stored must be made available in some form of display in order to use it.

Collimators for Scanning. In order to restrict the field of view of the detector to a particular region, we must absorb gamma rays coming towards the detector from all other regions. The processes by which gamma rays interact with matter have been described in Chapter 7. These are of course the processes by which the unwanted radiation is absorbed. At low ener-

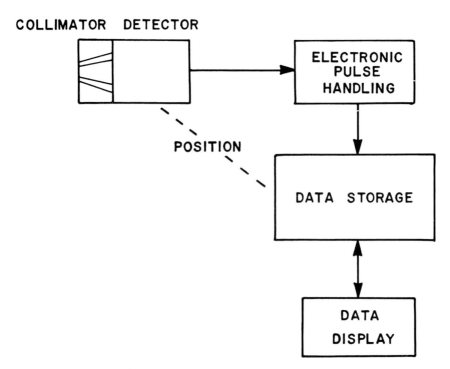

FIG. 19–5.   Generalized block diagram of a scintillation scanner. The various sections are common to all scanners.

gies the photoelectric effect is dominant and can be very large in high atomic number materials. At these energies even a thin layer of a material such as lead will easily absorb most gamma rays striking it. At energies above about 500 keV in lead, Compton scattering becomes the dominant process of gamma-ray attenuation. Unlike the photoelectric process, Compton scatter depends only upon the number of electrons in the absorber. Thus, the amount of Compton interaction in a layer of fixed *thickness* depends upon the density of the layer.

The absorption requirement of the collimator necessitates its fabrication from high atomic number material of high density. For most purposes lead is a satisfactory metal for collimator construction. Its atomic number is high (82) and its density is reasonable (11.4) so that good absorption is obtained at most energies. In addition lead is not expensive and is easily cast into the forms required for collimation. Special high energy collimators are sometimes machined from a tungsten alloy. While tungsten has a lower atomic number (74) than lead, it has a higher density (19.3) so that it is more absorbent in a given thickness. However, tungsten collimators must be machined individually rather than cast. This makes them very expensive compared to lead. Exotic materials such as gold (high atomic number, high density) have also been used for collimation, but are hardly of practical interest.

Gamma rays from the region of interest pass through holes in the collimator to reach the detector. Unfortunately we can not gather gamma rays with a lens as we do with light, so the more we restrict the view of a collimator the fewer the photons which strike the detector. An ideal collimator will transmit all the gamma rays coming from a small area towards the detector and reject all others. How closely a particular collimator will approach this ideal depends upon its design.

The design of collimators for scanning is a specialized subject, generally requiring the services of a digital computer. The majority of users merely purchase a commercially fabricated unit. Therefore, only the factors of interest in the selection of a collimator will be discussed, and no design information will be presented.

From Figure 19–2 it is obvious that a single straight hole collimator has a resolving power which is larger than the diameter of the hole and which broadens with increasing distance from the collimator. Neither property is desirable in a collimator used for scanning. Further, as the source is moved away from such a collimator, the counting rate drops off rapidly. This again is an undesirable property for scans of non-superficial distributions. Even the tapered, single hole, which has better resolving properties, suffers from this last deficiency.

For these reasons most collimators used for scanning are the multiple hole, focusing variety. Such a collimator is shown schematically in cross section in Figure 19–6a. Each hole is tapered. The axis of every off-center hole is inclined in such a way that, if extended, all of them cross the axis of the

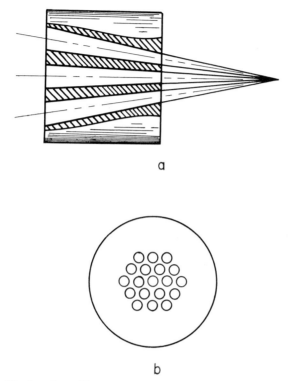

a

b

Fig. 19–6.   The focusing collimator.   View *a* is a cross section through the collimator showing the convergence to the focal point.   View *b* shows the close packed array of the holes.

center hole at a single point. This point is called the focal point. The taper of each hole is such that if tangents to its walls are extended they too pass through the focal point. These holes are positioned in rings in a close-packed array as is shown in Figure 19–6b. This arrangement achieves for the focusing collimator an axial response not found with the single hole devices. The counting rate increases as a source is moved along the central axis away from the face of the collimator until the source reaches the focal point. Thereafter it drops rapidly. The resolving power of a focusing collimator is much better than that of a single-hole collimator (comparing collimators which cover the same area of detector). Of course, the counting rate obtained with the focusing collimator is lower, but this sacrifice of counting rate must be allowed to gain the needed resolution.

Typical response curves for a focusing collimator are shown in Figure 19–7. One curve shows the relative counting rate as the source is moved across the face of the collimator at a fixed distance from the face. This called the lateral response curve. The other curve demonstrates the response as a source is moved away from the face of the collimator along the central axis. This is the axial response curve. The data for these curves

22

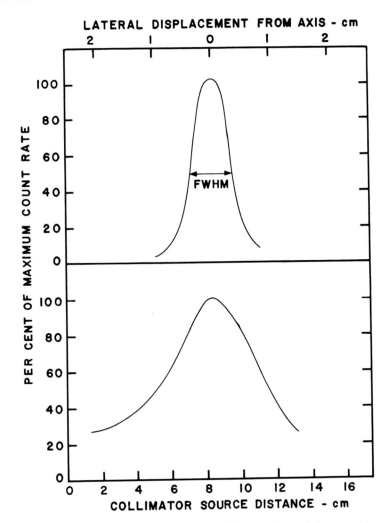

Fig. 19–7. Response curves of a focusing collimator to a point source in a water phantom. The upper curve is the lateral (across the face) response with the resolution of 0.9 cm (full width at half height) shown. The lower curve is the axial (away from the face) response. Notice that although the peak is at 8.5 cm from the face the design focal distance is 10 cm.

were obtained with the point source in a water phantom. This method of measurement is more realistic than to take the data in air. Contributions from small angle Compton scatter are included here as they are in scanning a patient. The details of this figure will in some degree depend upon the pulse height discrimination used. However, the general features will be maintained.

A method to specify resolving power (in addition to the one discussed above) is to give the full width of the lateral response curve at half of its maximum height. It is indicated in the figure. This specification is similar to optical resolution, and would be the true resolving power of the collimator if there were no background and no statistical fluctuations in the counting rate. In a practical situation background and fluctuations must be considered, and the actual resolving power is wider than the full width at half maximum. However, because lateral response data are easily obtained and because such specification serves well for comparing collimators, the width is frequently used.

The lateral response resolving power in Figure 19–7 is 0.9 cm which is typical of focusing collimators in common usage. The designed focal length of this collimator is 10 cm but the peak of the axial response curve appears at 8.5 cm. This is also a typical result, *i.e.* a peak response closer to the face than the focal point.

In addition to the better resolving power as compared to a single hole, the axial response of the focusing collimator makes it particularly desirable for scanning. In certain tests the superficial activity levels, though diagnostically unimportant, can be high and interfere with the determination of the distribution at a deeper, more significant, level. By having a response which increases with depth, the focusing collimator helps overcome this difficulty. Careful choice of the focal length and control of the height of the collimator above the scanned area permit the point of maximum response to occur at the desired distance below the scanned surface.

The design of a collimator involves factors other than the focal length. Detector size is one. It determines the area to be covered by the tapered holes. The gamma-ray energy is another. It influences the amount of absorber, termed septa, left between holes. These septa must be made thicker for higher gamma-ray energies to maintain the same degree of attenuation. Thicker septa reduce the open area and thereby the counting rate. The number of holes will also change the resolution. Since a close packed array is used, this number will be one of the series 1, 7, 19, 37 ... $[1 + 3n(n + 1)]$ where n is an integer. The designer must choose the most advantageous number. This is generally decided on the basis of resolution, sensitivity and the penetration through the septa. These factors are, to some extent, mutually opposing factors, *i.e.* better resolution usually means lower sensitivity. Therefore, the design must be a compromise.

The factors which a purchaser of collimator can specify are the detector diameter, the focal length and the energy of the gamma ray. He must then pick among the available models. However, data offered by the manufacturers do not always permit direct comparison among these models. Tests in air and in a phantom are, for example, not the same. Each manfuacturer tries to emphasize the best points of his design by giving his results in the most advantageous form. At times it may be necessary for the purchaser to conduct his own tests.

Detectors. This is the one area of scanning equipment where uniformity is the rule and choice minimal. With the exception of very few special systems, all scanners employ thallium-activated sodium iodide scintillation counters for detectors. This universal usage is a tribute to the high sensitivity of the counter to the commonly encountered gamma rays.

To specify the scintillation detector all that is usually required are the crystal diameter and thickness. The latter is determined, in large measure, by the energy of the gamma ray. For low energies (below 200 keV) a thickness of about one inch is sufficient. Thicker crystals will not produce greater sensitivity, but do increase background. At higher energies, thicker crystals intercept a significantly higher proportion of those gamma rays traversing the crystal. Also a higher precentage of the interacting gamma rays will be totally absorbed in the crystal. When energy analysis is employed to discriminate against scattered radiation, this latter factor results in a significant increase in sensitivity. However, cost increases with increasing thickness and a compromise is made. A 2-inch crystal is common although one 3 inches thick is sometimes used.

The diameter of the crystal not only affects the sensitivity of the system but also influences the resolution because it affects the design of the collimator. Generally, the larger the diameter the more sensitive the system can be made with other factors constant. Again, the cost of the system will be adversely influenced by such an increase. The cost rises very rapidly with diameter because of factors other than the actual detector cost. As the diameter increases the weight of the detector shielding also increases, and this involves strengthening mechanical parts, increasing motor sizes, etc. These costs rapidly reduce the desirability of increasing the diameter. Therefore, 5-inch crystals are usually the largest encountered in commercial systems. Three-inch detectors are more frequently used.

Present scintillation detectors are generally one-piece units with the crystal and phototube in a common, sealed housing. Such units have proved to be trouble-free, long-lasting and very stable over long periods of time.

The energy resolution of scanning detectors is not a crucial factor. Resolution is important only insofar as it affects the response of the system to scattered radiation. Small angle scatter (less than 30 degrees) cannot be discriminated against even using the best scintillation counter. (Solid state detectors offer promise in this area although their present sensitivity is far too low.) Therefore, acquiring a detector of especially low energy resolution hardly justifies its extra cost.

Pulse Circuitry. The electronic circuitry employed in scanning systems for pulse amplification and height selection is similar to that used for other scintillation counting applications. This circuitry has been described in previous chapters. Pulse height analysis of some form is generally accepted as mandatory in scanning. There is some question as to its efficacy at rejecting scattered photons but for large angle or multiple scatter it is certainly of help.

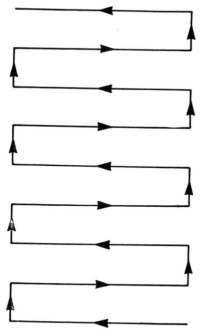

Fig. 19–8.   Scan pattern for a rectilinear scanner.   Direction of traversal is indicated by arrows.

The several different data storage and display methods used require additional circuitry of varying complexity. These will be described with the discussion of the particular scanning systems.

Motion in Scanners. The vast majority of scanners use a collimated detectors (or detectors) which is moved in a regular pattern over the surface of interest. Usually there are two motions at right angles to one another; hence these are termed rectilinear scanners. The pattern of motion is shown diagrammatically in Figure 19–8. The detector is moved back and forth in a series of rows from one edge of the field to the other. At the end of each row the detector position is incremented at right angles to the next row. The row length and spacing are preselected before beginning the scan as is the speed of traversal along the row. These factors are chosen from a knowledge of the area to be covered and the time available to complete the scan. However, other factors, such as the collimator resolving power, the patient dose, etc. must be considered.

The detector is generally moved continuously along a row. Step-by-step devices which move the detector rapidly from one point to the next with pauses between points have also been constructed. The data are taken during these pauses, *i.e.* at a discrete number of points over the area. The point to point method is useful when mathematical treatment of the acquired data is performed after completion of the scan.

There are several variations of the rectilinear scan, each designed to speed the data taking process. One involves the use of two separate, mechanically coupled detectors moved so that each covers only half the scanned area, thus halving the required time to obtain the data. Another also uses two detectors moved simultaneously, but each scans a separate area; for example the two sides of the head. A combination of these two detector methods has been employed to scan both sides of a head simultaneously, scanning each side with two detectors, *i.e.* a total of four.

A still more complex scanner is available which uses a number of detectors in a linear array. These are moved across the area of interest at right angles to the array line so that a single pass covers the entire area. The detectors can also be moved at right angles, *i.e.* along the line of the array. Thus, by scanning one or more additional rows, greater detail can be obtained.

Data Storage and Display in Moving Detector Systems. In moving detector systems two types of information must be supplied from the detector units to the storage-display portion of the scanner. The first, which we have already discussed, is detector event information. Of course if we have multiple detectors, we must have multiplicity in the pulse circuitry. The second kind of information required can be termed detector position information. With a single detector system the term is exact in that we supply, usually by direct mechanical connection between detector and storage unit, the coordinates of the detector's position. With multiple detectors the system must also note in which detector an event occurs. This is usually accomplished by having separate storage systems for each detector. Electronic sorting can also be employed.

There are two principal data storage systems in common usage today. These are the photographic and the count-marking methods. In the former a light source is moved by means of a mechanical linkage from the detector across a piece of photographic film contained in a light-tight box. Thus, the position of light on the film is in a one-to-one correspondence with the position of the detector over the patient. The intensity of the light is varied (modulated) by the counting rate from the detector. When this film is developed by standard photographic techniques, the blackening of the film will be a function of the activity distribution in the patient.

The degree of blackness or film density is not necessarily directly related to this distribution. It is possible to arrange to have no film blackening (light source turned off) in areas where the count rate is equal to the background count rate. This is called background suppression. Also, the blackening in areas of high count rate can be made darker than they would be if a directly proportional system were used. This is called contrast enhancement. Both background suppression and contrast enhancement are techniques used to assist in the visualization of abnormal activity distributions. By these means small differences in counting rate can be detected which, in a directly proportional system, would pass unnoticed.

Obviously, such a system, if not properly adjusted, can produce films in which variations due to statistical fluctuations appear as real differences in activity. Also, it is not a simple matter to insure that the system is correctly adjusted. Two controls are involved. One fixes the count rate to be considered as background and the other establishes the rate for maximum film blackening. The first is usually set with the detector viewing an area where there is little or no activity and the second fixed when the detector is positioned over the area of maximum activity. These positions can be found by a preliminary search of the area to be scanned. Such adjustments may seem to be an undue complication. but appropriate choice of control settings greatly enhances the probability of good visualization of abnormalities.

Data storage via count marking is a more straightforward technique The marker is moved over a piece of paper by a mechanical linkage to the detector in the same manner as is used to move the light source over the photographic film. Of course, a light-tight container for the paper is not required. Each time a scaler has received a preset number of counts from the detector, the marker is activated and an impression is made on the paper. The marker may be an electrical pen making an imprint on special paper. More commonly, it consists of a device operating somewhat like an electric typewriter. A piece of metal is made to strike an inked ribbon which strikes the paper and marks it.

With this system, each mark represents a fixed number of counts. Background suppression is provided by preventing the storage of counts when the count rate is below the chosen value. Another control setting required is the scaling factor selection, *i.e.* the number of counts per mark. The criterion here for appropriate selection is to insure that at the highest counting rate the marks are not so close together as to be indistinguishable from one another. However, the scaling factor should not be larger than that required to achieve this condition.

Both the photographic and count marking methods have been adopted to produce color displays, although in commercial equipment only the latter is generally available. In a color display the color of the mark on the paper or on the color film is varied according to the counting rate. Thus areas of high activity appear in a different color from those of low activity. This is purported to be of aid in the visualization of the activity distribution, although this is a matter of some controversy. The method of producing these color displays in count marking equipment is quite simple. A multi-color inked ribbon positioned by the output of a rate meter is used between the strike and the paper. Non-colored carbon paper copies can be obtained simultaneously with the color display.

The count-marked display is immediately available upon completion of the scan. The photographic method requires the film to be developed befor the display can be viewed. In either case when the display is available, there is little more which can be done to improve the presentation. Thus, if an improper choice of control settings was made, the information lost can not be recovered without redoing the entire scan.

A new group of instruments which permits post-scan manipulation of the data is now available. The data storage in such devices is quite different from both the count mark and photographic storage methods where the final image is made at the time of the scan. These newer devices do not create the final image immediately, but rather "remember" the image by storing the data in numerical form using digital computer techniques. The stored data are available after the scan and various levels of background suppression and contrast enhancement can be employed. The final display in such systems (made after the scan is completed) is usually photographic. Several pictures of each scan at various control levels can be made. Thus, an unusual distribution for which incorrect pre-scan control settings might be chosen using non-digital techniques, will not have to be rescanned when recorded digitally. Additionally, these digital systems have auxiliary equipment which permit the data to be stored permanently on magnetic tape. These tapes can be reread into the equipment when a further review is required.

While digital systems have obvious advantages, they are accompanied by a high purchase price, great complication in circuitry and a requirement for a highly trained operator. Where these drawbacks are not over-whelming, digital systems are undoubtedly preferable. If a digital computer is to be used to treat the scan data in order to improve image quality, digital recording is mandatory. However, these computer procedures are highly sophisticated, still experimental and are not widely used as yet.

Fixed Detector Scanning Systems. The scanning devices included in this category are undoubtedly the most complex instruments in the field of nuclear medicine. Only the basic principles will be described as a detailed description of their operation would require an entire textbook and serve little function here. Use of these scanners is becoming wide-spread despite their expense and complexity because of the advantages obtained from their use. These advantages stem primarily from the greater data acquisition rates of the fixed detector scanners compared to the moving detector systems.

The fixed detector scanner views the entire scan area at all times. This fact explains their greater speed. The view of a moving detector must be restricted to a small portion of the area. Therefore, a large fraction of the gamma rays emerging from the patient at any instant are not recorded. By viewing the entire area at once, a far smaller fraction of these gamma rays is wasted and hence a far greater speed obtained.

To obtain a large area of view requires a detector which is large. Also, the system must have the capability of signaling in which portion of the detector a gamma ray has been absorbed. Each such portion must only view a limited section of the scanned field. To accomplish this, a large, multi-hole collimator is employed, each hole of which acts as a separate single hole collimator for its section of the detector system.

Three different types of fixed detector scanners are currently available. The oldest is the Gamma Camera which was originally a pin hole camera device, *i.e.* a single hole formed an image on a large single crystal of sodium iodide. The camera has been modified to use a multi-holed collimator in order to increase its sensitivity. The light output from the crystal is viewed by a number of photomultiplier tubes optically connected to the face of the crystal opposite the collimator. Each event in the crystal causes light to strike each photomultiplier. The intensity of the light received by a photomultiplier will, of course, depend upon the energy absorbed in the crystal and also upon the distance from the photomultiplier to the point in the crystal where the event occurred. By adding the output of all photomultipliers together it is possible to determine if the event represents the full energy of the emitted gamma rays or if it is only a scattered photon. Thus, scattered events can be rejected. Note, however, rejecting scattered radiation is limited to scattering events of greater than thirty degrees even in a high energy resolution detector, and in the Camera the energy resolution is not as good as this.

By electronically examining the ratios of the outputs of the several photomultipliers it is possible to determine where in the crystal the event occurred. This information is used to position the beam of an oscilloscope to a point on the face of the cathode ray tube corresponding to this point in the crystal. The beam of the oscilloscope is then turned on for a short period if the full gamma-ray energy was absorbed. The oscilloscope face is viewed by a camera and the photographic film records all such events. The result is a picture of the distribution. It is also possible to digitize this information and to store it by using computer techniques. This yields similar advantages to the digital systems described above for moving detector scanners.

The Autofluoroscope is a similar instrument but instead of a single crystal it uses an array of small crystals packed together in a rectangular matrix (rows and columns). The light from each crystal is split into two parts by means of a complex light piping system and conducted to a set of photomultiplier tubes. From these are obtained the event position information (row and column) which is used for digital storage of the data. Again, as in the Gamma Camera, the total light is examined to discriminate against scattered radiation. The scan data in the Autofluoroscope are displayed on a cathode ray oscilloscope where they can be photographed and are also permanently recorded on magnetic tape.

A third fixed detector scanner utilizes an x-ray intensifier as its detector. This is the only widely used system which does not employ photomultipliers. The image intensifier converts the incoming gamma rays to light, the light to electrons and, after acceleration, the electrons back into light at the output screen. The light at the output screen is in one-to-one spatial correspondence with the input light. Still further amplification is obtained by means of a light amplifier; a device similar to a television camera. Originally the image intensifier system did not permit energy discrimination but this restriction has been removed by more recent developments. The final output of this device is usually a photographic image although magnetic tape recording is now available for permanent storage and after scan review.

The image-intensifier scanner is perhaps the least complex of the fixed detector systems. However, it is restricted to low gamma-ray energies because of its rapid falloff in efficiency with increasing photon energy. The Gamma-Camera and Autofluoroscope are extremely complex devices. Newer models of these devices will be still more complex owing to the development of additional features. This complexity should not be viewed as a drawback. The speed of data acquisition and the possibility of post scan manipulation of these data more than compensates for the complicated electronic circuitry required. Activity distributions can be determined in seconds, so that the short time changes of the activity distribution immediately after the administration of a radioactive tracer can be studied. Such studies can represent an important addition to other diagnostic techniques although spatial resolution in scanning can not begin to approach that available with diagnostic x rays.

Nuclides for Scanning. The choice of a nuclide to use for a particular scan is an important consideration but one, unfortunately, which is often not clear-cut. Conflicting claims of superiority of one nuclide over another are not infrequent, and the entire subject has generated a great deal of emotional debate. The controversies will not be discussed here, but rather a few general principles to assist in the choice of an appropriate nuclide will be given.

It is particularly desirable to use a drug which, owing to its chemical properties, will concentrate in the volumes we are seeking to visualize in a scan. The higher the uptake ratio in the volume the better. The best example of such chemical concentration is iodide in the thyroid. When such a drug exists the only choice required is the selection of the isotope of the tagging element. This is usually a limited choice and therefore uncomplicated.

Unfortunately chemical concentration is more the exception than the rule. More often concentration occurs because of differences in metabolic rate. These differences produce only small differential uptakes, and uptakes which differ but slightly among several drugs.

Aside from chemical considerations, several physical factors, such as half life, nuclear decay scheme, etc. enter into the choice of a nuclide. These factors influence the patient dose as well as the scan, and a choice should be made considering these factors.

To understand how physical factors influence the selection of a nuclide, let us consider an ideal and, unfortunately, non-existent radioactive chemical. In its decay, the radioactive nuclide of this chemical emits only one radiation, the gamma to be used in the scan. All other radiations (beta rays, other gamma rays, x rays, etc.) are not present in the ideal nuclide because they would contribute to the dose absorbed by the patient without contributing useful radiation to the scan. In addition, the effect of any other electromagnetic radiation, *i.e.* other gamma rays or x rays, must be eliminated by our shielding and electronic sorting equipment, an undesirable complication.

The gamma ray emitted by our ideal nuclide has an energy such that it is easily collimated, fully absorbed by a small thickness of detector and yet little absorbed in the patient's body. Unfortunately, this last specification is in direct opposition to the first two. If a gamma ray is easily absorbed by the collimator material and detector, it will also be absorbed by the patient. These contrary requirements do form the basis for an optimum choice in a real nuclide. Collimation and detection favor low energy while patient absorption favors high. This optimum is broad, depending on the depth of the volume within the patient, but is in the general range of 100 to 300 keV.

The elimination rate of our ideal chemical from the body (physical and biological half life) is long compared to the time required to establish the distribution and complete the scan, and yet is short enough so that it is quickly eliminated thereafter. Rapid post scan elimination helps decrease the dose to the patient without in any way affecting the scan. Retention of the activity until the scan is completed is assured by the first requirement.

Of course, no real chemical will behave in this fashion, but some will approximate the behavior more closely than others. Where the physical half life governs the decay rate, *i.e.* physical half life approximately equal to the effective half life, accurate assessment of the pre- and post-scan decay is simple. A very short physical half life, while desirable from dose considerations, presents problems of nuclide retention in the patient and of nuclide storage in the laboratory. In most practical cases the biological half life cannot be ignored.

Table 19–1 lists physical quantities of interest for nuclides which have been found useful in scanning procedures. While some of those listed have properties far from ideal, they have proved useful in scanning procedures.

Annihilation Radiation Scanning. When a positron combines with an electron, their combined mass is converted into annihilation radiation which consists of two 0.51 MeV photons emitted in opposite directions (see page 82). A positron emitter located in the body will produce this annihilation radiation in the near vicinity of the positron emission.

A technique particularly useful for brain scanning takes advantage of the directional relation between the two annihilation photons. Two counters are employed, arranged on opposite sides of the head and each equipped with a single straight hole collimator, the two holes pointed at one another.

*Table 19-1. Physical Properties of Some Nuclides Used in Scanning**

Nuclide	Half Life	Decay Mode	Principal Energy (MeV)	Gamma Per Cent	Other Radiations	Radioactive Daughter
^{51}Cr	27.8d	EC	0.32	9		
^{64}Cu	12.8 h	EC, β, β^+	0.511	38	β, β^+, e, γ	
^{72}As	26 h	EC, β^+	0.511	150	β^+, e, γ	
^{74}As	17.9 d	EC, β^+	0.511	59	β, β^+, γ	
^{85}Sr	64.0 d	EC	0.514	100	e**	^{85}Y
^{87m}Sr	2.83 h	IT, EC	0.388	80	e	
^{99}Mo	66.7 h	β	***		β, γ	^{99m}Tc
^{99m}Tc	6.05 h	IT	0.140	90	e	^{99}Tc
^{113m}In	99.8 m	IT	0.393	64	e	
^{125}I	60.2 d	EC	0.035	7	e	
^{131}I	8.05 d	β	0.364	82	β, e, γ	^{131m}Xe
^{141}Ce	32.5 d	β	0.145	48	β, e	
^{198}Au	2.70 d	β	0.412	95	β, e, γ	
^{197}Hg	65 h	EC	0.077	18	e, γ	
^{203}Hg	46.9 d	β	0.297	77	β, e	

    * Data from C. M. Lederer, J. M. Hollander, and I. Perlman: *Table of Isotopes*, 6th Ed. John Wiley & Sons, New York (1967).
  ** Other significant radiations from short-lived daughter.
*** Radiation from ^{99m}Tc daughter.

NOTES:

1. Abbreviations used above are: EC—Electron Capture, β—Beta Rays, β^+—Positrons, e—Conversion Electrons, IT—Isomeric Transition, h—hours, d—days, m—minutes
2. Gamma per cent is given as 100 × number of gammas observed ÷ number of decays. Thus, annihiliation radiation may exceed 100 per cent.
3. Characteristic x rays are produced in most decays. They are not mentioned above but often can not be ignored.

A single annihilation can cause an event in both detectors only if it occurs within a cylinder in the head whose radius is equal to the radius of the holes and whose axis is coaxial with that of the holes, *i.e.* the region of umbra of the two holes. Figure 19-9 demonstrates the truth of this statement.

    The two counters are used in coincidence (see page 215) to insure that only events occurring simultaneously in both counters, *i.e.* a single annihilation, will be registered. Further, a single channel analyzer is used with each detector so that only the 0.51 MeV photons will activate the circuitry. Thus, events in which an annihilation photon strikes one of the detectors but scattered radiation strikes the other are not registered. By these means very good spatial resolution can be achieved even with fairly large collimator holes. The use of large holes gives high sensitivity which is an obvious advantage. The depth of the holes will not change the spatial resolution as happens in gamma-ray scanning. In fact, collimators are unnecessary if hole-sized detectors are used, except as the collimators serve to reduce the number of false coincidence events in the detectors. Little shielding of the detectors is required and this greatly reduces the cost of the scanning mechanism through the resulting reduction in weight.

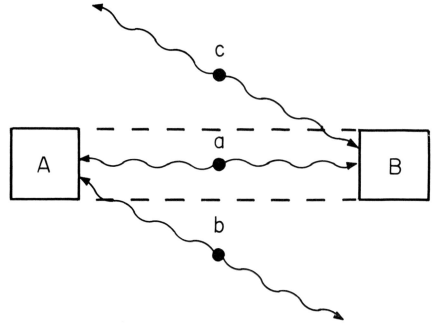

FIG. 19–9.   Detection of annihilation radiation.   Event *a*, within the cylinder of detection, strikes both detectors.   Event *b*, outside, strikes detector A but not B while event *c* strikes B but not A.

These advantages of positron scanning are offset at least in part by several disadvantages.   First, despite the use of two counters, which in a conventional scanner can provide both a right and a left lateral view and thereby distinguish the right or leftness of abnormalities, no such information is obtained in the positron scanner.   A tumor on the right side produces this same picture as a tumor on the left.   Second, for the most part positron emitters do not give particularly advantageous uptake ratios.   Third, the fairly high energy of the annihilation radiation is not conducive to high detector counting efficiency. Finally, most of the commonly used positron emitters are short-lived, limiting their use to the vicinity of installations where they can be produced.

20

Autoradiography

THE methods of obtaining information on the distribution of a radioactive nuclide in the body described in the preceding chapter have the advantage of high sensitivity and of the speed with which the result becomes available. They have, however, two disadvantages, complex instrumentation and a resolving power which is limited at best to a fraction of an inch. The limited resolving power makes scanning methods useless when information about nuclide distribution at the histological level is needed. This can be obtained by using photographic emulsions as radiation detectors. An image is formed on a photographic emulsion when it is placed in contact with the material containing a radioactive nuclide. This technique is called *autoradiography*. The low sensitivity of films, as compared to nuclear counters, can be offset by long exposure times which are limited only by the half life of the nuclide. Most of the radiation energy is emitted by radioactive disintegrations during the first and second half lives (after 2 half lives 75% of all disintegrations will have occurred). Longer exposures are, therefore, of no practical value. For nuclides with long half lives it may appear at first that the sensitivity of the autoradiographic method is limited only by the available time. This is not true for two reasons.

1. Photographic emulsions do not keep indefinitely, they gradually develop fogging which is due to chemical changes and to radiation background. Chemical fogging can be delayed by storage at low temperature and low humidity, but even at ideal conditions 2 years is about the longest time an emulsion remains useful.

2. The latent image in the emulsion fades with time exponentially like the decay of a radioactive substance. In prolonged exposure to a radioactive material this latent image grows and decays like a radioactive daughter in a radioactive parent. In such growth the activity of a daughter product reaches a maximum value after a definite time. If we call this time (at which the latent image also will reach a maximum) t, the half lives of the nuclide used T_r and of the latent image T_e, the optimal exposure time can be calculated from the equation :

$$t = 3.3 \frac{T_e T_r}{T_r - T_e} \log_{10} \left(\frac{T_r}{T_e} \right) \qquad 20-(1)^*$$

* From equation (4.2) on page 479 in Robley D. Evans, The Atomic Nucleus, McGraw-Hill Book Co., Inc., New York, 1955, by substituting half life for average life and $\log_{10}$ for $\log_e$.

338

The fading of the latent image depends on the photographic emulsion, and the storage conditions; it is quite variable. Ordinary photographic films have a half life of many months. The Kodak nuclear materials have as a rule a half life of 30 days and there are some emulsions with a half life of only 10 days. This information is usually available from the manufacturer.

As an example we shall determine optimal exposure time for ^{32}P (half life 14 days) with an emulsion of a half life of 30 days. From 20—(1):

$$t = 3.3 \times \frac{14 \times 30}{30\text{-}14} \times \log\left(\frac{14}{30}\right) = 3.3\ (-26)\ (-0.33) = 29 \text{ days}$$

For ^{131}I with $T_r = 8$ days we get in the same way optimal exposure at $t = 20$ days.

In these examples the optimal exposure time is about twice the half life of the nuclide, which is shorter than the half life of the latent image.

For critical work, when maximum sensitivity is required, equation 20—(1) should be used. For most practical work a simplified rule will suffice, which follows from this equation and from the consideration that most radiation (75%) will have been delivered in 2 half lives of the radioactive material*: *expose for 1½ to 2 times the half life of the radioactive material or of the half life of the latent image, whichever is shorter.*

Frequently the radioactivity will be so high that overexposure will result when optimal time is used. Under such conditions shorter times will have to be used which can be estimated from the Tables 20–2 and 20–3, or by a preliminary experiment. An alternate method is to prepare several autoradiographs of the same specimen and to develop them at short intervals one after the other.

The basic elements of the photographic process were discussed on page 199. It must now be considered how the distribution of the radioactive material becomes represented by the silver grains in the emulsion. If we examine a microscopically small deposit in a histological section (a point source) and consider the radiation emitted by this deposit impinging on an emulsion which is close to it, we shall expect to see an agglomeration of silver grains. The density of these grains will be highest over the deposit, decreasing outward from this center. The image of the point source will be not a point, but a diffused disk. The smaller this disk, the truer will be the image and the greater the resolution of a more complex source distribution, which can be considered as a multiplicity of point sources of varying intensity. The size of the diffusion disk will depend on several factors: 1, proximity of the film image to the histological section; 2, nature and range of the radiations emitted by the nuclide; 3, grain structure and thickness of the photographic emulsion; 4, the method of development.

* This applies approximately also for the build-up of an exponentially fading latent image.

A point source emits radiation in all directions. The photographic emulsion will be exposed to this radiation with an intensity inversely proportional to the square of the distance from this point. The better the contact between the emulsion and the section, the greater will be the gradient of radiation intensity between the silver halide molecules directly above the radiation source and those at increasing distances away from it.

With a radioactive source, a second factor will contribute to the sharpness of the image. Most radioactive materials used in autoradiography are beta-emitters, or emit beta together with gamma radiation. Beta and alpha radiations lose intensity not only because of increased distance between source and detector, but also because of their high absorption and limited range. On the other hand gamma radiation has no limited range, and its absorption in photographic emulsion is small. Beta rays show a much greater photographic effect than gamma rays. Both phenomena combine to help in improving the resolution in autoradiograms.

With soft beta radiation and good contact between film and section, the limits of resolving power in autoradiography are set by the range of the beta radiation and by the graininess of the photographic emulsion.

The ranges of some beta radiations are listed in Table 20–1, which indicates the limits of the resolution obtainable with the nuclides mentioned, even with the best possible photographic technique.

The graininess of the photographic image can be reduced to microscopic levels, but only at the expense of film sensitivity. It is a general property of emulsions that increased sensitivity is accompanied by a coarser grain structure. Most films have some natural fog level, which is in part inherent in the emulsion and in part due to background radiation, and increases with storage time. This fog interferes somewhat with the final resolution. Photographic processing (type of developer, developing time and temperature) also affect graininess and sensitivity. Most rigorous development increases sensitivity graininess and fog at the same time.

Consequently there are two ways of achieving optimal resolution in autoradiography with a given nuclide: optimal contact between section and emulsion and the use of highest resolution film with suitable processing. The first approach presents some technical difficulties, which however can be overcome, but the second has inherent limitations since low sensitivity

*Table 20-1. Estimated Mean Range of Electrons in Nuclear Emulsions**

Nuclide	$\bar{E}(Mev)$	Range (Microns)
^{32}P	0.69	800
^{131}I	0.187	100
^{14}C	0.049	10
^{3}H	0.006	1

* Based on curves given by R. H. Herz, Nucleonics, *9*:24–39 (1951).

Table 20-2. Autoradiographic Techniques

Method	Material	Resolution	Background Fog	Sensitivity* μCi/gm.
Contact autoradiography	Dental x-ray film	Low	High, visible	0.2–0.4
Emulsion painting and dipping	Kodak nuclear track pellicles NTB 2 and NTB 3	Medium	Medium, visible only under microscope	2
Emulsion flotation	Kodak scientific plates Code autoradiography Kodak Ltd (England) AR-10 stripping film	High	Negligible, even under microscope	20

* Lowest concentration of ^{131}I per gram of tissue which will produce a satisfactory autoradiogram after about 2 half-lives, when 5 μm thick sections are used (thicker section will require proportionally less exposure).

requires higher tracer doses which cannot always be used; a compromise has to be made. In the following, some typical methods used in autoradiography with a few frequently used photographic materials will be presented. Table 20–2 lists some of the typical data with ^{131}I for the techniques which will be discussed.

The simplest method of assuring contact between a photographic emulsion and a histological section is to press together mechanically by some clamping device a piece of dental x-ray film and the section mounted on a glass microscope slide; a coverglass should not be used. The film and slide are left together for a suitable exposure time; the film is then removed and processed; ordinary x-ray developing solutions, or a formula similar to the Kodak D 19 developer, are satisfactory. Fixation and drying are not critical. This simple technique is limited to macroscopic localization, since it is impossible to replace the film in original alignment over the section with precision. It is useful, however, when a particular area on the slide is large enough so that it can be identified visually after microscopic examination; this is frequently the case in thyroid lesions. The coarse grain of x-ray films is not objectionable in contact autoradiography.

Contact autoradiography is useful not only with tissue sections but also in paper chromatography. The paperstrip with separated protein fractions is left in contact with a photographic film in the same manner as a tissue section. After exposure and development, the blackening of the film indicates the location of the radioactivity on the paper. This method is particularly useful with two dimensional separation on paper.

Autoradiography is not limited to visual inspection; it can be used also as a quantitative method when the density of the photographic image is measured by a densitometer and compared to the densities obtained with the same photographic material exposed to different concentrations of the radioactive material for the same time as the autoradiograph and processed in the same way. Constant exposure time for the reference films and autoradiograph is essential, due to fading of the latent image. Such a quantitative use of autoradiography is the only method for estimating not only the average dose but the true dose to small tissue areas when the uptake of a radioactive nuclide is not uniform, as for instance the uptake of iodine in the thyroid gland.

In order to overcome the difficulty of correlating the photographic image with the slide, several methods have been worked out for maintaining the photographic emulsion in undisturbed alignment with the section throughout the whole sequence of exposure and processing.

1. *Emulsion painting* makes use of photographic emulsions which have not been hardened and can be liquefied by warming. They are available in the form of globules, pellicles, or they may be melted off from film. The liquid emulsion is applied over the histological section by a fine brush. It solidifies again on cooling and is developed after suitable exposure, without removing it from the slide. If no shrinkage has occurred,

the autoradiographic image will have remained in alignment with the histological section, and a microscopic comparison and correlation between the two is possible. While there are fine-grain emulsions available for emulsion painting, the main use of this technique is for low resolution purposes, since it is quite difficult to prepare uniform thin films by this method. When relatively coarse-grain emulsions are used, the requirements for thin films are less critical and adequate resolution is easily obtained with high sensitivity materials to distinguish, for instance, functioning and nonfunctioning follicles in the thyroid gland, which are visible only with magnification under a microscope.

2. *Section Dipping.* A modification of emulsion painting is to dip the section mounted on a glass slide into the liquefied emulsion (the emulsion deposited on the back of the slide is scraped off after processing). This modification is superior to the painting technique; it results in a thin and uniform emulsion layer and has been used successfully for high resolution work with Kodak NTB bulk emulsions.

3. *Section flotation* consists of picking up the histological section, floating on the surface of water, on a photographic plate or film. It has the advantage that practically any photographic film can be used. The best resolution is obtained with specially prepared nuclear emulsions. The disadvantage is that the photographic processing solutions have to penetrate the histological section and may damage it.

4. *Emulsion flotation* is the reverse of section flotation: a thin emulsion film is obtained by stripping the emulsion from specially prepared plates and floated on the surface of a water bath; this film is picked up by the glass slide on which the already stained histological section is mounted. The section can be covered first by a thin (about 1 micron) layer of collodion applied to it in a diluted solution (1 per cent, in a mixture of equal parts of ether and alcohol). This collodion layer protects the section and its stains from the effect of photographic chemicals. Stripping films are thin (4 to 5 microns) and quite uniform. Alignment between emulsion and section is excellent and very high resolution can be obtained with slow films of fine grain. With ^{131}I in the thyroid gland, it is possible to evaluate differences in the activity between single cells.

Table 20–2 contains some quantitative data on various techniques when used with ^{131}I. It is useful to interpret the listed sensitivities in terms of the minimal required tracer dose. For contact autoradiography of a somewhat enlarged thyroid gland of 100 grams weight, 20 to 40 μCi will be needed in the whole gland at the beginning of the exposure. If the uptake of this gland has been in the normal range, about 30 per cent, a tracer dose of 60 to 120 μCi would have been required. Usually, it takes several days between a preoperative administration of a tracer dose and the availability of the sections; if this interval is about a week, the tracer dose must be doubled, a total of 120 to 140 μCi will be needed. Similarly it will be found that for the emulsion painting technique one-tenth that amount, or about an ordinary tracer dose as used for uptake studies, would suffice. For the highest resolution obtainable with emulsion flotation material, on the other hand, 3 times the dose, 360 to 720 μCi, is needed, which approaches a therapeutic dose; in cases of complete thyroidectomy with suspected malignancy this is not prohibitive. It has to be remembered that for shorter exposures, when the information is urgently needed for a clinical decision, the tracer dose has to be increased accordingly.

Table 20-3. Approximate Specific Activity (μCi/gm) Required for Several Nuclides, with an Exposure of One to Two Weeks, Relative to ^{131}I. These Factors Are Applicable to Single Coated Films. For Double Coated X-ray Films, the Differences Are Less.

Nuclide	Relative Sensitivity	For Equivalent Exposure—$\mu Ci/gm$
^{3}H *	0.3	3.3
^{14}C	0.3	3.3
^{35}S *	0.3	3.3
^{45}Ca	0.6†	1.6
^{131}I	1.0	1.0
^{32}P	2.7	0.37

* assumed to have the same efficiency as ^{14}C.
† The authors have some doubts about this reported value, and estimate it to be closer to 0.4.

While the data in Table 20–2 refer to ^{131}I, they can be used for rough estimates of the specific activities required with other nuclides for comparable exposure times (one to two weeks). The photographic effect decreases with the energy of beta radiation; Table 20–3* gives the specific activity needed for several nuclides relative to ^{131}I.

Autoradiographs can yield information of biological significance not obtainable by any of the *in vivo* or *in vitro* techniques described above. Cell metabolism measured by uptake of a label in a heterogeneous population of cells can only yield some form of an average for the population. Such a measurement gives none of the details of the processes. An autoradiograph can be used to determine the uptake of each kind of cell. Details such as the fraction of cells of a given kind which are labeled, how much label is absorbed per cell, and where in the cell the label is concentrated are also obtainable. Various tagged agents can be employed to secure different kinds of information. Fairly complete metabolic studies have been performed in this fashion.

Autoradiographic techniques are simple in principle, but, except for contact methods, they require familiarity and facility with a considerable

* This table is based with some modifications on table 2 in *Autoradiography in Biology and Medicine* by George A. Boyd, page 49, Academic Press, Inc., New York, 1955. This book gives, in table 22 (pages 125–135) a comprehensive review of data on a variety of nuclides used with most available emulsions and techniques.

mass of minute details in order to avoid a variety of pitfalls and artifacts. While the reference (see footnote p. 344) attempts to give comprehensive instructions, it is recommended that reading be supplemented by some personal instruction and by practical supervised experience in the dark-room. While this remark applies to the whole section on instrumentation, it is particularly valid in connection with autoradiography.

21

Use of Radiation Detectors for Health Protection

THE aims of health protection in connection with radiological hazards were discussed in Chapter 11. The techniques used to eliminate or to reduce these hazards were also presented. The purpose of the present chapter is to describe the means of evaluating their effectiveness.

The two basic types of instruments used in this work are total dose and dose rate measuring devices. They are used for three types of radiation measurements: personnel, area, and process monitoring.

Total dose measuring devices are capacitor-type ionization chambers (see page 204ff), photographic film dosimeters and sometimes thermo-luminescent dosimeters (see page 199). Chemical radiation detectors are not suitable for the dose ranges of interest for health monitoring.

Capacitor-type ionization chambers are made as small fountain-pen-sized instruments which can be carried in the pocket. Their useful range is usually 50 to 250 mrad. When they are used to measure the dose accumulated over days or weeks, they show some spontaneous discharge even when they are not exposed to man-made radiation; this discharge is due partly to background radiation and partly to electrical leakage. It varies in different makes and even in individual instruments of the same manufacturer, and it can change in the course of time. Its order of magnitude is 0.5 to 5 mrad per day, and it must be determined for each chamber and checked at frequent intervals. This leakage limits the time intervals over which these chambers can be used without recharging. Daily reading and charging offer optimal reliability; a week is about the practical maximum. Leakage tests must be made regularly (at least once a month, particularly in humid weather). Early pocket chambers of this type had to be kept in a desiccator when not in use; modern improved devices do not require this. The scales on the built-in electrometers or on the external reading devices are calibrated in milliroentgens or millirads; this calibration can be accepted as sufficiently reliable for monitoring purposes with most gamma-ray energies encountered with radioactive nuclides (a significant deviation occurs below 100 keV). Because of relatively thick walls, these chambers are not sensitive to beta radiation.

Photographic film offers in many respects the best means to measure the total dose accumulated over an extended interval. The blackening of the exposed film after development can be easily measured quantitatively with a densitometer, and the observed density is linearly proportional to the exposure, that is to the total dose, over a considerable range. This range depends on the characteristics of the film emulsion and on processing. The smallest dose which can be detected by a film of high sensitivity to gamma radiation is about 5 mrad; the ratio between the maximum and minimum measurable dose (the dynamic range) is between 30:1 and 400:1. This means that when a film of high sensitivity is used, doses between 5 mrad and about 0.5 rad can be measured. When film is used for measurements of larger doses, less sensitive emulsions are required. By using two films of different sensitivities packed together, any required dose range can be covered.

Since these films keep over one or two years without developing objectionable fogging, they can be used for measurements extending over a period of weeks and months.

Another advantage of photographic measurement of dose is that it is easy to estimate the nature of radiation exposure. In Figure 21–1 parts of the film are covered by an aluminum and by a lead sheet, and a portion is left uncovered (except that it is wrapped, of course, in a lightproof material). If this film is exposed to beta radiation and the thickness of the aluminum sheet exceeds the range of this radiation, only the uncovered are of the film will show blackening. An exposure to gamma radiation of a few hundred keV will blacken not only the uncovered area, but also the area under the aluminum filter; the film behind the lead filter will show much lower density because of high absorption of the comparatively low-energy gamma radiation by lead. High-energy gamma radiation, of a few MeV, will be less absorbed by the lead filter and the differences between film areas behind the different filters will be reduced. The total density is therefore a measure of dose, and the relative densities an indication of type and energy of radiation.

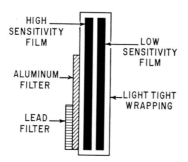

FIG. 21–1.   Schematic illustration of a film badge for monitoring personnel exposure. The filters permit the differentiation between exposure to beta, x-ray, and high energy gamma radiation. A film badge as illustrated will differentiate between radiation of different types only if the exposure occurs from the left. It is customary, therefore, to use identical filters on both sides of the film packet, which makes the badge bidirectional.

Below energies of 100 keV, the speed of film emulsions has strong energy dependence; it may increase 5 to 30 fold. In this region, therefore, films are useless for quantitative measurements. At higher energies this dependence is small, below 10 per cent up to several MeV.

Films for personnel monitoring are packed in the size of dental x-ray films and are carried in some sort of holder which usually contains the filters. The holders have clips for attaching to clothing. The complete assembly is called a film badge.

The disadvantage of film dosimetry is that films have to be processed (developed and so forth) before readings can be made. Film processing has to be done with great care to maintain reproducible results.* It is not advisable, therefore, to attempt to do these measurements in the individual laboratory; a commercial film-badge service is preferable. Periodic checks of the reliability of such services are advisable by exposing film badges to known doses of radiation, preferably of several energies. Such doses can be determined from the Γ factors and the known activities of the calibrating sources.

Dose-rate meters are ionization chambers, used in connection with transitor or other types of amplifiers, particularly battery-powered portable instruments (see page 203ff). Portable Geiger-Mueller or scintillation counter rate-meters are also used; they have a much higher sensitivity but lower precision and greater variation in response (calibration) for different energies.

The required sensitivity is determined by the permissible average weekly dose of 100 mrad. For a week of forty working-hours, this means a maximum continuous dose rate of 2.5 mrad per hour. For skin exposure the permissible dose is 3 times higher, and the corresponding dose rate here is 7.5 mrad per hour. Portable rate-meters have a selector switch, which permits a choice of several sensitivity ranges. The highest sensitivity of ionization chamber dose-rate meters is usually 20 to 25 mrad per hour full scale, so that a single division corresponds to between 0.5 and 1 mrad per hour. The ranges of lower sensitivity may go to several rad per hour full scale, which is useful in measuring high radiation levels of short duration.

Ionization chamber dose-rate meters usually have plastic walls of sufficient thickness to make them resistant to damage in handling. They have provisions to remove some section of this wall and to uncover a thin plastic window so as to make the instrument sensitive to beta radiation; the scale calibrations are not applicable for this type of use and the meter deflection can be interpreted only in a qualitative way. Usually the readings are low, *i.e.* the actual dose rate is much higher than is indicated by the meter.

The wave-length dependence of these ionization chambers is similar to that of pocket chambers; they are reliable for gamma-ray energies above

---

* Additional information can be found in the National Bureau of Standards Handbook 57: *Photographic Dosimetry of X and Gamma Rays.* For sale by the Superintendent of Documents, Washington, D.C., 20025. Price 15 cents.

100 keV. The precision of these devices is not high, about 25 per cent; this is, however, adequate for monitoring purposes.

Portable Geiger-Mueller counters have much higher inherent sensitivity than ionization chambers; however, their wave-length dependence is great. The meters are calibrated either in counts per minute or in milliroentgens. In the latter case this calibration is usually done with high-energy gamma radiation (^{60}Co or radium). When they are to be used with other radioactive nuclides for dose-rate determination, they must be recalibrated with a known source of the particular nuclide. Portable Geiger-Mueller counters frequently have thin walls or windows, so that some sensitivity in beta detection is available; this is again of little value for quantitative measurements, but very useful in finding low-level contamination. Many of these instruments have a light signal to indicate visually the occurrence of a counting event. Some have provisions for connecting a headphone, to make the counts audible. Portable scintillation counters have maximum sensitivity and they can detect small changes in natural radioactive background. This extreme sensitivity is of limited use in health protection measurements; their main application is in prospecting for radioactive minerals.

Application to Monitoring Problems. All measures of radiation protection have, of course, the final aim of limiting the radiation exposure of people to the permissible value. The final check of success or failure of these measures is *personnel monitoring,* that is the measurement of total dose received by individuals.

When daily information is required, pocket ionization chambers are the only practical device. Film badges are less expensive, and they can be worn over a period of a week to a month; further, they can give indication about the source of exposure (low or high energy gamma and x rays, or beta radiation); the results are not available immediately.

A common sense rule is to have all personnel working with radioactive nuclides wear film badges during working hours. At the beginning, daily measurements of key people with pocket chambers are highly advisable, until the health safety of the laboratory working conditions has been established; after that, the pocket chambers should be worn when an unexplained rise in film-badge reading is reported, or when techniques are changed, new nuclides are introduced or increased quantities are used.

The hands can easily get more than 3 times the dose indicated on the film badge worn on a coat, since they frequently come close to radioactive materials which are inside of shielding enclosures. However, a higher exposure level is permitted for hands than for the whole body (see page 158). Pocket chambers and film badges can be, for occasional use, taped to the hand, but this is usually inconvenient. Special ring type film badges are available for these purposes. They consist of small waterproof film packs, attached to plastic rings which can be worn on a finger.

This external monitoring will not reveal internal radiation exposure due to accidental ingestion or inhalation of radioactive material. This danger sometimes exists with ^{131}I. Such internal exposure is easily detected by standard uptake methods. It is advisable to do such uptake monitoring at regular intervals on everybody who handles this nuclide. Other nuclides are less easily detected, but internal exposure can usually be established, if not by external counting, then by occasional measurements by *in vitro* methods of excreta or expired air, depending on the metabolic behavior of the particular element.

Area Monitoring. In order to establish adequacy of shielding or, when radiation levels are high, to determine the permissible time for work in such areas, the dose rates at various working areas have to be established; this surveying is called area monitoring and can be done both by total dose and by dose-rate meters. Measurements are made at strategic points in workrooms; common sense will guide in their selection (sinks, desks, etc.). Records of such surveys by area monitoring should be kept. A convenient way to do this is to note the observed dose rates at the surveyed locations on a floor plan.

Dose-rate meters are convenient for a quick survey; they should be used for preliminary work and for checking of unusual situations (occasional shipments of large amounts of a short-lived nuclide, for instance). A better overall result is obtained by the slower method of total dose instruments, since they will average the possibly changing levels of radiation in a given room, for example, a hot laboratory, where shipments are unpacked, dilutions prepared and put behind storage shields.

Process monitoring is used for establishing the radiological safety of certain operations which are either part of routine or which have to be performed occasionally. If potential radiation levels are high, the actual dose rates must be known, in order to decide whether the operation is at all possible, or how much time can be allowed for its completion, and perhaps to organize work in relays, so that each person performs a share of the work within the permissible exposure time. An example of such a situation is the autopsy of a patient who received 100 millicuries of radioactive gold. For process monitoring, only dose-rate meters are useful; their reading permits a rapid estimate of time which can be spent by an individual at the particular job.

Waste disposal requires no special instruments. The amount of radioactivity to be disposed of can usually be determined by *in vitro* measurement of aliquot samples, or by improvising an adaptation of uptake measurement technique for the total bulk material. This is rarely feasible for the measurement of the radioactivity which is disposed of in the sink by washing of contaminated glassware. A rough, but practically adequate estimate is that less than 1 per cent of radioactive material used in a laboratory is washed out from glassware.

Finally, a special problem in health protection measurements should be mentioned briefly: checking for flaking or leaking of the radioactive material from an external radiation source (for instance a ^{60}Co teletherapy unit or a ^{90}Sr surface applicator).   For a γ-emitter this test is performed by wiping the housing as near to the source as possible (usually the part where treatment cones are inserted) with a cotton swab on an applicator stick and counting the swab in a well-type scintillation counter.   A β-emitter is tested by wiping the surface of the source on a piece of paper, which has been cut to fit a planchette, and counting with an end window counter.   At present significant leakage is considered to exist if activities exceeding 5 nanocuries are found.

22

Laboratory Design

In starting a radioactive nuclide program in a hospital or in a private office, the first question to be answered is how much space is required. The answer depends on the type of work planned, on the expected work-load, and on some general conditions set by the necessary measurement techniques.

A modest beginning will be to plan for diagnostic use of radioactive iodine only. This will require an uptake measuring apparatus and a well-type scintillation counter; both can be housed in a single room. But some other additional area will be needed for storage and handling of tracer doses and some processing of blood samples. If these auxiliary operations are done in the same room in which the measuring instruments are located, an erratic background will almost inevitably result, which will interfere with the accuracy of measurements. However good the shielding of nuclides in storage is, there will be some measurable contribution to background when storage containers are in the same room with counters; as the stored nuclides decay or are used up this background contribution will decrease, and it will rise again with the receipt of new shipments. In spite of the most careful handling, some minor spillage of radioactive material will occur; this may be negligible from the point of view of health hazards, but it may be detectable in the counting equipment. Glassware, bottles, and other materials which have been used for handling radioactive material, will create an addition to background counting rate which will change after washing and other disposal. These effects can be eliminated if the counting room proper is a separate unit and all operations except radioactivity measurements are carried out elsewhere and at some distance. The second area need not be large; it should contain a sink; it can be part of another laboratory, under the condition that sufficient bench space can be reserved for radioactive nuclide work. In this case, the whole room may become a radiation area in the sense of requirements for personnel monitoring, and everybody working there will have to be provided with film badges.

The two room set-up is sufficient only when the patients seen for tracer studies and therapy can be scheduled for either morning or afternoon visits, or if waiting rooms are available which are far enough removed from the counting rooms; otherwise the presence of a patient who has received a tracer dose may interfere with measurements, particularly in a well counter;

patients with therapeutic doses will certainly create an increased background. When a separation of patients and counting equipment is not feasible by scheduling or by remote waiting areas, it will become necessary to separate the less sensitive uptake-counting equipment from the more sensitive sample-counting instruments. This becomes almost imperative when the patient load is so great that sample counting must frequently be done at the same time as uptake measurements.

Increasing the variety of nuclides used and widening of the scope of diagnostic and therapeutic applications will make further additions to the available space necessary, but these requirements must be met according to the specific needs and no general rules can be formulated.

To summarize: 1. Minimal requirements are two rooms, one for handling radioactive materials and the second for measurements; 2. Increased work load will make a third room necessary, so that *in vivo* and *in vitro* counting can be separated.

There are no special structural requirements for a room where only measurements on patients are made. When samples are handled, the surfaces are likely to become occasionally contaminated. Trays and waxed paper covering table tops will allow easy decontamination. In addition it is helpful to have the table-top material itself non-absorbent and washable (stainless steel, plastic laminates) or to have it made of some easily replaceable, inexpensive material (composition boards). In areas where high activities are handled, it is advisable to have floors covered in such a way that they also can be easily washed and replaced in sections; composition tiles appear to be the best way to achieve both.* It is not economical to build a storage room or closet with lead-lined walls; storage shielding is accomplished much more easily by shielding individual containers or by constructing a small lead enclosure or box to hold the available containers. Enclosures can be economically assembled out of lead bricks. The effectiveness of the shield should be checked by measuring the dose rate outside of the enclosure, when a known amount of every nuclide to be stored is placed one at a time inside. This measurement will indicate the dose rate per millicurie of the nuclides stored, so that maximum amounts which may be kept in the enclosure can be easily calculated. When larger amounts must be stored, lead bricks can be added to increase the shielding or additional enclosures can be assembled.

Construction materials used in counting areas must be checked for natural radioactivity, since some paints, bricks and particularly tiles (with thorium-containing glaze) may significantly increase the background.

Since radioactive nuclide laboratories are frequently operated by radiologists or by the staff of a radiological department in a hospital, there is a tendency to locate the nuclide work in the vicinity of x-ray equipment.

---

* National Bureau of Standards Handbook 48: *Control and Removal of Radioactive Contamination in Laboratories,* pages 11 to 16. For sale by the Superintendent of Documents, Washington, D.C., 20025. Price 20 cents.

The possibility of interference of the x radiation with nuclear measurements has to be evaluated under these circumstances.

The starting point is the assumption that a diagnostic and radiotherapy area has adequate radiation protection. This means a radiation level of not more than 100 mrad per week. If a forty-hour working week is assumed, the average dose rate per minute will be about 0.05 mrad. If it is further assumed that equipment is on half the time and off half the time, the dose rate will vary between 0 and 0.1 mrad per minute. Counting equipment registers radiation bursts which accompany radioactive disintegration or, generally, high energy photons impinging on the detector (we are not concerned in this connection with beta radiation). We must know, therefore, to how many photons 0.1 mrad per minute corresponds; this varies with x-ray energy. Some illustrative values are listed in Table 22–1, where the

Table 22-1. Number of Photons per Minute Traversing an Area of 25 cm² (Cross Section of a Well Type Scintillation Counter), when the Dose Rate is 0.1 mrad per Minute*

Photon Energy (keV)	Photons per Minute (Millions)
50	76
100	62
200	26
500	9.5
1,000	5.0
2,000	3.0
5,000	1.6
10,000	1.0

* Dose rate in muscle. Absorption data from Physical Aspects of Irradiation, ICRU Report 10b. National Bureau of Standards Handbook 85 (1962).

number of photons per minute impinging on a 2 × 2 inch scintillation counter has been calculated for 0.1 mrad per minute. If we assume that the source of this radiation is for example a 400 kV constant potential machine and that the radiation detector is shielded with 2 inches of lead (attenuation factor about 10^{10}), there will be no significant increase of background counts, but if uptake is measured, scatter from the patient's neck into the detector may be appreciable. With an x-ray source of one million volts, the number of photons will be smaller, but the shielding effect of lead will be less, so that an appreciable counting rate may be observed. Precise quantitative evaluation of the effect on the counting rate is almost impossible because of the changes in radiation quality with absorption and scatter. In practice it appears that a distance of 100 feet between the counting room and a radio-therapy installation using conventional x-rays up to 400 kV is sufficient. When ^{60}Co machines and betatrons are used, 300 feet or more may be required.

Equipment. The equipment requirements are determined, as are space requirements, by the contemplated work. For diagnostic and therapeutic use of radioactive iodine, the minimum needs are a scaling circuit, radiation detectors for uptake and for sample measurements.

When nuclides are obtained from a manufacturer in prepared and standardized tracer and therapeutic doses, handling precautions are simple. Long forceps are usually all that is needed for administration to patients. Syringes with plastic shields are available for injection of β-emitting nuclides. Interstitial administration of larger activities calls for individual techniques (see for instance Silver: *Radioactive Nuclides in Medicine and Biology*, pages 454ff). If radioactive materials are obtained in bulk solution, the preparation of dilutions and the dispensing of individual doses requires some additional handling equipment. Depending on activity and the results of process monitoring (see Chapter 21) remote-pipetting devices, shielding of solutions while pipetting and ventilated hoods may be needed.

Remote-pipetting devices may be long (about 2 feet) holders for the pipette, with a syringe at the handle of the holder, and a rubber tube connecting the pipette and the syringe. This permits filling and emptying a pipette by visual control without bringing the hands close to the solution or the pipette. Usually it will be found sufficient to use pipetting devices which are attached directly to the pipette. This keeps the hands away from the active bulk solution by the length of the pipette. A considerable variety of such devices are available commercially. They are either a type of syringe with the plunger controlled by a screw motion or rubber bulbs with finger-operated valves to draw up and to dispense the solution. Pipetting of radioactive solutions by mouth should never be done, even when a length of rubber tube is used between pipette and mouth.

Some compounds may undergo chemical changes, particularly when dilutions are made, which volatilize the radioactive material so that it can be inhaled. Such volatilization must be prevented by suitable chemical measures (maintenance of proper pH, etc.) (see page 258).

Possibility of percutaneous absorption of many compounds makes the use of rubber or plastic gloves mandatory while handling glassware containing radioactive materials.

The body of the operator can be protected when necessary by keeping the bulk solutions in a lead shield (the shipping container or a shield assembled from lead bricks). If the activity in the pipette causes excessive body exposure, a vertical lead plate or a lead brick barrier must be used and inspection of the pipette done through a lead glass shield which forms the upper part of the vertical lead plate (the use of a mirror is rarely needed in biological work.) The table on which pipetting is done must also be shielded with a horizontal lead plate. Suitable assemblies of horizontal and vertical lead shields with lead glass are usually available commercially, as designed for handling of radium.

The selection of a scaling circuit is complicated by the great variety of manufacturers and models. It is not possible to recommend specific makes, but a visit to a few established laboratories, where work in this field has been carried out for some time, will give some guidance.

The beginner may be tempted to get the most elaborate scaling circuit which he can afford.

It must be considered, however, that all electronic equipment gets out of order occasionally, and the more complicated a piece of equipment the more probable a malfunction becomes. The modular construction of most modern equipment may weigh in favor of a simple unit along with a set of spare modules to use if the equipment should fail. In selecting a particular make the availability of local service including the stocking of component modules is an important factor. If service and stocking are available, spare modules need not be purchased thus reducing costs. Local service can even outweigh the superior engineering of another manufacturer.

An uptake measurement set-up, with a scintillation crystal as detector, a well-type scintillation counter and a Geiger-Mueller beta-ray counter will complete the basic instrumentation and permit the handling not only of ^{131}I, but also ^{32}P and of other nuclides for blood volume determination and tests using ^{60}Co or ^{58}Co tagged vitamin B_{12}.

The next step in expanding clinical instrumentation is a scanning device. This, of course, involves a great deal of additional equipment but permits liver function tests, brain scans, etc.

Measurements with low energy beta emitters require at the least a thin end window Geiger-Mueller counter or, if ^{3}H is to be used, a liquid scintillation counter. Usually ^{3}H counting is not a clinical procedure and research instrumentation is so specialized that general rules are usually of little value.

For monitoring radiation exposure, film badges, worn by every person participating in work with radioactive materials, are the first requirement. They are supplemented by pocket ionization chambers, which should be used whenever new techniques are introduced or unusual situations are expected, which may be accompanied by higher radiation levels than normally prevail.

A portable ionization chamber, designed as a dose-rate meter, is desirable for area monitoring and is essential for process monitoring. Every location where exposure to personnel for full-time occupancy may exceed the weekly permissible levels, must be surveyed periodically and if dose rates exceeding 2 to 2.5 mrad per hour are found, the locations should be posted with radiation signs indicating the radiation dose rate. Areas where radiation levels are below those permissible for occupational exposure but in excess of non-occupational levels should also be posted, but the dose rate need not be noted on them.

A portable Geiger-Mueller counter is not essential; it is, however, of great convenience in inspecting working areas and equipment for low-level contamination, which may be insignificant as a health hazard but will interfere with measurements.

The qualifications of professional personnel directing and participating in clinical radioactive nuclide work are of fundamental importance, but it is much more difficult to formulate them without ambiguity than to describe specifications and requirements for instrumentation. One of the original conditions for authorization to obtain radioactive nuclides from the Atomic Energy Commission was the establishing of a local committee in an institution. This committee had to have at least one member experienced in the use of radioactive materials. As additional members were recommended a radiologist, an internist, a hematologist, a pathologist or another basic scientist, preferably a physicist. The internist represented frequently, in the beginning, the driving force in starting radioactive nuclide program; at present, the interest in this field appears to be shifting to radiologists. Whatever the primary specialized professional field of the worker may be, he should have some solid background in the specialties represented on the committee, or be assisted by a team, representing such background.

Formal training requirements for licensing by the Atomic Energy Commission or the several state agencies in those states which have accepted control from the Commission differ somewhat from one another. Details can be obtained by writing to the Atomic Energy Commission or to the state agency. Training can be obtained through courses at a number of medical institutions.

When the patient load is small, the physician may be able to cope both with the medical and technical aspects, but at some stage, technical help will be required. Technicians trained in the field of nuclear medicine are not readily available but a number of institutions now offer training courses.* Professional as well as technician training is available. On-the-job training, particularly at the technician level, can be quite satisfactory and has been the main source of personnel in the past.

* A list of some of these institutions can be obtained from the Bureau of Radiological Health, Public Health Service, 12720 Twinbrook Parkway, Rockville, Md. 20852.

Appendix A

Useful Physical Constants

(New Values for the Physical Constants, as Recommended by the NAS–NRC. Physics Today, *17*, No. 2, 48, 1964.)

Avogadro's Number—N = 6.02252×10^{23} molecules per gram-mole.

Planck's Constant—h = 6.6256×10^{-27} erg-seconds.

Velocity of light—c = 2.997925×10^{10} cm per second.

Electron Charge—e = 4.80298×10^{-10} esu of charge.
$\quad\quad\quad\quad\quad\quad\ = 1.60210 \times 10^{-19}$ coulombs of charge

One Mass Unit—mu = 1.66044×10^{-24} grams.

Energy Equivalent of one Mass Unit = 1.492×10^{-3} ergs
$\quad\quad\quad\quad\quad\quad\quad\quad\quad\quad\quad\quad\quad\quad = 931.48$ MeV.

Electron Rest Mass—m_o = 9.1091×10^{-28} gm
$\quad\quad\quad\quad\quad\quad\quad\quad\ = 0.0005486$ mu
$\quad\quad\quad\quad\quad\quad\quad\quad\ = 0.511006$ MeV.

Proton Rest Mass—M_o = 1.67252×10^{-24} gm
$\quad\quad\quad\quad\quad\quad\quad\quad\ = 1.007251$ mu
$\quad\quad\quad\quad\quad\quad\quad\quad\ = 938.26$ MeV.

Neutron Rest Mass—M_n = 1.67482×10^{-24} gm
$\quad\quad\quad\quad\quad\quad\quad\quad\ = 1.008665$ mu
$\quad\quad\quad\quad\quad\quad\quad\quad\ = 939.55$ MeV.

Appendix B

Convenient Conversion Factors

1 ampere (amp) $= 3 \times 10^9$ esu of charge per second
$\qquad\qquad\quad = 6.25 \times 10^{18}$ electrons per second.

1 calorie (cal) $= 4.184 \times 10^7$ ergs.

1 curie (Ci) $= 3.7 \times 10^{10}$ disintegrations per second.
1 millicurie (mCi) $= 3.70 \times 10^7$ disintegrations per second.
1 microcurie (μCi) $= 3.70 \times 10^4$ disintegrations per second.
1 nanocurie (nCi) $= 37$ disintegrations per second.

1 day $= 1440$ minutes
$\qquad\quad = 86400$ seconds.

1 electron volt (eV) $= 1.602 \times 10^{-12}$ ergs.
1 million electron volts (MeV) $= 1.602 \times 10^{-6}$ ergs.

1 electrostatic unit of charge (esu) $= 2.083 \times 10^9$ electrons.
1 erg $= 6.24 \times 10^5$ MeV.

1 gram $= 5.60999 \times 10^{26}$ MeV.
$\qquad\quad = 6.0242 \times 10^{23}$ mu.

1 rad $= 100$ ergs absorbed per gram of any absorber
$\qquad = 6.24 \times 10^7$ MeV absorbed per gram.

1 roentgen (R) produces ionization $= 1$ esu of charge per 0.001293 gm
$\qquad\qquad\qquad\qquad\qquad\qquad\qquad$ dry air
$\qquad\qquad\qquad = 1$ esu of charge per cu cm air (NTP)
$\qquad\qquad\qquad = 1.61 \times 10^{12}$ ion pairs per gram of dry air
$\qquad\qquad\qquad = 2.083 \times 10^9$ ion pairs per cu cm air (NTP)
$\qquad\qquad\qquad = 5.47 \times 10^7$ MeV per gram of dry air
$\qquad\qquad\qquad = 7.08 \times 10^4$ MeV per cu cm air (NTP)
$\qquad\qquad\qquad = 93\text{–}98$ ergs per gram of water (or soft tissue) for photon
$\qquad\qquad\qquad$ energies from 200 kVp (hvl 0.5 mm Cu) to 1 MVp (hvl
$\qquad\qquad\qquad$ 3.3 mm Pb)

W $= 34$ electron volts per ion pair (average for radiations of interest in
$\qquad$ this book).

Wave length of photon of energy keV, $\lambda(\text{Å}) = \dfrac{12.40}{\text{keV}}$.

Appendix C

Physical Data for a Number of Radioactive Nuclides

In this table are listed a large number of radioactive nuclides currently used in medical or biological practice, or likely to be so used in the near future. The data represent a collection from a number of published sources, supplemented by computations by the present author. Material in the earlier edition of this book has been checked and updated. References used are listed below. Values for $\overline{E}_\beta$ and for Γ were taken from all of these except the two isotope tables. When several values were found for one of these constants, it was recalculated to determine the best one. When no values were found, calculations were made, on the basis of material in Chapters 6 and 9. For positron emitters the contribution from annihilation radiation is included in Γ. For nuclides of half life less than 4 hours, decay during the first hour is taken into account in the calculation. Abbreviation e.c. denotes electron capture and IT denotes isomeric transition (decay from an excited metastable state).

REFERENCES

ATTIX, F. H.: *Computed Values of the Specific Gamma-ray Constant* Γ *for* ^{137}Cs *and* ^{60}Co. Phys. in Med. and Biol., *13*, 119, 1968.
JOHNS, HAROLD: *Physics of Radiology*, Springfield, Charles C Thomas, 1964.
LEDERER, C. M., HOLLANDER, J. M. and PERLMAN, I.: *Table of Isotopes*. 6th Ed., New York, John Wiley & Sons, Inc., 1967.
Radiochemical Center, Amersham, England: *The Radiochemical Manual, Part One*.
SLACK, L. and WAY, K.: *Radiations from Radioactive Atoms in Frequent Use*. Washington, D.C., United States Atomic Energy Commission, 1959.
SMITH, E. M., HARRIS, C. C. and ROHRER, R. H.: *Calculation of Local Energy Deposition Due to Electron Capture and Internal Conversion*. J. Nuc. Med., *7*, 23, 1966.
STROMINGER, D., HOLLANDER, J. M. and SEABORG, G. T.: *Table of Isotopes*, Rev. Mod. Phys. April, *30*, 585, 1958.

Physical Data for a Number of Radioactive Nuclides

Element	Atomic Number Z	Mass Number A	Half Life	Radiation	$\overline{E}_\beta$ MeV per Disintegration	Γ R per mCi/Hr at 1 Cm
Antimony	51	122	2.8 d	β^-,e.c.	0.56	2.4
		124	60.4 d	β^-,γ	0.38	9.8
Argon	18	37	35.1 d	e.c.	0.003	
Arsenic	33	72	26 hr	β^+,e.c.,γ	0.91	8.9
		74	18 d	β^-,β^+,e.c.,γ	0.26	4.6
		76	26.5 hr	β^-,γ	1.14	2.4
Barium	56	131	12.0 d	e.c.,γ	0.007	2.04
		133	7.2 yr	e.c.,γ	0.012	3.27
with Lanthanum-140		140	12.8 d	β^-,γ	0.749	12.4
Beryllium	4	7	53 d	e.c.,γ	0.00011	0.3
Bismuth	83	206	6.2 d	e.c.,γ	0.06	18.2
		210	5.0 d	β^-	0.397	
Bromine	35	82	35.3 hr	β^-,γ	0.137	14.6
Cadmium	48	115m	43 d	β^-,γ	0.62	0.2
Calcium	20	45	165 d	β^-	0.076	
		47	4.5 d	β^-,γ	0.33	5.95
Carbon	6	11	20 min	β^+	0.38	2.5*
		14	5730 yr	β^-	0.049	
Cerium	58	141	32.5 d	β^-,γ	0.15	0.35
Cesium	55	131	9.7 d	e.c.	0.007	0.56
		134	2.05 yr	β^-,γ	0.116	8.7
with Barium 137-m .		137	30 yr	β^-,γ	0.242	3.26
Chlorine	17	36	3×10^5 yr	β^-,e.c.	0.27	
		38	37.3 min	β^-,γ	1.47	2.8*
Chromium	24	51	27.8 d	e.c.,γ	0.005	0.15
Cobalt	27	56	77 d	β^+,e.c.,γ	0.125	17.6
		57	270 d	e.c.,γ	0.023	0.99
		58	71 d	β^+,e.c.,γ	0.035	5.4
		60	5.27 yr	β^-,γ	0.093	13.0
Copper	29	64	12.8 hr	β^-,β^+,e.c.	0.130	1.1
		67	58.5 hr	β^-,γ	0.145	0.97
Fluorine	9	18	110 min	β^+,e.c.	0.279	4.4*
Gallium	31	66	9.4 hr	β^+,e.c.,γ	1.0	9.3
		67	78 hr	e.c.,γ	0.009	1.0
		72	14.1 hr	β^-,γ	0.4	11.6
Gold	79	198	2.7 d	β^-,γ	0.315	2.3
		199	3.15 d	β^-,γ	0.10	0.59
Hydrogen	1	3	12.26 yr	β^-	0.0055	

Physical Data for a Number of Radioactive Nuclides (Continued)

Element	Atomic Number Z	Mass Number A	Half Life	Radiation	$\overline{E}_\beta$ MeV per Disinte- gration	Γ R per mCi/Hr at 1 Cm
Indium	49	113m	1.7 hr	IT,γ	0.11	1.75
Iodine	53	123	13.0 hr	e.c.,γ	0.028	2.2
		124	4 d	β^+,e.c.,γ	1.62	7.2
		125	60 d	e.c.,γ	0.021	1.23
		126	13 d	β^-,β^+,e.c.,γ	0.16	2.5
		130	12.3 hr	β^-,γ	0.285	12.1
		131	8.04 d	β^-,γ	0.180	2.20
		132	2.26 hr	β^-,γ	0.483	9.4*
Iridium	77	192	74.4 d	β^-,e.c.,γ	0.20	5.1
		194	19 hr	β^-,γ	0.72	1.5
Iron	26	52	8.2 hr	β^+,e.c.,γ	0.195	4.6
		55	2.6 yr	e.c.	0.006	
		59	45 d	β^-,γ	0.116	6.4
Krypton	36	85	10.6 yr	β^-,γ	0.225	0.012
Lanthanum	57	140	40.2 hr	β^-,γ	0.48	11.3
Magnesium . . . . with Aluminum-28	12	28	21.2 hr	β^-,γ	0.140	15.7
Manganese	25	52	5.7 d	β^+,e.c.,γ	0.085	18.5
		54	303 d	e.c.,γ	0.005	4.7
Mercury	80	197	65 hr	e.c.,γ	0.079	0.31
		203	47 d	β^-,γ	0.100	1.20
Molybdenum . . .	42	99	66.7 hr	β^-,γ	0.400	1.29
Nickel	28	56	6.4 d	e.c.,γ	0.007	2.3
		63	92 yr	β^-	0.02	
Nitrogen	7	13	10 min	β^+	0.49	1.5*
Oxygen	8	15	2.0 min	β^+	0.72	0.25*
Palladium . with Silver 109m	46	109	13.6 hr	β^-,IT,γ	0.39	1.8
Phosphorus	15	32	14.2 d	β^-	0.694	
		33	25 d	β^-	0.08	
Potassium	19	42	12.4 hr	β^-,γ	1.42	1.4
		43	22.4 hr	β^-,γ	0.31	5.6
Praesodymium . . .	59	142	19.2 hr	β^-,γ	0.81	0.3
Radium . . . . in equilibrium with Rn, Ra A, B, C with 0.5 mm Pt filter	88	226	1620 yr	γ		8.25
Rhenium	75	186	3.7 d	β^-,IT,γ	0.34	0.16

Physical Data for a Number of Radioactive Nuclides (Continued)

Element	Atomic Number Z	Mass Number A	Half Life	Radiation	$\overline{E}_\beta$ MeV per Disinte- gration	Γ R per mCi /Hr at 1 Cm
Rubidium	37	84	33 d	$\beta^-,\beta^+,$e.c.,γ	0.125	4.46
		86	18.7 d	β^-,γ	0.62	0.49
Samarium	62	153	46.2 hr	β^-,IT,γ	0.26	0.32
Scandium	21	46	84 d	β^-,γ	0.12	11.0
		47	3.4 d	β^-,γ	0.166	0.7
Selenium	34	75	120 d	e.c.,γ	0.019	1.76
Silver	47	110m	253 d	β^-,γ	1.27	14.3
		111	7.5 d	β^-,γ	0.35	0.14
Sodium	11	22	2.6 yr	β^+,e.c.,γ	0.214	13.0
		24	15.0 hr	β^-,γ	0.553	18.7
Strontium	38	85	64 d	e.c.,γ	0.014	3.0
		87m	2.8 hr	IT,γ	0.082	1.3*
		89	52 d	β^-	0.56	
with Yttrium-90 . .		90	28 yr	β^-	0.200+ 0.93	
Sulfur	16	35	87.9 d	β^-	0.048	
Tantalum	73	182	115 d	β^-,γ	0.92	6.8
Technecium	43	99m	6.04 hr	IT,γ	0.014	0.7
Tellurium	52	121	17 d	e.c.,γ	0.007	4.2
		132	78 hr	β^-,γ	0.06	2.2
Thallium	81	204	3.8 hr	β^-,e.c.	0.238	
Thulium	69	170	134 d	β^-,γ	0.35	0.025
Tin	50	113	115 d	e.c.,γ	0.006	1.3
with Indium-113m .				+IT	0.12	3.05
		121	27.5 hr	β^-	0.11	
Tungsten.	74	185	75 d	β^-	0.124	
		187	24 hr	β^-,γ	0.24	3.0
Vanadium	23	48	16.2 d	β^+,e.c.,γ	0.16	15.6
Xenon	54	133	5.3 d	β^-,γ	0.12	0.73
Yttrium . . . . . with Strontium-87m	39	87	80 hr	IT,e.c.,γ	0.03	2.9
		90	64 hr	β^-	0.93	
		91	59 d	β^-	0.585	
Zinc	30	65	245 d	β^+,e.c.,γ	0.10	2.9
Zirconium . . . . with Niobium-95m	40	95	65 d	IT,β^-,γ	0.102	4.1

* When the half life is less than 4 hours, decay must be taken into account in the calculation of Γ, as discussed on page 108.

Appendix D

Some Characteristics of the Standard Man

(From Recommendations of the International Commission on Radiological Protection; Report of Committee II on Permissible Dose for Internal Radiation, 1959.)

Mass of Organs of the Adult Human Body;
Total Body Weight, 70,000 Grams.

Organ	Weight in Grams	Organ	Weight in Grams
Muscle	30,000	Urinary Bladder	150
Skin and Subcutaneous		Pancreas	70
Tissue*.	6,100	Salivary Glands (6)	50
Fat	10,000	Testes (2)	40
Skeleton		Spinal Cord	30
Bones	7,000	Eyes (2)	30
Red Marrow	1,500	Thyroid Gland	20
Yellow Marrow	1,500	Teeth	20
Blood	5,400	Prostate Gland	20
Gastrointestinal Tract	2,000	Adrenal Glands	
Contents of G-I Tract*	1,635	or Suprarenal (2)	20
Liver	1,700	Thymus	10
Brain	1,500	Ovaries	8
Lungs (2)	1,000	Pituitary	0.6
Lymphoid Tissue	700	Parathyroids (4)	0.15
Kidneys (2)	300	Miscellaneous	390
Heart	300	(Blood vessels, cartilage,	
Spleen	150	nerves, etc.)	

* The mass of the skin alone is taken to be 2000 grams. The mass of the G-I tract does not include its contents.

365

Chemical Composition of the Body

Element	Percentage of Total Body Weight	Weight Grams	Element	Percentage of Total Body Weight	Weight Grams
Oxygen	65.0	45,500	Zinc	0.0033	2.3
Carbon	18.0	12,600	Rubidium	0.0017	1.2
Hydrogen	10.0	7,000	Strontium	0.0002	0.14
Nitrogen	3.0	2,100	Copper	0.00014	0.1
Calcium	1.5	1,050	Aluminum	0.00014	0.1
Phosphorus	1.0	700	Lead	0.00011	0.08
Sulfur	0.25	175	Tin	0.000043	0.03
Potassium	0.2	140	Iodine	0.000043	0.03
Sodium	0.15	105	Cadmium	0.000043	0.03
Chlorine	0.15	105	Manganese	0.00003	0.02
Magnesium	0.05	35	Barium	0.000023	0.016
Iron	0.0057	4			

Water Balance

Daily Water Intake	ml	Daily Water Output	ml
In food (including 300 ml water of oxidation)	1300	Sweat	600
As fluids	1200	From Lungs	300
Total water intake	2500	In feces	200
		Urine	1400
		Total water output	2500

Respiration

8 Hours at work . . .	10^7 cm³ air
16 Hours not at work . .	10^7
Total in 24 Hours . . .	2×10^7

Appendix E

Total Radiation Dose in Critical Organ, for 100 µCi Administered (Intravenous or Oral as Indicated.)

Element	Mass No.	Route of Adm	Critical Organ	% of Adm. Dose in Crit. Org.	T_{eff} Days	Dose in Rads		
						1 Week	13 Weeks	1 Year
Arsenic	74	I.V.	Kidneys	10	17	3	12.7	13
	76	"	"	"	1	2.9	2.9	2.9
Bromine	82	P.O.	Total Body	100	1.3	0.14	0.14	0.14
Calcium	45	P.O.	Bone	50	162	0.19	2.3	5.2
	47	"	"	"	5	0.67	1.1	1.1
	45	I.V.	"	90	162	0.34	3.3	9.2
	47	"	"	"	5	1.2	2.0	2.0
Carbon	14	Either	Fat	50	12	0.07	0.22	0.22
Cesium	131	Either	Muscle	40	9	0.02	0.04	0.04
	137	"	"	40	138	0.46	4.8	11.0
Chlorine	38	Either	Total Body	100	0.026	0.005	0.005	0.005
Chromium	51	I.V.	Total Body	100	26.6	0.006	0.036	0.04
Cobalt	58	P.O.	Liver	4	61	0.2	1.4	2.2
	60	"	"	"	365	0.4	5.4	16.5
Copper	64	I.V.	Spleen	7	0.5	0.25	0.25	0.25
Gallium	72	I.V.	Bone	30	0.6	0.12	0.12	0.12
Gold	198	I.V.	Kidneys	3	2.7	0.58	0.7	0.7
Hydrogen	3	Either	Total Body	100	12	0.002	0.007	0.007
Iodine	125	Either	Thyroid	30	17	9.5	38.0	38.6

Element	Isotope	Route	Organ					
Iodine	131	Either	Thyroid	30	6	44.0	87.5	87.5
	132	"	"	"	0.1	4	4	4
	125	I.V.	Total Body	100	17	0.04	0.17	0.17
		(RISA)						
	131	"	"	"	7	0.13	0.26	0.26
	131	"	"	100	1	1	1	1
		(RoseBengal)						
Iron	55	I.V.	Spleen	2	388	0.06	0.8	2.33
	59	"	"	"	42	1.0	6.6	8.5
Mercury	197	I.V.	Kidneys	35	2.3	1.45	1.65	1.65
	203	"	"	"	11	4	11	11
Phosphorus	32	I.V.	Bone	20	14	0.6	2.0	2.0
		P.O.	"	40	"	1.2	4.0	4.0
Potassium	42	Either	Muscle	65	0.5	0.12	0.12	0.12
Selenium	75	Either	Kidneys	4	10	0.16	0.4	0.4
Silver	111	I.V.	Kidneys	2	4	0.5	0.7	0.7
Sodium	22	Either	Total Body	100	11	0.6	1.5	1.5
	24	"	"	"	0.6	0.2	0.2	0.2
Strontium	85	I.V.	Bone	70	65	0.05	0.42	0.76
	87m	"	"	0.013	0.12	0.01	0.01	0.01
Sulfur	35	Either	Testes	1	76	0.05	0.5	0.9
Technecium	99m	I.V.	Kidneys		0.25	0.002	0.002	0.002
Zinc	65	I.V.	Liver	35	66	1.4	12.3	20

Appendix F

Fluorescent Yields[1], Critical Absorption Energies,[2] and K and L Emission Energies[3] for a Wide Range of Elements

Z	Element	ω	Binding Energy—keV		Emission Energy—keV		
			K	L_1	$K\alpha$	$K\beta$	$L\alpha$
12	Mg	0.02	1.30		1.25	1.30	
14	Si	0.03	1.84		1.74	1.84	
16	S	0.05	2.47		2.31	2.46	
18	Ar	0.08	3.20		2.96	3.19	
20	Ca	0.12	4.04		3.69	4.01	
22	Ti	0.17	4.97		4.51	4.93	
24	Cr	0.23	5.99		5.41	5.95	
26	Fe	0.29	7.11		6.40	7.06	
28	Ni	0.36	8.33		7.48	8.27	
30	Zn	0.43	9.66		8.64	9.57	
32	Ge	0.49	11.10		9.89	10.98	
34	Se	0.55	12.66		11.22	12.50	
36	Kr	0.60	14.33		12.65	14.11	
38	Sr	0.65	16.10	2.22	14.17	15.84	1.81
40	Zr	0.70	18.0	2.53	15.8	17.7	2.04
42	Mo	0.73	20.0	2.87	17.5	19.6	2.29
44	Ru	0.77	22.1	3.22	19.3	21.7	2.56
46	Pd	0.79	24.4	3.60	21.2	23.8	2.84
48	Cd	0.82	26.7	4.02	23.2	26.1	3.13
50	Sn	0.84	29.2	4.46	25.3	28.5	3.44
52	Te	0.86	31.8	4.94	27.5	31.0	3.77
54	Xe	0.87	34.6	5.45	29.8	33.6	4.11
56	Ba	0.88	37.4	5.99	32.2	36.0	4.47
58	Ce	0.89	40.4	6.55	34.7	39.3	4.84
60	Nd	0.90	43.6	7.13	37.4	42.3	5.23
62	Sm	0.91	46.8	7.74	40.1	45.4	5.64
64	Gd	0.92	50.2	8.38	43.0	48.7	6.06
66	Dy	0.93	53.8	9.05	46.0	52.1	6.50
68	Er	0.93	57.5	9.75	49.1	55.7	6.95
70	Yb	0.94	61.3	10.49	52.4	59.4	7.42
72	Hf	0.94	65.4	11.27	55.8	63.2	7.90
74	W	0.94	69.5	12.10	59.3	67.2	8.40
76	Os	0.95	73.9	12.97	63.0	71.4	8.91
78	Pt	0.95	78.4	13.88	66.8	75.8	9.44
80	Hg	0.95	83.1	14.84	70.8	80.3	9.99
82	Pb	0.96	88.0	15.86	75.0	84.9	10.55

[1] Lederer, C. M., Hollander, J. M. and Perlman, I.: Table of Isotopes, 6th ed., 1967.
[2] Bearden, J. A. and Burr, A. F.: Reevaluation of X-Ray Atomic Energy Levels. Rev. Mod. Phys. *39*, 125 (1967).
[3] Bearden, J. A.: X-Ray Wavelengths. Rev. Mod. Phys. *39*, 78 (1967).

Appendix G
Four Place Logarithms

N	0	1	2	3	4	5	6	7	8	9
10	0000	0043	0086	0128	0170	0212	0253	0294	0334	0374
11	0414	0453	0492	0531	0569	0607	0645	0682	0719	0755
12	0792	0828	0864	0899	0934	0969	1004	1038	1072	1106
13	1139	1173	1206	1239	1271	1303	1335	1367	1399	1430
14	1461	1492	1523	1553	1584	1614	1644	1673	1703	1732
15	1761	1790	1818	1847	1875	1903	1931	1959	1987	2014
16	2041	2068	2095	2122	2148	2175	2201	2227	2253	2279
17	2304	2330	2355	2380	2405	2430	2455	2480	2504	2529
18	2553	2577	2601	2625	2648	2672	2695	2718	2742	2765
19	2788	2810	2833	2856	2878	2900	2923	2945	2967	2989
20	3010	3032	3054	3075	3096	3118	3139	3160	3181	3201
21	3222	3243	3263	3284	3304	3324	3345	3365	3385	3404
22	3424	3444	3464	3483	3502	3522	3541	3560	3579	3598
23	3617	3636	3655	3674	3692	3711	3729	3747	3766	3784
24	3802	3820	3838	3856	3874	3892	3909	3927	3945	3962
25	3979	3997	4014	4031	4048	4065	4082	4099	4116	4133
26	4150	4166	4183	4200	4216	4232	4249	4265	4281	4298
27	4314	4330	4346	4362	4378	4393	4409	4425	4440	4456
28	4472	4487	4502	4518	4533	4548	4564	4579	4594	4609
29	4624	4639	4654	4669	4683	4698	4713	4728	4742	4757
30	4771	4786	4800	4814	4829	4843	4857	4871	4886	4900
31	4914	4928	4942	4955	4969	4983	4997	5011	5024	5038
32	5051	5065	5079	5092	5105	5119	5132	5145	5159	5172
33	5185	5198	5211	5224	5237	5250	5263	5276	5289	5302
34	5315	5328	5340	5353	5366	5378	5391	5403	5416	5428
35	5441	5453	5465	5478	5490	5502	5514	5527	5539	5551
36	5563	5575	5587	5599	5611	5623	5635	5647	5658	5670
37	5682	5694	5705	5717	5729	5740	5752	5763	5775	5786
38	5798	5809	5821	5832	5843	5855	5866	5877	5888	5899
39	5911	5922	5933	5944	5955	5966	5977	5988	5999	6010
40	6021	6031	6042	6053	6064	6075	6085	6096	6107	6117
41	6128	6138	6149	6160	6170	6180	6191	6201	6212	6222
42	6232	6243	6253	6263	6274	6284	6294	6304	6314	6325
43	6335	6345	6355	6365	6375	6385	6395	6405	6415	6425
44	6435	6444	6454	6464	6474	6484	6493	6503	6513	6522
45	6532	6542	6551	6561	6571	6580	6590	6599	6609	6618
46	6628	6637	6646	6656	6665	6675	6684	6693	6702	6712
47	6721	6730	6739	6749	6758	6767	6776	6785	6794	6803
48	6812	6821	6830	6839	6848	6857	6866	6875	6884	6893
49	6902	6911	6920	6928	6937	6946	6955	6964	6972	6981
50	6990	6998	7007	7016	7024	7033	7042	7050	7059	7067
51	7076	7084	7093	7101	7110	7118	7126	7135	7143	7152
52	7160	7168	7177	7185	7193	7202	7210	7218	7226	7235
53	7243	7251	7259	7267	7275	7284	7292	7300	7308	7316
54	7324	7332	7340	7348	7356	7364	7372	7380	7388	7396
N	0	1	2	3	4	5	6	7	8	9

FOUR PLACE LOGARITHMS—Continued

N	0	1	2	3	4	5	6	7	8	9
55	7404	7412	7419	7427	7435	7443	7451	7459	7466	7474
56	7482	7490	7497	7505	7513	7520	7528	7536	7543	7551
57	7559	7566	7574	7582	7589	7597	7604	7612	7619	7627
58	7634	7642	7649	7657	7664	7672	7679	7686	7694	7701
59	7709	7716	7723	7731	7738	7745	7752	7760	7767	7774
60	7782	7789	7796	7803	7810	7818	7825	7832	7839	7846
61	7853	7860	7868	7875	7882	7889	7896	7903	7910	7917
62	7924	7931	7938	7945	7952	7959	7966	7973	7980	7987
63	7993	8000	8007	8014	8021	8028	8035	8041	8048	8055
64	8062	8069	8075	8082	8089	8096	8102	8109	8116	8122
65	8129	8136	8142	8149	8156	8162	8169	8176	8182	8189
66	8195	8202	8209	8215	8222	8228	8235	8241	8248	8254
67	8261	8267	8274	8280	8287	8293	8299	8306	8312	8319
68	8325	8331	8338	8344	8351	8357	8363	8370	8376	8382
69	8388	8395	8401	8407	8414	8420	8426	8432	8439	8445
70	8451	8457	8463	8470	8476	8482	8488	8494	8500	8506
71	8513	8519	8525	8531	8537	8543	8549	8555	8561	8567
72	8573	8579	8585	8591	8597	8603	8609	8615	8621	8627
73	8633	8639	8645	8651	8657	8663	8669	8675	8681	8686
74	8692	8698	8704	8710	8716	8722	8727	8733	8739	8745
75	8751	8756	8762	8768	8774	8779	8785	8791	8797	8802
76	8808	8814	8820	8825	8831	8837	8842	8848	8854	8859
77	8865	8871	8876	8882	8887	8893	8899	8904	8910	8915
78	8921	8927	8932	8938	8943	8949	8954	8960	8965	8971
79	8976	8982	8987	8993	8998	9004	9009	9015	9020	9025
80	9031	9036	9042	9047	9053	9058	9063	9069	9074	9079
81	9085	9090	9096	9101	9106	9112	9117	9122	9128	9133
82	9138	9143	9149	9154	9159	9165	9170	9175	9180	9186
83	9191	9196	9201	9206	9212	9217	9222	9227	9232	9238
84	9243	9248	9253	9258	9263	9269	9274	9279	9284	9289
85	9294	9299	9304	9309	9315	9320	9325	9330	9335	9340
86	9345	9350	9355	9360	9365	9370	9375	9380	9385	9390
87	9395	9400	9405	9410	9415	9420	9425	9430	9435	9440
88	9445	9450	9455	9460	9465	9469	9474	9479	9484	9489
89	9494	9499	9504	9509	9513	9518	9523	9528	9533	9538
90	9542	9547	9552	9557	9562	9566	9571	9576	9581	9586
91	9590	9595	9600	9605	9609	9614	9619	9624	9628	9633
92	9638	9643	9647	9652	9657	9661	9666	9671	9675	9680
93	9685	9689	9694	9699	9703	9708	9713	9717	9722	9727
94	9731	9736	9741	9745	9750	9754	9759	9763	9768	9773
95	9777	9782	9786	9791	9795	9800	9805	9809	9814	9818
96	9823	9827	9832	9836	9841	9845	9850	9854	9859	9863
97	9868	9872	9877	9881	9886	9890	9894	9899	9903	9908
98	9912	9917	9921	9926	9930	9934	9939	9943	9948	9952
99	9956	9961	9965	9969	9974	9978	9983	9987	9991	9996
N	0	1	2	3	4	5	6	7	8	9

Appendix H

Exponentials

x	e^{-x}	x	e^{-x}	x	e^{-x}
0.00	1.000	0.40	0.670	1.0	0.368
0.01	0.990	0.41	0.664	1.1	0.333
0.02	0.980	0.42	0.657	1.2	0.301
0.03	0.970	0.43	0.651	1.3	0.273
0.04	0.961	0.44	0.644	1.4	0.247
0.05	0.951	0.45	0.638	1.5	0.223
0.06	0.942	0.46	0.631	1.6	0.202
0.07	0.932	0.47	0.625	1.7	0.183
0.08	0.923	0.48	0.619	1.8	0.165
0.09	0.914	0.49	0.913	1.9	0.150
0.10	0.905	0.50	0.607	2.0	0.135
0.11	0.896	0.52	0.595	2.1	0.122
0.12	0.887	0.54	0.583	2.2	0.111
0.13	0.878	0.56	0.571	2.3	0.100
0.14	0.869	0.58	0.560	2.4	0.0907
0.15	0.861			2.5	0.0821
0.16	0.852	0.60	0.549	2.6	0.0743
0.17	0.844	0.62	0.538	2.7	0.0672
0.18	0.835	0.64	0.527	2.8	0.0608
0.19	0.827	0.66	0.517	2.9	0.0550
		0.68	0.507		
0.20	0.819			3.0	0.0498
0.21	0.811	0.70	0.497	3.2	0.0408
0.22	0.803	0.72	0.487	3.4	0.0334
0.23	0.795	0.74	0.477	3.6	0.0273
0.24	0.787	0.76	0.468	3.8	0.0224
0.25	0.779	0.78	0.458		
0.26	0.771			4.0	0.0183
0.27	0.763	0.80	0.449	4.2	0.0150
0.28	0.756	0.82	0.440	4.4	0.0123
0.29	0.748	0.84	0.432	4.6	0.0101
		0.86	0.423	4.8	0.0082
0.30	0.741	0.88	0.415		
0.31	0.733			5.0	0.0067
0.32	0.726	0.90	0.407	5.5	0.0041
0.33	0.719	0.92	0.399	6.0	0.0025
0.34	0.712	0.94	0.391	6.5	0.0015
0.35	0.705	0.96	0.383	7.0	0.0009
0.36	0.698	0.98	0.375	7.5	0.0006
0.37	0.691			8.0	0.0003
0.38	0.684			8.5	0.0002
0.39	0.677			9.0	0.0001

(Courtesy of Editors of Handbook of Chemistry and Physics.
Published by Chemical Rubber Company)

Appendix I

Table for f = e$^{-0.693\ t/T}$ (see page 31)

T = half life   t = decay time

f

t/T		0.00	0.01	0.02	0.03	0.04	0.05	0.06	0.07	0.08	0.09	t/T
0.0	0.		9931	9862	9794	9727	9659	9593	9526	9461	9395	0.0
0.1		9330	9266	9202	9138	9075	9013	8950	8888	8827	8766	0.1
0.2		8706	8645	8556	8526	8467	8409	8351	8293	8236	8179	0.2
0.3		8123	8066	8011	7955	7900	7846	7792	7738	7684	7631	0.3
0.4		7579	7526	7474	7423	7371	7320	7270	7220	7170	7120	0.4
0.5		7071	7022	6974	6926	6878	6830	6783	6736	6690	6643	0.5
0.6		6598	6552	6507	6462	6417	6373	6329	6285	6242	6199	0.6
0.7		6156	6113	6071	6029	5987	5946	5905	5864	5824	5783	0.7
0.8		5743	5704	5664	5625	5586	5548	5510	5471	5434	5396	0.8
0.9		5359	5322	5285	5249	5212	5176	5141	5105	5070	5035	0.9
1.0		5000	4965	4931	4897	4863	4830	4796	4763	4730	4698	1.0
1.1		4665	4633	4601	4569	4538	4506	4475	4444	4414	4383	1.1
1.2		4353	4323	4293	4263	4234	4204	4175	4147	4118	4090	1.2
1.3		4061	4033	4005	3978	3950	3923	3896	3869	3842	3816	1.3
1.4		3789	3763	3737	3711	3686	3660	3635	3610	3585	3560	1.4
1.5		3536	3511	3487	3463	3439	3415	3391	3368	3345	3322	1.5
1.6		3299	3276	3253	3231	3209	3186	3164	3143	3121	3099	1.6
1.7		3078	3057	3035	3015	2994	2973	2952	2932	2912	2892	1.7
1.8		2872	2852	2832	2813	2793	2774	2755	2736	2717	2698	1.8
1.9		2679	2661	2643	2625	2606	2588	2570	2553	2535	2517	1.9
2.0		2500	2483	2466	2449	2432	2415	2398	2382	2365	2349	2.0
2.1		2333	2316	2300	2285	2269	2253	2238	2222	2207	2192	2.1
2.2		2176	2161	2146	2132	2117	2102	2088	2073	2059	2045	2.2
2.3		2031	2017	2003	1989	1975	1961	1948	1934	1921	1908	2.3
2.4		1895	1882	1869	1856	1843	1830	1817	1805	1792	1780	2.4
2.5		1767	1756	1743	1732	1719	1708	1696	1684	1672	1661	2.5
2.6		1649	1638	1627	1615	1604	1593	1582	1571	1560	1550	2.6
2.7		1539	1528	1518	1507	1497	1487	1476	1466	1456	1446	2.7
2.8		1436	1426	1416	1406	1397	1387	1377	1368	1358	1349	2.8
2.0		1340	1330	1321	1312	1303	1294	1285	1276	1267	1259	2.9
3.0		1250	1241	1233	1224	1216	1207	1199	1191	1183	1174	3.0
3.1		1166	1158	1150	1142	1134	1127	1119	1111	1103	1096	3.1
3.2		1088	1081	1073	1066	1058	1051	1044	1037	1029	1022	3.2
3.3		1015	1008	1001	*9944	*9876	*9807	*9740	*9672	*9606	*9539	3.3
3.4	0.0	9473	9401	9343	9278	9214	9151	9087	9025	8962	8900	3.4
3.5		8839	8778	8717	8657	8597	8538	8479	8420	8362	8304	3.5
3.6		8247	8190	8133	8077	8021	7966	7911	7856	7802	7748	3.6
3.7		7695	7642	7589	7536	7484	7432	7381	7330	7280	7229	3.7
3.8		7179	7130	7080	7032	6983	6935	6887	6839	6792	6745	3.8
3.9		6699	6652	6606	6561	6515	6470	6426	6381	6337	6294	3.9
4.0		6250	6207	6164	6121	6079	6037	5994	5940	5913	5872	4.0
4.1		5832	5791	5751	5711	5672	5633	5594	5555	5517	5479	4.1
4.2		5441	5403	5366	5329	5292	5256	5219	5183	5147	5112	4.2
4.3		5077	5042	5007	4972	4938	4904	4870	4836	4803	4770	4.3
4.4		4737	4704	4671	4639	4607	4575	4544	4512	4481	4450	4.4
4.5		4419	4389	4359	4328	4299	4269	4239	4210	4181	4152	4.5
4.6		4124	4095	4067	4039	4011	3983	3956	3928	3901	3874	4.6
4.7		3847	3821	3794	3768	3742	3716	3691	3665	3640	3615	4.7
4.8		3590	3565	3540	3516	3492	3467	3444	3420	3396	3373	4.8
4.9		3349	3326	3303	3280	3258	3235	3213	3191	3169	3147	4.9
t/T		0.00	0.01	0.02	0.03	0.04	0.05	0.06	0.07	0.08	0.09	t/T

f

t/T		0.00	0.01	0.02	0.03	0.04	0.05	0.06	0.07	0.08	0.09	t/T
5.0	0.0	3125	3103	3082	3061	3040	3019	2998	2977	2956	2936	5.0
5.1		2916	2896	2876	2856	2836	2816	2797	2778	2758	2739	5.1
5.2		2721	2702	2683	2665	2646	2628	2610	2592	2574	2556	5.2
5.3		2538	2521	2503	2486	2469	2452	2435	2418	2401	2385	5.3
5.4		2368	2352	2336	2320	2304	2288	2272	2256	2241	2225	5.4
5.5		2210	2194	2179	2164	2149	2134	2120	2105	2090	2076	5.5
5.6		2062	2048	2033	2019	2005	1992	1978	1964	1950	1937	5.6
5.7		1924	1910	1897	1884	1871	1858	1845	1833	1820	1807	5.7
5.8		1795	1782	1770	1758	1746	1734	1722	1710	1698	1686	5.8
5.9		1675	1663	1652	1640	1629	1618	1606	1595	1584	1573	5.9
6.0		1562	1552	1541	1530	1520	1509	1499	1489	1478	1468	6.0
6.1		1458	1448	1438	1428	1418	1408	1398	1389	1379	1370	6.1
6.2		1360	1351	1342	1332	1323	1314	1305	1296	1287	1278	6.2
6.3		1269	1260	1252	1243	1234	1226	1217	1209	1201	1192	6.3
6.4		1184	1176	1168	1160	1152	1144	1136	1128	1120	1112	6.4
6.5		1105	1097	1090	1082	1075	1067	1060	1052	1045	1038	6.5
6.6		1031	1024	1017	1010	1003	*9958	*9889	*9820	*9753	*9685	6.6
6.7	0.00	9618	9552	9486	9420	9355	9291	9227	9163	9099	9037	6.7
6.8		8974	8912	8851	8790	8729	8669	8609	8549	8490	8431	6.8
6.9		8373	8315	8258	8201	8144	8088	8032	7977	7922	7867	6.9
7.0		7812	7759	7705	7652	7599	7546	7494	7442	7391	7340	7.0
7.1		7289	7239	7189	7139	7090	7041	6992	6944	6896	6848	7.1
7.2		6801	6754	6708	6661	6615	6570	6524	6479	6434	6390	7.2
7.3		6346	6302	6258	6215	6172	6130	6087	6045	6003	5962	7.3
7.4		5921	5880	5839	5799	5759	5719	5680	5640	5601	5563	7.4
7.5		5524	5486	5448	5411	5373	5336	5299	5263	5226	5190	7.5
7.6		5154	5119	5083	5048	5013	4979	4944	4910	4876	4843	7.6
7.7		4809	4776	4743	4710	4678	4645	4613	4581	4550	4518	7.7
7.8		4487	4456	4425	4395	4364	4334	4304	4275	4245	4216	7.8
7.9		4187	4158	4129	4100	4072	4044	4016	3988	3961	3933	7.9
8.0		3906	3879	3852	3826	3799	3773	3747	3721	3696	3670	8.0
8.1		3645	3619	3594	3570	3545	3521	3496	3472	3448	3424	8.1
8.2		3401	3377	3354	3331	3308	3285	3262	3240	3217	3195	8.2
8.3		3173	3151	3129	3108	3086	3065	3044	3023	3002	2981	8.3
8.4		2960	2940	2920	2899	2879	2860	2840	2820	2801	2781	8.4
8.5		2762	2743	2724	2705	2687	2668	2650	2631	2613	2595	8.5
8.6		2577	2559	2542	2524	2507	2489	2472	2455	2438	2421	8.6
8.7		2405	2388	2371	2355	2339	2323	2307	2291	2275	2259	8.7
8.8		2244	2228	2213	2197	2182	2167	2152	2137	2123	2108	8.8
8.9		2093	2079	2064	2050	2036	2022	2008	1994	1980	1967	8.9
9.0		1953	1940	1926	1913	1900	1887	1874	1861	1848	1835	9.0
9.1		1822	1810	1797	1785	1773	1760	1748	1736	1724	1712	9.1
9.2		1700	1689	1677	1665	1654	1642	1631	1620	1609	1597	9.2
9.3		1586	1575	1565	1554	1543	1532	1522	1511	1501	1490	9.3
9.4		1480	1470	1460	1450	1440	1430	1420	1410	1400	1391	9.4
9.5		1381	1372	1362	1353	1343	1334	1325	1316	1307	1298	9.5
9.6		1289	1280	1271	1262	1253	1245	1236	1228	1219	1211	9.6
9.7		1202	1194	1186	1178	1169	1161	1153	1145	1137	1130	9.7
9.8		1122	1114	1106	1099	1091	1084	1076	1069	1061	1054	9.8
9.9		1047	1039	1032	1025	1018	1011	1004	*9971	*9902	*9834	9.9
10.0	0.000	9766	9698	9631	9565	9499	9433	9368	9303	9239	9175	10.0
t/T		0.00	0.01	0.02	0.03	0.04	0.05	0.06	0.07	0.08	0.09	t/T

25

Author Index

A

Abbatt, J. D., 14
Abelson, P., 4
Alexander, Peter, 154
Anderson, D. C., 4, 35
Andrews, H. L., 6, 32, 34, 35, 51, 97
Attix, F. H., 5, 361
Avogadro, Amadeo, 3, 13

B

Bacq, Z., 154
Bancroft, M., 242
Barkla, C. G., 3
Bearden, J. A., 371
Becker, A., 34
Becquerel, Henri, 3, 7, 17
Berman, M., 227, 230
Blackett, P. M. S., 34
Bohr, Niels, 4, 7
Bothe, W., 34
Boyd, G. A., 344
Braestrup, C. B., 176
Brownell, G. L., 5, 63, 64, 77, 103, 107, 122, 127, 139, 140
Brucer, M., 5
Burr, A. F., 371
Bush, F., 116, 140

C

Chadwick, James, 4, 6, 34, 77, 97
Chase, G. D., 5
Cockroft, J. D., 4
Comar, C. L., 5
Corrigan, K. E., 6, 38, 77, 97, 177
Crooks, W., 9
Curie, Eve, 32
Curie, Irene, 4
Curie, Marie, 3, 17, 32
Curie, Pierre, 3, 17
Curie-Joliots, 20, 34, 36

D

Dalton, John, 3, 7
Davidson, W. C., 6, 38, 77
Du Sault, L., 154
Dyche, G. M., 140

E

Eisenbud, M., 5
Ellet, W. H., 122, 140

Ellis, C. D., 97
Ellis, R. H., 103, 104, 105, 113, 140
Elmore, Wm., 5
Errera, M., 154
Evans, Robley, 5, 241, 338

F

Failla, G., 176
Fermi, Enrico, 4, 52, 55
Fermi, Laura, 5
Ferran, H. E., 140
Focht, E., 116, 140
Forssberg, A., 154
Friedlander, G., 5, 14, 32, 38, 41, 47, 51, 91, 97
Frisch, O., 4, 53

G

Gershowitz, M., 116, 140
Glaser, D. A., 87
Glasser, O., 5, 16, 32, 38, 77, 97, 139, 176
Gleason, A. I., 280
Godwin, J. T., 140
Gray, L. H., 154

H

Hahn, O., 4, 53
Halliday, D., 5, 52
Harris, C. C., 118, 140, 361
Harriss, E. B., 140
Herz, R. H., 340
Hess, Victor, 3
Hill, R. F., 140
Hine, G. J., 5, 63, 64, 77, 103, 107, 139, 140, 274
Hoecker, F., 111, 140
Hollaender, A., 154
Hollander, J. M., 6, 11, 336, 361
Hull, G. F., 5

J

Johns, Harold, 6, 97, 361
Joliot, F., 4

K

Kennedy, J. W., 5, 14, 32, 38, 41, 47, 51, 91, 97

L

Lamerton, L. F., 140
Lapp, R. E., 6, 32, 38, 51, 97
Lawrence, E. O., 4, 36
Lawrence, John, 130, 140
Lea, D. E., 154
Lederer, C. M., 6, 11, 336, 361
Lees, D. S., 34
Loevinger, Robt., 102, 122, 140, 227, 230

M

Mackay, N. R., 140
MacMillan, 4
Mann, W. B., 260
Marinelli, L. D., 140
Meitner, Lise, 4, 52, 53
Mendeleev, D., 3, 8
Miller, A., 275
Miller, J. M., 5, 14, 32, 38, 41, 47, 51, 97
Minski, M., 139, 177
Morgan, R. H., 5, 6, 16, 32, 38, 77, 97, 139, 176, 177
Moseley, H. G. J., 4

N

Needham, J., 16

P

Pagel, W., 16
Perlman, I., 11, 336, 361
Pizzarello, D. J., 154
Pollard, E. C., 6, 38, 77
Powsner, E. R., 127, 140
Prout, Wm., 3, 9

Q

Quimby, E. H., 5, 6, 16, 32, 38, 77, 97, 139, 140, 177

R

Rabinowitz, J. L., 5
Reddy, A. R., 122, 140
Robertson, J., 140
Roentgen, Wm. C., 3, 17
Roesch, W. C., 5
Rohrer, R. H., 140, 361
Roofe, P. G., 111, 140
Rossi, H. H., 103, 104, 105, 113, 140
Rutherford, Ernest, 3, 4, 6, 7, 20, 33, 34, 36, 77, 97

S

Sayre, E., 51
Scott, W. G., 177
Seaborg, G. T., 361
Seidlin, S. M., 134, 140
Seliger, H. H., 263
Semat, Henry, 6, 51
Siegel, E., 134, 140
Sinclair, Warren, 133, 140
Slack, L., 6, 361
Smith, E. M., 118, 140, 361
Soddy, F., 3, 9
Spiers, F. W., 111, 140
Stern, Curt, 154
Strassman, F., 4, 52, 53
Strominger, D., 361

T

Tabern, D. L., 280
Taylor, J. D., 280
Taylor, L. S., 5, 16, 32, 38, 77, 97, 139, 176
Thompson, J. J., 3, 4

U

Urey, Harold, 4

V

Vennart, J., 139, 177
Villard, P., 3, 18

W

Wagner, H. N., 6, 139
Walton, E. T. S., 4
Way, K., 6, 361
Weatherwax, J. L., 5, 16, 32, 38, 77, 97, 139, 176
Werner, S. C., 274
White, H. E., 6, 51
Widman, J. C., 127, 140
Wilson, C. T. R., 4, 87
Witcofski, R. L., 154
Witten, V. H., 140
Wood, W. S., 140
Wyckoff, H. O., 176

Y

Yalow, A. A., 134, 140

Subject Index

A

Absolute activity, 257
Absorbed fraction, 122 ff
Absorption coefficient, Compton, 94, 95
  effective, 115
  linear, 88, 93
  mass, 89, 93
  pair, 94, 95
  photoelectric, 94, 95
  total, 94
  true, 107
Absorption curve, 88 ff
Absorption, of beta radiation, 88, 280, 282,
  290 ff
  of photons, 93
  of radiation, 88 ff
Absorption, percutaneous, 355
Accelerators, 36
Actinium series, 68
Activated water, 152
Activation analysis, neutron, 49
Activity, 24
  absolute, 257
  background equivalent, 351
  specific, 31, 257
Addition of beta and gamma doses, 118
  of rads and roentgens, 118
Administration of radioactive material to
  patients, 166
Advisory Commission on Biology and
  Medicine, 176
Alpha decay, 61
Alpha particles (rays), 3, 18, 34, 78
  as bombarders, 33, 44
  interactions with matter, 81
  magnetic deviation, 18
  range, 61, 81
  sources, 102
Amplifiers, 208
  linear, 208
Analyzers, see Pulse height analyzer
Anemia following irradiation, 141, 145
Annihilation radiation, 82, 95, 97
  scanning, 335 ff
Anticoincidence circuit, 215 ff
Antineutrino, 63
Area monitoring, 350
Artificial radioactivity, 4, 19, 36
  transmutation, 33
Assay, 257
Atomic bomb, 4, 57

Atomic bomb, (continued)
  Casualty Commission, 144
  fallout from, 58, 157
  radiation effects from, 144
Atomic, building blocks, 7
  concept, 7
  disintegration, 19
  energy, 39
  hypothesis, 3, 7
  mass, 8, 13
    mass unit, 13
  models, 7
  pile, 55
  structure, 7, 9, 13, 19
  weight, 8, 9, 13
Atomic Energy Commission (AEC), 5, 357
  requirements in radionuclide program,
    175
  in waste disposal, 178
Atoms, 3, 7 ff, 18
  number in one curie, 26
Attenuation (photon beam), 93
  coefficient, 94
  factor, for barriers, 164
  vs. half value layer, 114
Autofluoroscope, 333
Autopsy, radioactive body, 172
Autoradiograph (radioautography), 111,
  133, 338 ff
  exposure, 339
  quantitative, 342
  techniques, 339
Avalanche, 189, 191
Average life, radioactive, 21, 112
Avogadro's hypothesis, 47

B

Back scatter, 91
Background equivalent activity, 251 ff
Background, radioactive, 225 ff
  counting, 233 ff
  reduction, 286 ff
  rule for neglecting, 231
  statistics, 225 ff
Barn, 47
Barriers, examples of calculation, 165
  for radiation protection, 163, 164
  position of, 165
Beta, decay, 61 ff
  emitters, in nuclear reactions, 46, 61

Beta, (*continued*)
  particles (rays), 3, 18, 79, 82
    absorption of, see Absorption, beta
      radiation
    counting, see Counting, beta
    energy, 63, 88
      average, 63, 111
      maximum, 63
    interactions with matter, 82
    magnetic deviation, 18
    range, 90
    scattering, 91
    self-absorption, 92
    -scattering, 92
  spectrum, 20, 62, 63
Bikini, atom bomb information, 144
Binding energy, nuclear, 40, 42
  of electrons in orbit, 85
Binary, coding, 211
  numbers, 209 ff
Biological effects of ionizing radiation,
    141 ff
  genetic, 148 ff
  somatic, 142 ff
    delayed, 142
    doses to produce, 144
    factors influencing, 142
    latent period, 142
    sources of information, 143 ff
Biological half-life, 127
Blood, dose from I–131 therapy, 135
  effects of radiation on, 145
Body burden, 136
  dose from, 136
  permissible, 172
Bombarders, nuclear, 44 ff
  alpha particles, 44
  deuterons, 45
  neutrons, 45
  photons, 46
  protons, 44
Bone-seeking radionuclides, 110, 146
Bremsstrahlung, 83, 89, 90, 161
  counting, 292
British Medical Research Council, 154, 176
Bromine, radioactive, dosage example, 136
Bubble chamber, 87
Building blocks, atomic, 7
Burial, of bodies containing radioactive
    material, 172
  of radioactive waste, 179

C

Cadmium, as moderator in reactor, 55
Calculation, of permissible dose of radio-
    active material, 173
  of quantity of radioactive material to
    deliver specified radiation dose, 132

Calculation, (*continued*)
  of radiation dose, alpha sources,
    external, 102
    internal, 110
  beta sources, external, 103
    in radioactive solutions, 114
    internal, 111
      in small regions, 113
  gamma sources, external, 106
    internal, 115 ff
Calibration, 248, 260 ff
  factor, 260
  standards, 260 ff
Camera, gamma, 333
Cancer, following irradiation, 142, 146, 175
  thyroid, following irradiation, 147
Capture, electron, 64, 118 ff
Carrier, 31, 50, 179
  -free, 31, 258, 284
Cataract following irradiation, 144, 147
Cells, effects of radiation on, 141
Chain reaction, nuclear fission, 5, 53
Characteristic radiation, 86, 119 ff
Charts, isotope, 67
Chi square method, 241
Chromatography, 277, 293 ff
Cloud chamber, 4, 34, 87
  tracks, 34, 87
Coefficient of variation, 223 ff
Coincidence, circuits, 215 ff
  counters, 336
Collimators, 313, 315 ff, 323 ff
  depth sensitivity, 325 ff
  focussing, 324 ff
  resolving power, 316 ff, 325 ff
Collision (atomic interaction), 81 ff
  Compton, 84
  photoelectric, 85
  radiative, 190 ff
Combined counting rate, 225
Compton absorption, 84, 96
  coefficient, 94
  collision, 84
  electron, 84
Confidence limit, 225
Contamination, radioactive, 166 ff
  internal (of personnel), 182, 350
  of sample containers, 233, 258, 350,
    352
  removal of, 180 ff
  rules for dealing with, 180
  test for, 350
Controls, electronic, 262 ff, 287 ff
Conversion electrons, 66
Co-precipitation, 52
Cosmic rays, 3, 156, 225
Counters, anticoincidence, 215 ff
  binary, 209 ff
  calibration of, 248, 260 ff
  coincidence, 215 ff

Counters, (*continued*)
  decade, 209, 211
  dip, 276
  efficiency of, 247 ff, 281
  electromechanical, 209
  electronic, 209 ff
  end window, 280
  flow gas, 291 ff
  gas, 292
  Geiger-Mueller, 190 ff, 260 ff, 263 ff, 315, 348, 356
  Marinelli, 276
  non-paralyzing, 243
  paralyzing, 243
  portable, 203 ff, 348 ff, 356
  precision, 249 ff
  printing, 213 ff, 309 ff
  proportional, 188 ff, 260 ff, 266 ff
  response, 247 ff
  ring, 349
  scintillation, 193 ff, 260 ff, 267 ff, 285 ff, 328
  selection, 251, 327 ff
  semiconductor, see Counters, solid state
  sensitivity, 247 ff
  solid state, 197 ff
  well type, 277 ff
  windowless, 291
  whole body, 279, 306
Counting (See also Counters)
  Bremsstrahlung, 292
  beta, 279 ff, 291 ff
    low energy, 285 ff
  circuits, 207 ff
  gamma, 272 ff
  gas, 292
  geometry, 272 ff
  losses, 242 ff
  mechanism, 209 ff
  mixed sources, 266 ff
  printers, 213 ff, 309
  rate, background, 225 ff, 233 ff
    combined, 225
    correction, 243
    gross, 225
    net, 225
  rate-meter, see rate meters and recorders
  recorder, see rate meters and recorders
  statistics, see statistics of counting
  time, 226
"Cow," radioactive, 67, 76
Cremation of bodies containing radioactive material, 180
Critical organ, 174
  size, in chain reaction, 57
Cross-section, nuclear, 47
Curie (Ci), 25, 248
  number of atoms in, 26
  weight of, 26
Cyclotron, 4, 36 ff

D

Dead time, 192, 242 ff
Death resulting from irradiation, 142, 144
Decay, radioactive, 19 ff
  constant, 21, 22, 27
  curve, 23, 24, 29
    complex (for mixture of radionuclides), 30
  formula, 21
  modes of, 61 ff
    alpha, 61
    beta, 61
    gamma, 65
  rates, 20
  schemes, 65
Deceased patients with radioactive burdens, 180
Decontamination, 180 ff
Dees, of cyclotron, 38
Detectors, See Counters
Deuterium, 4
Deuteron, 13, 78
  as nuclear bombarder, 45
  interaction with matter, 82
Deviation, standard, 222 ff, 240
Dilutions, 258, 355
Dimensions of atoms and nuclei, 15
Discriminator, 208, 267
  setting, 269 ff
    for background reduction, 287 ff
Disintegration, atomic or nuclear, 19, 20
  constancy of type and rate, 20
  constant, 21, 22, 23, 27
  law, 21
  rate, 21
Disposal of radioactive waste, 178 ff, 350
  AEC regulations, 179
  burial, 178
  garbage, 178
  incineration, 179
  return to Atomic Energy Commission, 178
  sea, 178
  sewage, 178
  stable isotope dilution, 179
Disruption of stable nitrogen, 33
  of stable nuclei, 35
Distance as radiation protection, 162
Dominant mutations, 149
Dosage calculations, 102 ff
  examples, 129 ff
  external, beta radiation, 102
    gamma radiation, 106
  from constant body burden, 136
  internal, alpha radiation, 110
    beta radiation, 111 ff
    gamma radiation, 115 ff
      very low energy, 118
Dose, 102 ff

Dose, (continued)
  doubling, for mutations, 150 ff
  in objects floating in radioactive solu-
    tion, 114
  in small region, 113, 114
  maximum permissible, 155, 156
  measurement of, 203 ff
  meters, 204 ff
  permissible, 155, 156
  rate, 188, 199, 203, 348, 356
  rate meters, 203 ff, 348, 350, 356
  specified quantity of radionuclide to
    deliver, 132, 133
  tolerance, 155
  total, 188, 199, 204 ff
  units, rad, 102, 110, 111, 142
    rem, 110, 157
    roentgen, 102, 106
Dose-effect relationships, 144
Dosimeter, solid state, 199
Double nuclide technique, 295 ff
Doubling dose for mutations, 150 ff
Dummy runs for new procedures, 174

E

Effective half-life, 127
Efficiency of counters, 247 ff
Electromagnetic radiation (see also
  photon), 79, 185
Electromechanical counters, 209
Electrometer, string, 205 ff
Electron, 7
  capture, 64, 118 ff
  Compton, 84
  conversion, 66
  extranuclear, 3
  mass, 40
  multiplication, 189
  orbital, 4, 8
  orbits, 7
  photo, 85
  recoil, 84
  secondary, 87, 189, 194
  volt, 37, 40
Electrophoresis, 293
Electrostatic voltmeter, 204
Elements, 7
Encapsulated sources, 102 ff
End window counters, 280
Endoergic reaction, 39
Energy, atomic, 39
  binding, of nucleus, 40
    of orbital electrons, 85
  of the radiations, particle, 78, 79
    photon, 79
  of reactions, endoergic, 39
    exoergic, 39
Energy-mass equivalence, 3, 39
Epilation following irradiation, 141, 144

Equilibrium, radioactive, 68 ff
  secular, 73
  transient, 72
Equipment performance test, 239
Equivalence of mass and energy, 3, 39
Erg, 40
Errors, see uncertainty
  timing, 233
Erythema following irradiation, 141, 144
Exchange forces, 16
Excited state of nucleus, 42, 60
Excreta, radioactive, 167
Exoergic reaction, 39
Exponential decay law, 21
Exposure, occupational, 157, 349
  permissible, 156, 157
  population, 158
Exposure in autoradiography, 339
External monitoring, 349
External sources of radiation, 102 ff
  alpha, 102
  beta, 103
  gamma, 106

F

Fading of latent image, 338
Fallout, radioactive, from nuclear weapons,
  58, 157, 175
Federal Register, 175, 178
Film badge, 347
  ring, 349
Filter, 88
Fission, nuclear, 4, 52 ff
  products, 53, 57
  spontaneous, 67
Floor covering, 353
Flow gas counters, 291 ff
Fluctuations in rate meter, 236 ff
Fluorescence, 17
Focussing collimator, 324 ff
Fog, photographic, 338
Forces, exchange, 16
  nuclear, 15
Formulae of counting statistics, table,
  254 ff
Frequency of electromagnetic radiation, 80
Fuel, reactor, 55
Full width, at half maximum, 269
  of collimators, 326 ff
Fusion reactions, 58

G

Gamma constant (Γ), 106, 107, 108, 348
  decay, 65
  dosage calculations, 106 ff
    implants, 109
    internal, 115 ff
      geometrical constant, g, 116
        table of values, 117
  rays, 3

Gamma, radiation, counting, 272 ff
  spectrometry, 291
Garbage disposal of radioactive waste, 178
Gas amplification, 189
Gas counting, 292
Geiger-Mueller counters, see Counters,
  Geiger-Mueller
Genetic mutations, due to radiation, 148 ff
  spontaneous, 149
Geometrical factor, g, in gamma dose cal-
  culations, 116, 117
Geometry in counting, 272 ff
Gloves, 355
Gold, radioactive, rate of production in
  pile, 47
Grains, radioactive, 103
Gross counting rate, 225
Ground state of nucleus, 60
Growth of radionuclide in neutron flux, 74

H

Half-life, biological, 127
  effective, 127
  physical, 21
  radioactive, 21
  determination of, 27
Half value layers, 88, 93, 163, 290
  in barrier construction, 163
Handling of radioactive samples, 257 ff
  carrier-free, 258, 284
Hazards, radiation, 155 ff
  genetic, 148 ff
  somatic, 142 ff
Health protection, 155 ff, 346
Helium, 8
Hiroshima, atomic bomb information, 144
Homogeneous beam, photons, 93
Hydrogen, 8, 13, 18, 33
  bomb, 8, 58, 59

I

Identification of radionuclides, 290 ff
Implants, radioactive, 101, 109
Incineration of radioactive waste, 179
Induced radioactivity, 4, 19, 33 ff
Integral counting rate, 293
Interaction of radiation and matter, 78 ff
  alpha particles, 81
  beta particles, 82
  neutrons, 83
  photons, 84 ff
Internal conversion, 66
  emitters, permissible doses, 158
  sources, dosage, 109 ff
    alpha, 110
    beta, 111 ff
    gamma, 115 ff
Internal exposure, 349

Internally administered radioactive material, dosage calculation, 109 ff
  permissible dose, 158
International Commission on Radiological
  Protection, 155
Inverse square law, 162, 274, 315
Iodine, radioactive, dosage examples, 129,
  131
  various isotopes, 131
Ion, 81, 186 ff
  negative, 81
  pair, 81, 82
  positive, 81
Ionization, 81, 82
  specific, 82, 187
Ionization chambers, 186 ff, 203 ff, 258 ff,
  285 ff
  capacitor (condenser), 205 ff
  pocket, 346
  portable, 204
Ionizing radiations, biological effects of,
  141 ff
Irradiation, external, 102 ff
  internal, 102, 109 ff
Isobars, 3, 14, 67
Isomers, 14, 66, 67
Isomeric transition, 65, 66
Isotones, 14
Isotope charts, 67, 68
Isotopes, 9, 14
  of iodine, 62, 131
  radioactive, 3
  stable, 4, 45

J

Jamming, 243

K

K-electron capture, 64
K fluorescent yield, 114
Kick-sorter, 218
Kilocurie (kCi), 25
Kiloelectron volt (keV), 40
Kinetic energy of particle radiation, 78

L

Laboratory, radionuclide, 159 ff, 352 ff
Latent image, 199, 338
Latent period for radiation reaction, 142
Lead bricks, 286 ff, 353
  filters, 347
  half value layers, for various radio-
    nuclides, 163
  in barrier construction, 163, 286 ff, 353
Leakage of radioactive sources, 350
Length of plateau, 265
Lethal dose, median (MLD), 153

Leukemia following irradiation, 145
Life shortening by irradiation, 148
Linear absorption coefficient, beta rays, 88
  photons, 93
Linear energy transfer, 152
Liquid drop model of nucleus, 60
Liquid scintillation counters, 285 ff
Lithium, 8
Local effects of radiation, 141 ff
Logarithmic response, 312
Losses in counting, 242 ff
Low energy gamma rays, 118
Luminescence, 199, 315
Luminous markers, 157

M

Magnetic field, deflection of charged parti-
    cles, 3, 35, 36
  separation of radiations, 18
Malignant degeneration following irradia-
    tion, 142, 145
Manhattan Project, 4, 55
Marinelli counter, 276
Mass, absorption coefficient, beta rays, 89
    photons, 93
  number, 9, 14
  rest, 79
  unit, 8, 40
    energy equivalent of, 40
    variation with velocity, 79
Mass-energy equivalence, 3, 39, 65
Maximum permissible dose (MPD), 155 ff
  internal emitters, 158
  occupational conditions, 157
  whole population, 158
Median lethal dose (MLD), 153
Medical uses of radionuclides, 98 ff
  diagnostic, 98
    localization or transport of radio-
        nuclide, 101
  therapy, 98, 101
    implants, 101
    telecurie sources, 101
  tracer, 98
    limitations of, 99
    reutilization of metabolic products,
        100
    turnover studies, 100
Mesons, 16
Metastable state, 66
Mica windows, 280
Microcurie (μCi), 25
Millicurie (mCi), 25
  number of atoms in, 25
  weight of, 26
Million electron volts (MeV), 40
Mock-iodine, 262
Moderator, in nuclear reactor, 55
Molecules, 3

Molybdenum-technetium "cow," 76, 77
Momentum, conservation in beta decay, 63
Monitoring, 346 ff
  area, 350
  external, 349
  hands, 349
  internal, 350
  personnel, 349
  process, 350
Monoenergetic beam, photons, 93
Multichannel analyzer, 220
Mutations, dominant, 149
  produced by irradiation, 148 ff
  recessive, 149

N

Nagasaki, atomic bomb information, 144,
    145, 147
Nanocurie (nCi), 25, 250
National Bureau of Standards Handbooks,
    6, 156, 166, 172, 177
National Council on Radiation Protection
    and Measurements, 6, 167
Natural radioactivity, 17 ff, 225
Negative ion, 81, 186 ff
Negatron, 62
Neptunium, 4, 56
  series, 68
Net counting rate, 225
Neutrino, 62
Neutron, 4, 7, 35
  activation analysis, 49
  as bombarder, 45
  capture, 45
  emission, not in radioactivity, 67
  excess, 14
  interaction with matter, 83
  number, 14
  -proton ratio, 15
Nitrogen, stable, disruption of, 33, 41
Noise, 208, 264
Nomenclature, nuclear, 14
Non-uniformity of irradiation, 133
Nuclear chain reaction, 4, 5, 53, 54
  charges, 9
  cross-sections, 47
  fission, 4, 52
  forces, 15, 42
  masses, 9
  nomenclature, 14
  potential barrier, 42, 43
  reactions, 39 ff
    mechanism, 43
    notation, 41
    yield, 47
  reactor (or pile), 4, 55, 56
  transmutation, 4
  weapons, 57, 175
  well, 43

Nuclei of atoms, 3, 7
  dimensions, 15
  mass, 40
  structure, 42
Nucleon, 7
  mass, 40
Nuclide, radioactive, 20 ff
  scanning, 334 ff
  stable, 14
Nursing attendance rules, 168

O

Occupational exposure, 143
  maximum permissible dose, 157
Operating voltage, 265
Orbital electrons, 8
Oxygen, 33

P

Pair, absorption coefficient, 96
  formation, 86
  positron-electron, 86
Particle radiation, 18, 78 ff
Patients, administration of radioactive
    material, 167, 169
  precautions after administration, 167
  autopsy, 172
  emergency surgery, 172
Penumbra, 317
Percutaneous absorption, 355
Performance standard, 261
Periodic table, 3, 8, 10, 12
Permissible body burden, 173
  dose, maximum, 157 ff
    internal emitters, 158, 173
    occupational exposure, 157, 348
    times with radioactive patients, 162
    tracer doses, 170
Personnel monitoring, 349
Phantom, 302
Phosphorus, radioactive, dosage example,
    112, 130
Photocathode, 195
Photoelectric absorption, 85
  coefficient, 94
  collision, 85
Photoelectron, 85, 195
  in internal conversion, 66
Photographic emulsions, 338, 342 ff
  film, 346 ff
  process, 199
Photoluminescence, 199
Photomultiplier tube, 194 ff
Photon, 18, 78
  energy 79
  in nuclear reactions, 46
  interaction with matter, 84 ff
Photopeak, 267 ff

Picocurie (pCi), 25
Pile, atomic (or nuclear), 5, 55, 56
Pinhole camera, 315
Pions, 16
Pipetting, remote, 258, 355
Planchette, 281
Planck's constant, 80
Plaques, surface irradiation dose calcula-
    tions, 103
Plastic scintillators, 279
Plateau, 263 ff, 271
Plutonium, 4, 56
Poisson distribution, 222
Polonium, 3, 17, 102
Positive ion, 81, 186 ff
Positron, 4, 35, 62
  -electron pair, 86
  emitters, 44, 62
  scanning, 335 ff
Potential barrier, nuclear, 42, 43
  well, 43
Preamplifiers, 208
Precautions against radiation, 155 ff
  against radioactive patients, 167
Precision, 238, 249 ff
Pregnancy, effects of irradiation during,
    147
Preset count and time counting, 213, 229,
    232 ff
Printing counter, 213 ff, 309
Printing timer, 213 ff, 309
Probe detectors, 314
Process monitoring, 350
Production of radionuclides, 57
Proportional counters, see Counters,
    proportional
Protection supervisor, radiation, 159
Protons, 4, 7, 13
  as bombarders, 44
  emission in radioactivity not found, 67
  interaction with matter, 84
  number, 15
Protyle, 3
Pulse height analyzer, 217 ff
  for background reduction, 285
  multichannel, 220
  setting of, 271 ff
Pulse height spectrum, 267 ff
Purification, chemical, 292

Q

Quantitative autoradiography, 342
Quartz string electrometer, 205 ff
Quenching, 193, 286

R

Rad, per roentgen, 118
  unit of dose, 102, 111, 118

Radiation, annihilation, 82, 95, 97
dose, calculation, 101, 102 ff
  to produce specific biologic effects, 144
  effect produced by, 141 ff
  sources of information, 143
  effects at molecular level, 152 ff
    direct, 152
    indirect, 152
  electromagnetic, 14
  hazards, 155 ff
    genetic, 148 ff
    somatic, 142 ff, 155 ff
  natural, 156
    cosmic rays, 156
    environmental, 157, 233
    internal, 157
  particle, 78 ff
  protection, 155 ff
    supervisor, 159
  safety, procedures, 155 ff
  sources for human exposure, 156 ff
    man-made, 157
      luminous markers, 157
      medical and dental, 157
      nuclear installations, 157
      nuclear weapon fallout, 175
Radiations from radioactive nuclides, 17 ff, 60 ff
  magnetic deflection, 18
  origins of, 60 ff
Radioactive, contamination, 166
  removal of, 180 ff
  "cows," 67, 76
  decay or disintegration, 20, 60 ff
    constant, 21
    curves, 23, 24
    law, 21
    modes of, 60 ff
    rate, 20
  equilibrium, 68 ff
    secular, 73
    transient, 72
  fallout, 59, 175 ff
  patients, care of, 167
  radiations, 19, 60 ff
  series, 68
  spill, 166
  waste disposal, 178 ff
Radioactivity, 3, 17 ff
  induced, 4, 19, 36, 225
  natural, 17 ff, 225
Radioautography (autoradiography), 111, 133, 338 ff
Radiochromatography, 293 ff
Radionuclide laboratory, 159 ff, 352 ff
Radiological Protection, International Commission, 155
Radionuclides, 19, 41
  artificially produced, 44 ff

Radionuclides, artificially produced, (cont.)
    example of growth in neutron flux, 74
  identification of, 290 ff
Radium, 3, 17
Range of alpha rays, 61, 81
  beta rays, 90
Rate meters and recorders, 214 ff, 293, 311, 340, 348
  statistics, 234 ff
Reactions, nuclear, 39 ff
  energy of, 39, 46
  endoergic, 39
  exoergic, 39
  in alpha particle bombardment, 44
    deuteron bombardment, 55
    neutron bombardment, 45
    proton bombardment, 44
  produced by photons, 46
Reactor, nuclear (or atomic), 4, 55, 56
Recessive mutations, 149
Recombination, 86
Recorders, see rate meters and recorders
  logarithmic, 312
  rectilinear, 312
Reference books, general, 6
Reference sample, 261
Relative biological effectiveness (RBE), 110, 157
Reliability, 224 ff
Rem, unit of dose, 110, 157
Remote pipetting, 258, 355
Resolution, in autoradiography, 340
  of scintillation counters, 269
Resolving power, 317 ff, 326 ff
  time, 242 ff
    correction for, 243 ff
    determination of, 245 ff
Response, speed, 234
  time, 234 ff, 242 ff
Rest mass of electron, 79
Ring counter, 349
  film badges, 347
Roentgen, unit of dose, 106
Routines, safety, 174 ff

S

Safety procedures against radiation, 160 ff, 174
  external beta-ray emitters, 160
  gamma-ray emitters, 174
  general routines, 174
  internal emitters, 172
Sample, changers, automatic, 232
  dry, 281 ff
  measurements in vitro, 272 ff
  volume, 275 ff
Saturation voltage, 187
Scalers, 207 ff
Scanner, 321 ff

Scanner, (continued)
    collimators for, 323 ff
    count marking, 330 ff
    digital, 332
    fixed detectors, 332 ff
    instrumentation, 322 ff
    manual, 314 ff
    motion of, 329 ff
    moving detectors, 329 ff
    paper strip, 293 ff
    photographic, 330
    positron, 335 ff
    whole body, 279, 306
    x-ray intensifier, 333 ff
Scanning, nuclides, 334 ff
    time for, 321
Scatter of radiation, 88
    effect on counting, 275, 282, 301, 328
    of beta particles, 91
        self-scatter, 92
    of gamma rays (protection), 166
    of photons, 84
Scintillation counters, see Counters,
        scintillation
    liquid, 285 ff
    plastic, 279
    scanning, 328 ff
    well type, 277 ff
Sea disposal of radioactive waste, 178
Secondary electrons, 84 ff
    photons, 84
Secular equilibrium, 73
Seeds, radioactive, 103
Selection of counters, 251, 327 ff
Self-absorption, beta rays, 92, 282, 283 ff
    gamma radiation, 306
    methods to overcome, 292 ff
    photons (large sources), 109
    -scatter, 92
Self-discharge, 191
Self-quenching, 193, 286
Sensitivity of radiation detectors, 235,
    247 ff
Series, radioactive, 19, 68
    actinium, 68
    in beta decay, 68
    neptunium, 68
    thorium, 68
    uranium, 69
Sewage disposal of radioactive waste, 78
Shielding for radiation protection, 162 ff
    of counters, 233, 286 ff, 312 ff
Shortening of life span by radiation, 148
Single channel analyzer, 217 ff
Skin, effects of radiation on, 145
Slope of plateau, 265
Smallest detectable amount, 249
Sodium, radioactive, dosage example, 130
Solid state counters, 197 ff
Somatic radiation effects, 142 ff

Somatic radiation effects, (continued)
    delayed, 145
    doses to produce, 144 ff
    factors influencing, 142
    sources of information, 143 ff
Sources of radiations, 60 ff
    for irradiation, 102 ff
        alpha rays, external, 102
            internal, 110
        beta rays, external, 103
            internal, 111
        gamma rays, external, 106
            internal, 115 ff
Space requirements, 352 ff
Spallation, 46
Specific activity, 31, 257
    concentration, 257
    ionization, 82
Specified dose, calculation of mCi to
    deliver, 132
Spectrometer, see pulse height analyzer
Spectrometry, gamma ray, 291
Spectrum, beta ray, 20, 63
Stability curve, 15
    relation to radioactive decay, 61
Stable isotope dilution of radioactive
    waste, 179
Stable isotopes, 4, 14
    nuclei, 14
        disruption of, 33 ff
Standard deviation, 222 ff
    in rate meters, 234 ff
    of a difference, 226
Standardized samples, 260, 275
Standardization of radionuclides, 257 ff
    absolute, 260 ff
Standards, calibration, 260 ff
    performance, 261
    reference, 261
Starting voltage, 263
Statistics of counting, 221 ff
    table of formulae, 254 ff
    to determine performance, 239 ff
Sterility produced by radiation, 148
String electrometer, 205 ff
Strip chart recorder, 214
Structure of atom, 7, 8
    of nucleus, 60
Substitution of one radionuclide for
    another, 137
Summary of dosage formulae, 139
Surgery, emergency, on radioactive
    patient, 172
Survey instruments, 204, 215
Systemic effects of radiation, 147

T

Table top materials, 253
Tamper, in atomic bomb, 58

Target area, nuclear, 47
Therapy, with radionuclides, 101 ff
    differential uptake for adequate, 138
    examples, 134 ff
Thermoluminescence, 199
Thermonuclear reactions, 58
Thick samples, 283
Thorium, 17, 19, 34
    series, 68
Thorium X as alpha source, 102
Threshold voltage, 191, 263
Thyroidal uptake, 299 ff, 308
Time, constant, 214 ff, 238
    factor, 307 ff
    printers, 213, 309 ff
Timing errors, 233
    mechanisms, 212 ff
Total dose, 188, 199, 204 ff
Trace elements, 49, 307 ff
Transient equilibrium, 72
Transistors, 202
Transmutation, artificial, 33
    nuclear, 4
Transportation of radioactive material in
    hospital, 166
Transuranic elements, 4, 56
True counting rate, 225

U

Umbra, 317
Uncertainty, 221 ff
    percent, 224
United States Atomic Energy Commission
    (AEC), 5, 175
National Academy of Sciences, 154
Units, activity of radioactive nuclides, 25
    radiation dose, 102, 118
Uptake, differential, 314, 321 ff
    adequate for radiation therapy, 138
    measurements, 260, 308
    monitoring, 350
    thyroid, 299 ff, 308

Uranium, 3, 17, 19
    in fission, 53
    in reactor, 55
    series, 69

V

Velocity of particles, 78, 79
    photons, 79
Voltage, characteristic, 263
    noise, 264
    operating, 265
    saturation, 187
    self-discharge, 191
    stabilization, 265
    starting, 263
    supply, 207 ff
    threshold, 191, 263
Voltmeter, electrostatic, 204
Vomitus, radioactive, 180

W

Waste, radioactive, disposal of, 178 ff, 350
    Atomic Energy Commission rules, 178
    methods, 178
Wave-length dependence, 348
Wave length, photons, 80
Weapons, nuclear, 57
Weight of one curie, 25
Well-type counter, 277
Whole body counter, 279, 306
Window, sill, 219
    width, 219, 272
Work factor, 164

X

X-rays, discovery, 3
    electromagnetic radiation, 78
    scattered, 84

Y

Yield of a nuclear reaction, 47